Crohn's Disease

Editor

EDWARD V. LOFTUS Jr

GASTROENTEROLOGY
CLINICS OF NORTH AMERICA

www.gastro.theclinics.com

September 2017 • Volume 46 • Number 3

ELSEVIER

1600 John F. Kennedy Boulevard • Suite 1800 • Philadelphia, Pennsylvania, 19103-2899
http://www.theclinics.com

GASTROENTEROLOGY CLINICS OF NORTH AMERICA Volume 46, Number 3
September 2017 ISSN 0889-8553, ISBN-13: 978-0-323-54554-9

Editor: Kerry Holland
Developmental Editor: Alison Swety

Gastroenterology Clinics of North America (ISSN 0889-8553) is published quarterly by Elsevier Inc., 360 Park Avenue South, New York, NY 10010-1710. Months of issue are March, June, September, and December. Business and Editorial Offices: 1600 John F. Kennedy Blvd., Suite 1800, Philadelphia, PA 19103-2899. Customer Service Office: 6277 Sea Harbor Drive, Orlando, FL 32887-4800. Periodicals postage paid at New York, NY and additional mailing offices. Subscription prices are $330.00 per year (US individuals), $100.00 per year (US students), $616.00 per year (US institutions), $361.00 per year (Canadian individuals), $220.00 per year (Canadian students), $756.00 per year (Canadian institutions), $458.00 per year (international individuals), $220.00 per year (international students), and $756.00 per year (international institutions). Foreign air speed delivery is included in all *Clinics* subscription prices. All prices are subject to change without notice. **POSTMASTER**: Send address changes to *Gastroenterology Clinics of North America*, Elsevier Health Sciences Division, Subscription Customer Service, 3251 Riverport Lane, Maryland Heights, MO 63043. **Telephone: 1-800-654-2452 (U.S. and Canada); 314-447-8871 (outside U.S. and Canada). Fax: 314-447-8029. E-mail: journalscustomerservice-usa@elsevier.com (for print support); journalsonlinesupport-usa@elsevier.com (for online support).**

Reprints. For copies of 100 or more, of articles in this publication, please contact the Commercial Reprints Department, Elsevier Inc., 360 Part Avenue South, New York, New York 10010-1710. Tel. 212-633-3874, Fax: 212-633-3820, E-mail: reprints@elsevier.com.

Gastroenterology Clinics of North America is also published in Italian by Il Pensiero Scientifico Editore, Rome, Italy; and in Portuguese by Interlivros Edicoes Ltda., Rua Commandante Coelho 1085, 21250 Cordovil, Rio de Janeiro, Brazil.

Gastroenterology Clinics of North America is covered in *MEDLINE/PubMed (Index Medicus), Excerpta Medica, Current Contents/Clinical Medicine, Science Citation Index, ISI/BIOMED*, and *BIOSIS*.

Contributors

EDITOR

EDWARD V. LOFTUS Jr, MD
Professor of Medicine, Director, Inflammatory Bowel Disease Interest Group, Division of Gastroenterology and Hepatology, Mayo Clinic, Co-Director, Advanced Inflammatory Bowel Disease Fellowship, Rochester, Minnesota, USA

AUTHORS

WAQQAS AFIF, MD, MSc, FRCPC
Assistant Professor of Medicine, Division of Gastroenterology, McGill University Health Center, Montreal General Hospital, McGill University, Montreal, Quebec, Canada

BADR AL-BAWARDY, MD
Instructor of Medicine, Division of Gastroenterology and Hepatology, Mayo Clinic, Rochester, Minnesota, USA

SATIMAI ANIWAN, MD
Division of Gastroenterology and Hepatology, Mayo Clinic, Rochester, Minnesota, USA; Division of Gastroenterology, Thai Red Cross Society, King Chulalongkorn Memorial Hospital, Chulalongkorn University, Bangkok, Thailand

JOHN M. BARLOW, MD
Assistant Professor, Department of Radiology, Mayo Clinic, Rochester, Minnesota, USA

BRIGID S. BOLAND, MD
Assistant Professor, Division of Gastroenterology, Department of Medicine, Inflammatory Bowel Disease Center, Altman Clinical & Translational Research Institute, University of California, San Diego, La Jolla, California, USA

DAVID H. BRUINING, MD
Associate Professor of Medicine, Division of Gastroenterology and Hepatology, Mayo Clinic, Rochester, Minnesota, USA

PARAKKAL DEEPAK, MBBS, MS
Division of Gastroenterology, Assistant Professor, John T. Milliken Department of Medicine, Washington University School of Medicine, St Louis, Missouri, USA

WILLIAM A. FAUBION, MD
Professor of Immunology and Medicine and Pediatrics, College of Medicine, Division of Gastroenterology and Hepatology, Mayo Clinic, Rochester, Minnesota, USA

BRIAN G. FEAGAN, MD
Professor, Departments of Medicine and Epidemiology and Biostatistics, University of Western, London, Ontario, Canada

JEFF L. FIDLER, MD
Professor, Department of Radiology, Mayo Clinic, Rochester, Minnesota, USA

JOEL G. FLETCHER, MD
Department of Radiology, Mayo Clinic, Rochester, Minnesota, USA

JILL K.J. GAIDOS, MD
GI/Hepatology Service, Hunter Holmes McGuire VA Medical Center, Virginia Commonwealth University, Richmond, Virginia, USA

SUSHIL K. GARG, MBBS
Department of Internal Medicine, University of Minnesota, Minneapolis, Minnesota, USA

STEPHANIE L. HANSEL, MD, MS
Assistant Professor of Medicine, Division of Gastroenterology and Hepatology, Mayo Clinic, Rochester, Minnesota, USA

VALÉRIE HERON, MD, FRCPC
Division of Gastroenterology, McGill University Health Center, Montreal General Hospital, McGill University, Montreal, Quebec, Canada

VIPUL JAIRATH, MD, PhD
Associate Professor, Departments of Medicine and Epidemiology and Biostatistics, University of Western, London, Ontario, Canada

SUNANDA V. KANE, MD MSPH
Division of Gastroenterology and Hepatology, Mayo Clinic, Rochester, Minnesota, USA

REENA KHANNA, MD
Assistant Professor, Department of Medicine, University of Western, London, Ontario, Canada

SAHIL KHANNA, MBBS, MS
Assistant Professor of Medicine, Division of Gastroenterology and Hepatology, Mayo Clinic, Rochester, Minnesota, USA

JOHN B. KISIEL, MD
Division of Gastroenterology and Hepatology, Mayo Clinic, Rochester, Minnesota, USA

AMY L. LIGHTNER, MD
Division of Colon and Rectal Surgery, Mayo Clinic, Rochester, Minnesota, USA

EDWARD V. LOFTUS Jr, MD
Professor of Medicine, Director, Inflammatory Bowel Disease Interest Group, Division of Gastroenterology and Hepatology, Mayo Clinic, Co-Director, Advanced Inflammatory Bowel Disease Fellowship, Rochester, Minnesota, USA

GEOFFREY C. NGUYEN, MD, PhD
Joseph and Wolf Lebovic Health Complex, Associate Professor of Medicine, Mount Sinai Hospital Centre for Inflammatory Bowel Disease, Mount Sinai Hospital, University of Toronto, Institute for Clinical Evaluative Sciences, Toronto, Ontario, Canada

KONSTANTINOS A. PAPADAKIS, MD
Professor of Medicine, Division of Gastroenterology and Hepatology, Mayo Clinic, Rochester, Minnesota, USA

DARRELL S. PARDI, MD
Professor of Medicine, Division of Gastroenterology and Hepatology, Mayo Clinic, Rochester, Minnesota, USA

SANG HYOUNG PARK, MD
Division of Gastroenterology and Hepatology, Mayo Clinic, Rochester, Minnesota, USA; Department of Gastroenterology, Asan Medical Center, University of Ulsan College of Medicine, Seoul, Korea

MICHAEL F. PICCO, MD, PhD
Department of Gastroenterology and Hepatology, Mayo Clinic Jacksonville, Jacksonville, Florida, USA

LAURA E. RAFFALS, MD
Associate Professor of Medicine, Division of Gastroenterology and Hepatology, Mayo Clinic, Rochester, Minnesota, USA

GUILHERME PIOVEZANI RAMOS, MD
Department of Internal Medicine, Mayo Clinic, Rochester, Minnesota, USA

WILLIAM J. SANDBORN, MD
Professor of Medicine and Adjunct Professor of Surgery, Chief, Division of Gastroenterology, Vice Chair for Clinical Operations, Department of Medicine, Director, Inflammatory Bowel Disease Center, University of California, San Diego, UC San Diego Health System, La Jolla, California, USA

RAINA SHIVASHANKAR, MD
Instructor of Medicine, Division of Gastroenterology, University of Pennsylvania, Philadelphia, Pennsylvania, USA

SIDDHARTH SINGH, MD, MS
Assistant Professor of Medicine, Divisions of Gastroenterology and Biomedical Informatics, University of California, San Diego, La Jolla, California, USA

FERNANDO S. VELAYOS, MD
Division of Gastroenterology, University of California San Francisco, San Francisco, California, USA

SÉVERINE VERMEIRE, MD, PhD
Staff Member, Department of Gastroenterology, University Hospitals Leuven, Professor of Medicine Chair, Department of Clinical and Experimental Medicine, KU Leuven, Leuven, Belgium

MING-HSI WANG, MD, PhD
Senior Associate Consultant/Assistant Professor, Department of Gastroenterology and Hepatology, Mayo Clinic Jacksonville, Jacksonville, Florida, USA

Contents

Preface: Crohn's Disease: Etiology, Complications, Assessment, Therapy, and Management xiii

Edward V. Loftus Jr

Crohn's Disease: Genetics Update 449

Ming-Hsi Wang and Michael F. Picco

Since the discovery of the first Crohn's disease (CD) gene *NOD2* in 2001, 140 genetic loci have been found in whites using high-throughput genome-wide association studies. Several genes influence the CD subphenotypes and treatment response. With the observations of increasing prevalence in Asia and developing countries and the incomplete explanation of CD variance, other underexplored areas need to be integrated through novel methodologies. Algorithms that incorporate specific genetic risk alleles with other biomarkers will be developed and used to predict CD disease course, complications, and response to specific therapies, allowing precision medicine to become real in CD.

Epidemiology, Natural History, and Risk Stratification of Crohn's Disease 463

Satimai Aniwan, Sang Hyoung Park, and Edward V. Loftus Jr

Crohn's disease (CD) is a chronic condition that can result in significant morbidity and disability. By studying the association between demographics and initial clinical features and subsequent natural history, one may be able to stratify patients by their risks of clinical relapse, hospitalization, and surgery. Understanding the potential environmental risk factors and natural history of CD in a given patient guides the physician when counseling the patient and selecting a treatment strategy. In this review, updated data regarding the incidence and prevalence of CD, important environmental risk factors, natural history of the disease, and important prognostic factors are discussed.

The Microbiome in Crohn's Disease: Role in Pathogenesis and Role of Microbiome Replacement Therapies 481

Sahil Khanna and Laura E. Raffals

Individuals with a genetic predisposition to Crohn's disease develop aberrant immune responses to environmental triggers. The gastrointestinal microbiota is increasingly recognized to play an important role in the development of Crohn's disease. Decrease in global gut microbial diversity and specific bacterial alterations have been implicated in Crohn's disease. Advances in sequencing techniques and bioinformatics and correlation with host genetics continue to improve insight into the structure and function of the microbial community and interactions with the host immune system. This article summarizes the existing literature on the role of the gut microbiome and its manipulation in the development and management of Crohn's disease.

Endoscopic and Radiographic Assessment of Crohn's Disease 493

Badr Al-Bawardy, Stephanie L. Hansel, Jeff L. Fidler, John M. Barlow, and David H. Bruining

Crohn's disease is a chronic inflammatory disorder that can progress to obstructive and penetrating complications. Although clinical symptoms are an important component of therapy, they correlate poorly with objective measures of inflammation. The treatment targets have evolved from clinical improvement only to the addition of more objective measures, such as endoscopic mucosal healing and radiologic response, which have been associated with favorable long-term outcomes, including reduced hospitalizations, surgeries, and need for corticosteroids. There are multiple endoscopic and radiologic scoring systems that can aid in quantifying disease activity and response to therapy. These modalities and scoring tools are discussed in this article.

Intestinal and Nonintestinal Cancer Risks for Patients with Crohn's Disease 515

Sushil K. Garg, Fernando S. Velayos, and John B. Kisiel

Crohn's disease (CD) is a chronic inflammatory disease that confers a higher risk of cancer than in the general population. New, large, population-based studies in the past decade show that patients with CD are at higher risk of colorectal, small bowel, melanoma, and cervical cancer. Patients who use thiopurines are at additional risk of development of lymphoma and nonmelanoma skin cancer. Preventive surveillance for cancers of the colorectum, skin, and uterine cervix is advised.

Sexuality, Fertility, and Pregnancy in Crohn's Disease 531

Jill K.J. Gaidos and Sunanda V. Kane

Many factors influence the sexual health of people with Crohn's disease, but active disease and depression play key roles. The fertility rate in nonoperated patients with inflammatory bowel disease with quiescent disease is similar to that in the general population. Crohn's disease can increase the risk for adverse pregnancy outcomes, but being in remission on a stable, steroid-free medication regimen for at least 3 months before conception and adhering to the treatment throughout pregnancy can improve outcomes. Infants with intrauterine exposure to anti–tumor necrosis factor medications should avoid live vaccines for the first 9 months or until drug concentrations are undetectable.

Interdisciplinary Management of Perianal Crohn's Disease 547

Amy L. Lightner, William A. Faubion, and Joel G. Fletcher

Perianal disease is a common manifestation of Crohn's disease (CD) that results in significant morbidity and decreased quality of life. Despite several medical and surgical options, complex perianal CD remains difficult to treat. Before the advent of biologic therapy, antibiotics were the mainstay of medical treatment. Infliximab remains the most well-studied medical therapy for perianal disease. Surgical interventions are limited by the risk of nonhealing wounds and potential incontinence. When treatment options fail, fecal diversion or proctectomy may be necessary. Stem cell therapies may offer improved results and seem to be safe, but are not yet widely used.

Management of Crohn's Disease After Surgical Resection 563

Siddharth Singh and Geoffrey C. Nguyen

Approximately 25% to 35% of patients with Crohn's disease (CD) who undergo surgery require repeat surgery. Active smoking, multiple prior surgeries, and penetrating or perianal disease are risk factors for recurrence of CD after surgical resection. Early initiation of prophylactic therapy is effective in decreasing the risk of recurrence. Active colonoscopic surveillance for the early detection of endoscopic recurrence within 6 to 12 months of surgery is recommended. In symptomatic patients without evidence of endoscopic recurrence, noninflammatory causes should be sought.

Targeting Specific Immunologic Pathways in Crohn's Disease 577

Guilherme Piovezani Ramos, William A. Faubion, and Konstantinos A. Papadakis

Understanding the immunologic pathways in intestinal inflammation is crucial for the development of new therapies that can maximize patient response and minimize toxicity. Targeting integrins and cytokines is intended to control leukocyte migration to effector sites or inhibit the action of proinflammatory cytokines. New approaches to preventing leukocyte migration may target integrin receptors expressed on the intestinal vascular endothelium. The interleukin (IL)-12/IL-23 pathway has been a therapeutic target of interest in controlling active Crohn's disease (CD). New therapeutic approaches in CD may involve the enhancement of anti-inflammatory cytokine pathways and modulation of cellular responses and intranuclear signals associated with intestinal inflammation.

Use of Anti–Tumor Necrosis Factors and Anti-Integrins in the Treatment of Crohn's Disease 589

Raina Shivashankar and Darrell S. Pardi

In patients with Crohn's disease (CD), anti–tumor necrosis factor (TNF) therapy is efficacious for the induction and maintenance of clinical remission, mucosal healing, reducing rates of surgery and hospitalizations, and improving health-related quality of life. The decision between anti-TNFs and anti-integrins as first-line treatment in CD depends on disease severity, safety concerns, and prescription coverage. Given the existing data on long-term outcomes and safety, anti-TNFs are often preferred to anti-integrins. Additional clinical experience and preferably prospective, head-to-head studies will be important to determine whether vedolizumab should be considered more often for first-line therapy in CD.

Ustekinumab and Anti-Interleukin-23 Agents in Crohn's Disease 603

Parakkal Deepak and William J. Sandborn

This article reviews the available data regarding the efficacy of ustekinumab across published randomized clinical trials and open-label experience from tertiary medical centers, safety data, including in pregnancy, and its use in patients who have failed tumor necrosis factor (TNF) antagonists as well as patients who have not failed TNF antagonists. We have proposed an algorithm for positioning the use of ustekinumab among other agents (TNF antagonists, vedolizumab) in moderate-severe Crohn's disease. The article also enumerates drugs that are specific interleukin-23 blockers, including brazikumab (MEDI2070), risankizumab, LY3074828, tildrakizumab, and guselkumab, and the current status of their clinical trials.

Janus Kinase Antagonists and Other Novel Small Molecules for the Treatment of Crohn's Disease **627**

Brigid S. Boland and Séverine Vermeire

There is an ongoing, unmet need for effective therapies for Crohn's disease. Treatments for Crohn's disease continue to evolve from the traditional biologics to novel small molecules, with targeted mechanisms directed toward pathways that are dysregulated in Crohn's disease. There are multiple emerging mechanisms of action, including Janus kinase inhibition, Smad7 inhibition, and sphingosine-1-phosphate receptor modulators, that are administered as oral medications, and small molecules represent the next generation of therapies for Crohn's disease.

Update on Therapeutic Drug Monitoring in Crohn's Disease **645**

Valérie Heron and Waqqas Afif

In patients with Crohn's disease on biologic medications, the use of therapeutic drug monitoring leads to a personalized approach to optimize treatment. Using an algorithmic approach, measurement of drug concentrations and anti–drug antibodies can be used to improve treatment outcomes. Therapeutic drug concentrations and absence of antibodies are associated with improved clinical and endoscopic outcomes. In clinical practice, therapeutic drug monitoring has been shown to be clinically useful and cost-effective in patients experiencing a loss of response to treatment. This review highlights the available data on therapeutic drug monitoring in the treatment of patients with Crohn's disease on biologic medications.

The Evolution of Treatment Paradigms in Crohn's Disease: Beyond Better Drugs **661**

Reena Khanna, Vipul Jairath, and Brian G. Feagan

Despite advances in care, most patients with Crohn's disease (CD) develop complications, such as fistulas, or require surgery. Given the recent advances in drug therapy, an opportunity exists to optimize the management of this chronic disease through early use of effective therapies, clear definition of treatment targets, and application of the principles of personalized medicine. In this article, the authors discuss the evolution of treatment algorithms for CD to incorporate these strategies.

GASTROENTEROLOGY CLINICS OF NORTH AMERICA

FORTHCOMING ISSUES

December 2017
Complementary and Alternative Medicine in Inflammatory Bowel Disease
Ali Keshavarzian and Ece A. Mutlu, *Editors*

March 2018
Nutritional Management of Gastrointestinal Disease
Andrew Ukleja, *Editor*

June 2018
GastrointestinalTransplantation
Enrico Benedetti and Ivo G. Tzvetanov, *Editors*

RECENT ISSUES

June 2017
Liver Pathology
Jay H. Lefkowitch, *Editor*

March 2017
The Gut Microbiome
Eamonn M.M. Quigley, *Editor*

December 2016
Obesity and Gastroenterology
Octavia Pickett-Blakely and Linda A. Lee, *Editors*

RELATED INTEREST

Gastrointestinal Endoscopy Clinics
October 2016 (Vol. 26, Issue 4)
Endoscopy in Inflammatory Bowel Disease
Maria T. Abreu, *Editor*
Available at: http://www.giendo.theclinics.com

Preface

Crohn's Disease: Etiology, Complications, Assessment, Therapy, and Management

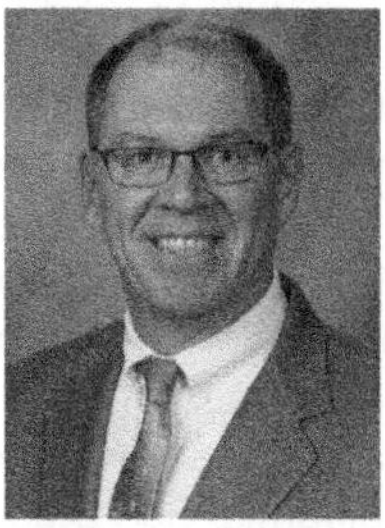

Edward V. Loftus Jr, MD
Editor

It has been over 100 years since the Scottish surgeon Sir T. Kennedy Dalziel described several cases of "chronic interstitial enteritis" resulting in diarrhea, abdominal pain, and intestinal obstruction, and 75 years since Drs Burrill B. Crohn, Leon Ginzburg, and Gordon Oppenheimer from Mount Sinai Hospital in New York published their case series of "terminal ileitis" in the *Journal of the American Medical Association*. What we now call "Crohn's disease" has evolved from a rare medical curiosity to an all-too-common diagnosis in not only North America and Europe but also the rest of the world. In this issue of *Gastroenterology Clinics of North America*, we have brought together a group of expert physicians to provide a wide-ranging update on the epidemiology, pathogenesis, natural history, disease assessment, and treatment of this vexing condition.

Drs Ming-Hsi Wang and Michael Picco of Mayo Clinic Florida review what is known about the most common genetic polymorphisms associated with Crohn's disease, including NOD2, IL-23, and ATG16L1, and what implications these have on the risk, phenotype, and prognosis of this illness. Drs Satimai Aniwan, Sang Hyoung Park, and I of Mayo Clinic Rochester provide an update on the epidemiology and natural history of Crohn's disease. Clinical and demographic features that are associated with more adverse outcomes are highlighted so that the clinician can target the level of therapy based on perceived risk. Drs Sahil Khanna and Laura Raffals of Mayo Clinic Rochester describe the complex changes in the intestinal microbiome

Gastroenterol Clin N Am 46 (2017) xiii–xv
http://dx.doi.org/10.1016/j.gtc.2017.06.001

in patients with Crohn's disease and discuss how this may be addressed with interventions such as prebiotics, probiotics, and fecal microbial transplantation.

Drs Badr Al-Bawardy and his gastroenterologic and radiologic colleagues from Mayo Clinic Rochester review the various endoscopic and radiologic means by which we assess the severity of inflammation and complications in Crohn's disease, including endoscopic and radiographic scoring systems.

Crohn's disease can cause complications. Dr Sushil Garg from the University of Minnesota, Dr Fernando Velayos of Kaiser Permanente Northern California, and Dr John Kisiel of Mayo Clinic Rochester provide an update on cancer risks, both intestinal and nonintestinal, in Crohn's disease patients, and how this relates to chronic intestinal inflammation as well as various medical therapies. Dr Jill Gaidos of Virginia Commonwealth University and Dr Sunanda Kane from Mayo Clinic Rochester review the impact that Crohn's disease has upon sexuality and fertility in both men and women and the impact of both disease activity and medications on pregnancy outcomes. Drs Amy Lightner, William Faubion, and J.G. Fletcher of Mayo Clinic Rochester describe the complexity of perianal Crohn's disease and highlight how an interdisciplinary approach (GI, radiology, surgery) can improve outcomes.

One of the particularly frustrating challenges of Crohn's disease is its tendency to recur after bowel resection. Dr Siddharth Singh of University of California–San Diego and Dr Geoff Nguyen of Mount Sinai Hospital (Toronto) review the evidence for efficacy of medications in the postoperative setting for preventing or at least decreasing the risk of recurrence and provide a management strategy for (it is hoped) earlier detection of endoscopic recurrence.

Drs Guilherme Piovezani Ramos, Faubion, and Konstantinos Papadakis of Mayo Clinic Rochester review immunologic alterations in Crohn's disease and highlight which receptors or molecules have been targeted in drug development. Dr Raina Shivashankar from the University of Pennsylvania and Dr Darrell Pardi of Mayo Clinic Rochester provide a succinct review of the evidence of efficacy and safety of anti-TNF agents and anti-integrins in Crohn's disease and compare and contrast the two drug classes. Dr Parakkal Deepak of Washington University in Saint Louis and Dr William Sandborn of University of California–San Diego review the evidence for efficacy and safety of ustekinumab in Crohn's disease and highlight an upcoming class of drugs, the anti-IL-23 agents (brazikumab and risankizumab), currently in development. Dr Brigid Boland of University of California–San Diego and Prof Severine Vermeire of University Hospitals Leuven provide an update on various oral small molecules such as the selective Janus kinase 1 inhibitors (eg, filgotinib and upadacitinib), Smad 7 inhibitors (eg, mongersen), and sphingosine-1 phosphate 1 receptor modulators (eg, ozanimod).

The protein-based biologic agents are "tricky" drugs to use due to their immunogenicity and extreme variation in pharmacokinetics. Drs Valerie Heron and Waqqas Afif of McGill University Health Center review the recent literature on the utility of therapeutic drug monitoring of biologics in Crohn's disease. In the final article, Drs Reena Khanna, Vipul Jairath, and Brian Feagan of the University of Western Ontario emphasize that it is neither disease assessment nor therapies alone that will alter the natural history of Crohn's disease, but the combination of these two in a "treat to target" approach may get us there.

It is gratifying to look back and see the advances in assessment and management of Crohn's disease over the past 25 years, but we need to press forward, build upon these gains, and continue to work toward a goal of abolition of intestinal complications and ultimately cure of this enigmatic condition.

Edward V. Loftus Jr, MD
Inflammatory Bowel Disease Interest Group
Division of Gastroenterology and Hepatology
Mayo Clinic
200 First Street, Southwest
Rochester, MN 55905, USA

E-mail address:
loftus.edward@mayo.edu

Crohn's Disease

Genetics Update

Ming-Hsi Wang, MD, PhD*, Michael F. Picco, MD, PhD

KEYWORDS

• Crohn's disease • Genetics • GWAS • Phenotypes • Behavior • TNF • NOD2
• Genetic score

KEY POINTS

- Since the discovery of first Crohn's disease (CD) gene *NOD2*, at least additional 140 genetic loci have been found associated with CD.
- Several CD-related genes can influence the CD disease location, behavior, need for surgery, extra-intestinal manifestations, and response to anti-tumor necrosis factor.
- Many CD genes known in Caucasians are shared across several non-European populations.
- The globally increasing prevalence of inflammatory bowel disease for the past decade, especially in Asia and developing countries, suggests the role of gene-environment interaction factors.
- In the future, algorithms incorporating genome, microbiome, environmental factors, and epigenome will be used to predict disease course, prognosis, and personalized therapeutic strategies in CD.

INTRODUCTION

Inflammatory bowel diseases (IBD) are chronic, relapsing intestinal inflammatory diseases affecting more than 2.5 million Caucasians (European descent), with increasing prevalence in Asia and developing countries.[1,2] The observation of familial clustering (roughly 1 of 5 Crohn's disease [CD] patients report having at least 1 affected family member), the role of ethnicity (Ashkenazi Jews are at 2- to 4-fold higher risk of IBD than non-Jews), and the relatively high concordance rate in monozygotic twins (eg, respective monozygotic vs dizygotic twin concordance for CD are 20%–50% vs 4%) begins the argument for a genetic disposition for CD. Through family-based genome-wide linkage studies, comparing the frequency of shared segments of human chromosomes among affected relative pairs with those expected by chance, the first

Disclosure: The authors have no financial disclosure.

Department of Gastroenterology and Hepatology, Mayo Clinic Jacksonville, 4500 San Pablo Road, Jacksonville, FL 32224, USA
* Corresponding author.
E-mail address: Wang.Ming-Hsi@mayo.edu

Gastroenterol Clin N Am 46 (2017) 449–461
http://dx.doi.org/10.1016/j.gtc.2017.05.002
gastro.theclinics.com

CD genetic locus at pericentromeric region of chromosome 16 was first identified in 1996, where the *NOD2* (nucleotide-binding oligomerization domain containing 2, also known as *CARD15* [caspase-recruitment domain 15]), was later identified after further gene fine-mapping approaches.[3,4] This landmark discovery further supported the previously proposed pathogenetic mechanism of CD, which was the abnormal inflammatory response directed against enteric microflora in a genetically susceptible host. It was estimated that 20% to 30% of CD patients carry an abnormal variant in *NOD2* and the penetrance of *NOD2* is not more than 5% and 0.5% for carrying 2 copies and 1 copy of CD-associated variants, respectively.[5] This finding suggests that there are other genes influencing the risk of CD. The advances in microarray-based biotechnology allowed investigators to genotype efficiently enormous numbers of single nucleotide polymorphisms (SNPs) and facilitated the development of genome-wide association study (GWAS) in human complex diseases. GWAS began in 2005 and the first IBD GWAS was conducted in Japanese CD patients and healthy controls using 80,000 SNPs and identified the tumor necrosis factor (TNF) superfamily member 15 (*TNFSF15*) as the highest risk for CD among Pacific Asian populations. This association was further confirmed in 2 European cohorts and confirmed that the genetic variations in the *TNFSF15* contribute to the susceptibility to CD.[6]

A landmark study, combining 75,000 cases of CD, ulcerative colitis (UC), and controls across 15 previously conducted adolescent- and adult-onset GWAS, identified 163 loci (110 shared between CD and UC; 30 CD specific and 23 UC specific) and supports a connection between disease risk and host interactions with microbes such as mycobacterial infections.[7] Additionally, the majority of IBD genes (113 of the 163 loci) are common to other immune-mediated diseases, such as type 1 diabetes, ankylosing spondylitis, and psoriasis. Twenty-seven IBD loci are located in chromosomal regions containing genes associated with primary immunodeficiencies of Mendelian inheritance, which supports the observation that individuals with primary immunodeficiency syndromes have a higher rate of Crohn's-like disease. With increasing prevalence in Asia and developing countries,[1,2] a trans-ethnicity international collaborative study, composed of 86,640 European individuals and 9846 individuals of East-Asian, Indian, or Iranian descent, increased the number of IBD loci from 163 to 200.[8] These studies identified several new genetic regions with key candidate genes validated in functional studies, but also left a substantial number of genetic loci located in chromosomal (noncoding or "gene desert") regions without knowing the candidate genes and the underlying biological meaning.

Genetic heterogeneity underpinning the natural history of IBD and the continuum of IBD subphenotypes (ie, ileal CD, colonic CD, and UC) using genetic risk scores was demonstrated in a recent international and the largest so far genotype–subphenotype study.[9] Composed of 30,000 patients with IBD, this study demonstrated for the first time in the clinical care of CD patients, genetic associations with disease onset, that clinical manifestations, disease behaviors, and clinical outcomes are potentially important to treatment strategies and prognosis.[9] This article summarizes the current understanding of the most important CD risk genes and how the currently identified genetic markers can influence the CD clinical behavior, disease location, need of surgery, response to CD therapy like anti-TNF, and clinical outcomes (**Table 1**).

THE TOP INFLUENTIAL CROHN'S DISEASE RISK GENES

NOD2

The most influential gene for susceptibility to CD identified thus far is *NOD2*. The 3 most common CD-associated mutations in *NOD2* (*Arg702Trp*, *Gly908Arg*, and *Leu1007fsinsC*) play an essential role of microbial recognition and sensing.[3,4] With the binding of microbial ligands, *NOD2* activates the transcription factor nuclear factor–κB and positively regulates the host innate immune defense. Carrying homozygous or compound heterozygous mutations among the 3 *NOD2* variants has been associated with reduced activation of nuclear factor-κB and the subsequent clearance of invading microbes, compared with wild-type *NOD2*.[10] In individuals of European ancestry, heterozygous carriage of 1 risk variant confers a 2- to 4-fold increase in risk for CD; homozygous or compound heterozygous carriage confers a 17- to 40-fold increase in risk for CD.[5,11]

IL-23

GWAS in CD found a functional variant Arg381Gln in the interleukin-23 receptor (*IL23R*) on chromosome 1p31, and carrying the uncommon glutamine allele (6% in Caucasians) has a reduced risk for CD by 3-fold (odds ratio [OR], 0.26 in non-Jewish whites).[12] IL-23 is a proinflammatory heterodimeric cytokine, composed of 2 linked subunits (p19 and p40) and produced by dendritic cells and macrophages in response to diverse microbial signals, acting together with other cytokines (IL-12, composed of p35 and p40 subunits; and IL-17) and transcription factors (JAK2, STAT3) have been associated with CD susceptibility. Ustekinumab, a humanized IgG1κ monoclonal antibody that binds to the p40 shared unit of IL-12 and Il-23, prevents IL-12/23 cytokine binding with IL-12R and IL-23R receptors, thereby reducing immune cell activation. It has been shown recently in clinical trials as a safe and an important therapeutic option for adult patients with moderate to severe CD.[13]

HLA

HLA (human leukocyte antigen) encodes cell-surface proteins responsible for the regulation of the immune system. In CD, HLA, risk alleles include *DRB1*07* (OR, 1.4) and *DRB*0301* (OR, 2.2). *DRB*03* is protective for CD (OR, 0.70). Certain *HLA* alleles are more important for specifying phenotype pattern; for example, *HLA-DRB1*0103* is risk factor for colonic disease in both UC and CD, whereas *DRB1*1502* is a risk factor for UC but protective for CD.[14]

ATG16L1, IRGM, and LRRK2/MUC19

Autophagy is a self-destructive mechanism of the cell that disassembles damaged organelles and degrades microorganisms that invade intracellularly. GWAS in CD have identified several autophagy-related genes that predispose individuals to a higher CD risk. The first, the Thr300Ala functional variant in autophagy-related 16-like 1 (*ATG16L1*), encodes an amino acid substitution from alanine to threonine. This reduces CD risk (OR, 0.69).[15,16] *ATG16L1* is expressed in intestinal epithelial Paneth cells, antigen-presenting cells, and T cells.[17] Functional knock down *ATG16L1* in cell lines abrogates autophagy of *Salmonella typhimurium*.[15] Furthermore, carrying a defective alanine allele in Thr300Ala reduced the ability to capture bacteria.[18]

The second autophagy-related CD gene is *IRGM* (immunity-related GTPase family member M).[19] Although the CD-associated variants of *IRGM* do not affect the amino acid sequence of its product, they more likely alter its expression.[20] *IRGM* seems to be important in resistance to intracellular pathogens such as mycobacteria, *Listeria monocytogenes*, and *Toxoplasma gondii*.[21]

Another 2 autophagy-related CD genes are *LRRK2* (leucine-rich repeat kinase 2) and *MUC19* (mucin 19).[22] Impairments in shuttling of autophagosomes into lysosomes and increase of apoptosis and oxidative damage were observed in *LRRK2* knockout mice.[23]

Table 1
Summary of the associations between currently identified genes/loci in whites (European descent) and CD susceptibility risk and its subphenotypes, disease location, EIMs, need of surgery, and response to anti-TNF

		CD Subphenotypes and Clinical Outcomes				
Gene	**CD Risk**	**Location**	**Stricturing or Penetrating**	**EIMs**	**Need for Surgery**	**Anti-TNF Response**
NOD2 (Arg702Trp, Gly908Arg, Leu1007fsinsC)	One allele, OR, 2–4 Two alleles, OR, 17–40	Ileal OR, 1.90	Stricturing OR, 1.82 Penetrating OR, 1.25 Complicated OR, 2.96		OR, 1.73	
IL23R	OR, 0.26 Arg381Gln					Poor response RR, 2.0[a]
OCTN/SLC22	OR, 1.7–2.0 L503F, rs2631367, rs17622208		Complicated OR, 1.43	OR, 1.32		
HLA loci	OR, 1.4–2.2 (DRB1*07, DRB*0301)	Colonic OR, 3.12[b]		Ocular[c] RR, 3.2–13		
ATG16L1 Thr300Ala	OR, 0.69					
LRRK2, MUC19[d]	OR, 1.54					
IRGM[e]	OR, 1.33					
PTPN22[f]	OR, 1.31			OR, 1.86–2.00		
TNFSF15	OR, 1.22 OR, 2.17[h]			EN[i] OR, 1.8	OR, 1.29[g]	Good response[j] OR, 1.7–2.0

JAK2[k]	OR, 1.12	Ileal OR, 1.44			OR, 1.28
TRAF3IP2[l]				PG/EN: OR, 2.54	
Genetic scores			Stricturing HR, 1.29[m] Penetrating HR, 1.43[o]		HR 1.35[n]

Abbreviations: CD, Crohn's disease; EIM, extraintestinal manifestations; EN, erythema nodosum; HR, hazard ratio; PG, pyoderma gangrenosum; RR, relative risk; TNF, tumor necrosis factor.

[a] IBD risk-increasing IL23R variants (rs1004819, rs2201841, rs10889677, rs11209032, and rs1495965) were more likely to respond to infliximab than were homozygous carriers of IBD risk-decreasing IL23R variants (rs7517847, rs10489629, rs11465804, and rs1343151) (74.1 vs 34.6%; RR, 2.2).

[b] HLA-DRB1*01:03 compared with ileal (OR, 3.12).

[c] HLA-B*27, HLA-B*58, HLA-DRB1*0103.

[d] rs11747270.

[e] rs1175593.

[f] rs2476601.

[g] rs4263839.

[h] Japanese GWAS: 14,340 T→C in intron 3 of TNFSF15.

[i] TNF-α −1031C.

[j] In TNF-α −308 G allele, TNF-α −238 G allele, and TNF-α −857 C allele.

[k] rs10758669.

[l] rs33980500 (TRAF3IP2).

[m] Genetic score (NOD2, JAK2, ATG16L1).

[n] Genetic score (IRGM, TNFSF15, C130RF31, NOD2).

[o] Genetic score (IL23R, LOC441108, PRDM1, NOD2).

SLC22/OCTN on 5q31

Linkage study for CD on chromosome 5q31 was first reported in the Canadian population[24] and further fine mapping refined the region to a risk haplotype (surrounding the carnitine/organic cation transporter *SLC22A4/A5* or called *OCTN1/N2*). In a population-based study, variant in *SLC22A4/A5* was associated with CD risk (OR, 1.7–2.0).[25]

TNF

The first CD GWAS, in Japanese CD patients,[6] identified a highly significant associations (OR, 2.17) of SNPs and haplotypes within the *TNFSF15* (TNF superfamily, member 15), which encodes TNF ligand–related molecule. Distinct patterns of association have been observed in IBD patients of European ancestry, and studies of Asian and European ancestry-associated polymorphisms indicate that disease-associated haplotypes might affect expression of *TNFSF15*. The use of anti-TNF agents such as infliximab, certolizumab, and adalimumab has revolutionized the clinical care of patients with CD during the last decade[26] and genetic associations may help target these therapies to appropriate patients.

GENES ASSOCIATED WITH PEDIATRIC OR EARLY ONSET OF CROHN'S DISEASE

Approximately 20% to 25% of IBD patients develop intestinal inflammation during childhood and adolescence. Early onset (younger than 10 years of age) IBD patients tend to have pancolitis, severely ulcerating perianal disease, higher rate of first-degree relatives with IBD, higher rate of resistance to conventional antiinflammatory and immunomodulatory therapy, and a higher risk of underlying primary immunodeficiency and underlying monogenic disorders.[27] Rare forms of very early onset IBD can be transmitted through Mendelian inheritance. For example, autosomal recessive missense mutations (with complete penetrance) of the IL-10 receptor gene causes severe Crohn's-like disease through loss of function and failure of IL-10 to downregulate inflammation.[28] Other monogenic genetic defects that disturb intestinal epithelial barrier function (eg, X-linked ectodermal dysplasia and immunodeficiency) or affect innate and adaptive immune function (eg, common variable immunodeficiency) have incomplete penetrance of the CD-like phenotype.

Compared with adult-onset CD, pediatric-onset CD patients have more frequent occurrence of polymorphisms, 3020insC (homozygosity rate of 4.2% in pediatric CD vs 0.6% in adult CD) in *NOD2* and rs3792876 (homozygous rate of 6.1% in pediatric CD vs 1.1% in adult CD) in *SLC22A4/5*.[29]

CLINICAL IMPLICATIONS OF GENETIC VARIANTS FOUND IN CROHN'S DISEASE

Genes Related to the Clinical Behavior of Crohn's Disease, Disease Location, and Need for Surgery

Earlier studies[30] suggested the association between ileal disease, ileal stenosis, and the need for surgery in CD patients and homozygosity for the *NOD2* Leu1007fsinsC variant. The recent European IBDchip project identified *NOD2* as one of the most influential genetic predictors for ileal disease (OR, 1.90), ileal stenosis (OR, 1.82), fistula (OR, 1.25), and CD-related surgery (OR, 1.73).[31] The overall OR for complicated disease behavior was 4.87 for CD patients homozygous for the NOD2 Leu1007fsinsC mutation.[31] However, this subgroup represents less than 3% of all CD patients of European descent so that its clinical usefulness is limited.

A metaanalysis of 36 studies showed that the presence of any *NOD2* mutant allele (*R702W*, *G908R*, and *Leu1007fsinsC*) was associated with complicated (ie, stricturing or penetrating) disease (relative risk [RR], 1.17). The RR of surgery for G908R was 1.58. The risk of complicated CD was increased by 8% for those with a single *NOD2* risk allele and 41% for those carrying 2 *NOD2* risk alleles. Carrying any *NOD2* risk allele also increased CD surgery risk by 58%, but not perianal disease risk.[32]

In a pediatric-onset CD cohort, *Leu1007fsinsC* in *NOD2* was associated with ileal involvement (1.9% in noncarriers vs 13.3% in carriers; RR, 12.2) and *DLG5* (discs large MAGUK scaffold protein 5, proposed function in the transmission of extracellular signals to the cytoskeleton and in cell–cell contact) was significantly associated with perianal disease (RR, 2.4).[29]

Janus kinase 2 (JAK2), a key component of signal transduction pathway of several cytokines including IL-12 and IL-23, was another gene associated with ileocolonic disease involvement and stricturing disease behavior in CD.[31] Interestingly, a recent clinical trial found that tofacitinib, an oral inhibitor of the JAK, was effective in the treatment of UC[33] but not in CD.[34]

A novel study[31] created genetic scores by comparing significant genes with CD subphenotypes and outcomes. Higher genetic scores were associated with higher probability of developing penetrating disease (*IL23R*, *LOC441108*, *PRDM1*, *NOD2*; composite scores hazard ratio, 1.43), need for surgery (*IRGM*, *TNFSF15*, *C13ORF31*, *NOD2*; composite scores hazard ratio, 1.35), and stricturing disease (*NOD2*, *JAK2*, *ATG16L1*; composite scores hazard ratio, 1.29). Similarly, among the previously identified 163 IBD-related loci,[7] only 3p21 (*MST1*, macrophage stimulating-1), *NOD2*, and the *HLA* were significantly associated with age of onset and disease location.[9] The strongest signal for CD location was a colonic association with *HLA-DRB1*01:03* compared with ileal (OR, 3.12) or ileocolonic disease (OR, 2.12). SNP rs77005575 in *HLA* was significantly associated with CD behavior, independent of disease location.[9] Although the associations between ileal CD and *NOD2*, and those between colonic CD and the *HLA*, have been previously described,[11,31,35] the most recent study suggested that the association between *NOD2* and stricturing CD behavior could be reduced and further influenced by CD location.[9] These findings suggest that the CD location is more representative of the disease's biological aspect than CD behavior, whereas CD behavior is more representative of the progression of disease.

Through a powerful approach of genetic risk scores, derived from subgroups of IBD associated SNPs instead of individual SNPs, the genetic architecture of colonic Crohn's disease is intermediate between ileal CD and UC.[9] This finding suggests that IBD may be redefined and divided into a 3-group continuum (ileal CD vs colonic CD vs UC), rather than the current division between CD and UC.

Genes Related to Extraintestinal Manifestations of Crohn's Disease

Extraintestinal manifestations in patients with CD are more frequently observed in patients with *HLA-A2*, *HLA-DR1*, and *HLA-DQw5*.[36,37] Distinct *HLA-B* and *HLA-DR* are associated with IBD-related arthropathy. For example, type 1 arthritis (large joint arthritis) was found to be associated with *HLA-B*27*, *B*35* and *HLA-DRB1*0103*, and type 2 arthritis (small joint polyarthritis) was found to be associated with *HLA-B*44* and *MICA*008*.[37,38] Ankylosing spondylitis was found to be associated with *HLA-B*27* and *DRB1*0101*.[37] Acute anterior uveitis was found to be associated with genes in the *HLA-B*27*.[39] Ocular inflammation was strongly associated with *HLA-B*27*, *B*58*, and *HLA-DRB1*0103*. There is a weak association between erythema nodosum and *HLA-B*15* but a strong association with the *-1031 TNF-*α.[36] Extraintestinal manifestations are also more common among the carriers of the *PTPN22* variant with an almost 2-fold increased risk.[31]

A GWAS-derived novel gene, *TRAF3IP2*, modulating the humoral immunity and involving in the IL-17–mediated cellular immune responses, is involved in the susceptibility to psoriasis.[40] In CD, a significant association was observed between *TRAF3IP2* and pyoderma gangrenosum and erythema nodosum (OR, 2.54). Among patients with primary sclerosing cholangitis and UC 2 genetic loci are significant: (1) rs38904 (*WNT2,CFTR*; OR, 2.78) and (2) rs11209026 (*IL23R*; OR, 4.08).[41] This finding warrants replication in a larger study.

Genes Related to Anti-Tumor Necrosis Factor Response in Crohn's Disease

Although with relatively low predictive power for a single mutation, a recent metaanalysis found a 98% high specificity of carrying 2 *NOD2* mutations for complicated CD course and may support the use of "aggressive" therapeutic strategies in this subgroup of patients.[32] Regarding the influence of *NOD2* on anti-TNF therapy, conflicting results from prior studies were found with some suggesting the need for more intensified therapy, poorer response to TNF agents, or no impact at all, depending on the variants studied.[42–44]

Similarly, in rheumatoid arthritis, 3 genetic variants (rs1568885, rs1813443, and rs4411591) were found possibly associated with the response to anti-TNF agents.[45] In a pilot study,[46] certain *IL23R* gene variants were associated with a better response to infliximab. Prior studies have suggested that homozygosity for a *TNF* polymorphism and carriers of *TNFR1* 36G mutations in the *TNFR1* gene were poor anti-TNF responders[43,47] but results are conflicting.[48,49] A recent metaanalysis examining the TNF polymorphisms and anti-TNF response in spondyloarthropathy, psoriasis, and CD suggested a significant increase of anti-TNF response in several TNF-α alleles.[50]

CROHN'S DISEASE GENETICS IN NON-WHITE POPULATIONS

In African Americans, *NOD2* mutations are much less common and only heterozygous, occurring at 20% the frequency observed in Americans of European ancestry—proportionate to the degree of European admixture.[51] However, the risk for CD among carriers of heterozygous mutations in African Americans is similar (OR, 4.1) to that observed in European ancestry cohorts. The *NOD2* mutations associated with CD are not observed in Asian or sub-Saharan African populations. Several other previously established Caucasian associations were replicated in African Americans at *IL23R*, *5p15.3*, and *IKZF3* in a recent GWAS among African Americans.[51]

The largest IBD GWAS cohort of 9846 non-European samples (East Asian, Indian, or Iranian descent)[8] revealed a male predominance in CD (67% of non-European CD vs 45% in Europeans), more stricturing behavior, and more perianal disease in non-Europeans. A highly positive correlation was observed between European and East Asian cohorts across 231 IBD SNPs, suggesting that the majority of IBD genes are shared across different populations.

REMAINING CHALLENGES IN CROHN'S DISEASE GENETICS

Unexplored Regions: Chromosome X, Mitochondrial DNA, and Rare Variants

The observations of higher IBD incidence among Turner's syndrome patients who lack 1 chromosome X[52] and the predominance of mother/child affected pairs than father–child affected pairs[53] support the role of chromosome X in IBD. The lack of attention of IBD genetic study on chromosome X is not only the lack of gene, but also the technical challenges of performing analysis. One of the histopathologic hallmarks in IBD includes a destruction of the intestinal epithelial barrier, increased gut permeability, and an influx of immune cells, which could be related to dysfunction of mitochondria. Several lines of evidence have linked the mitochondrial stress and alterations in mitochondrial function with human IBD.[54] Rare genetic variants, often defined as a minor allele frequency of less than 1%, are likely to have arisen from mutation events in the last 20 generations, and tend to be ethnic specific and carrying larger effect than common variants and may play a role in the genetics of CD.

Complex Gene–Gene and Gene–Environmental Interactions

Despite advances in IBD genetics, only 13.1% in CD and 8.2% in UC of total disease variance has been explained by the recently identified 200 genetic loci.[8] Furthermore, the genetic influence on the disease susceptibility goes beyond the number of risk alleles an individual carries.[41,55] Gene–gene and gene–environment interactions could uncover some of the missing explained disease variance left out from the conventional genetic additive models. For example, through a novel methodology, a high-order genetic interaction between genes *NOD2*, *IL10*, and *C13orf31* was identified and further validated in an independent cohort.[55]

The recent observed increasing incidence of IBD during the 20th century[1] may be explained at least partially by environmental exposures, including increased urbanization, industrialization, and changes in diet, which can be associated with changes in gut microbiome, improved sanitation, and possibly more frequent use of antibiotics in childhood. Immigration studies have observed a rising incidence of IBD in the first and second generations of Asian migrants to the West,[56] further suggested the critical interrelationships between host gene and environmental factors in IBD. As a recent example of gene–environment interactions in CD, a suggested interaction between smoking and *HDAC* (histone deacetylase) was recently reported. The effect of smoking on the CD risk was enhanced among carriers of *HDAC7* (OR, 4.23), whereas the risk became insignificant among noncarriers (OR, 1.31).[57]

SUMMARY AND FUTURE DIRECTIONS

This article provides a concise summary of current understanding of CD genetics and its potential clinical implications (eg, genes related to the CD subphenotypes, disease location, need of surgery, and anti-TNF response) (see **Table 1**). A recent genotype–subphenotype study[9] has challenged our current understanding by suggesting that IBD may be redefined and divided into a 3-group continuum (ileal CD vs colonic CD vs UC). Additionally, using the informative genetic risk scores can indeed identify some clinically misclassified IBD cases and reapply a more appropriate treatment strategy.

The quest to identify biomarkers, including genetic markers, may allow clinicians to determine the risk of CD and its complications, which has profound implications for prognosis and choice of therapy It is also increasingly apparent that no single biomarker will be able to perform such a task in CD without taking into account of complex gene and environmental interactions. System biology methodology can be applied to understand the complex molecular interactions of IBD and identify novel therapeutic targets.[58] Likely, in the future, algorithms that incorporate specific genetic risk alleles with other biomarkers (eg, antimicrobial markers, specific proteomic signature, microRNAs, and gut microbiome) will be used to predict complications, response to specific therapies, risk for surgery, and so on, allowing true precision medicine to become real in IBD.

REFERENCES

1. Molodecky NA, Soon IS, Rabi DM, et al. Increasing incidence and prevalence of the inflammatory bowel diseases with time, based on systematic review. Gastroenterology 2012;142(1):46–54.e42 [quiz: e30].

2. Ng SC, Tang W, Ching JY, et al. Incidence and phenotype of inflammatory bowel disease based on results from the Asia-pacific Crohn's and colitis epidemiology study. Gastroenterology 2013;145(1):158–65.e2.
3. Hugot JP, Chamaillard M, Zouali H, et al. Association of NOD2 leucine-rich repeat variants with susceptibility to Crohn's disease. Nature 2001;411(6837):599–603.
4. Ogura Y, Bonen DK, Inohara N, et al. A frameshift mutation in NOD2 associated with susceptibility to Crohn's disease. Nature 2001;411(6837):603–6.
5. Brant SR, Wang MH, Rawsthorne P, et al. A population-based case-control study of CARD15 and other risk factors in Crohn's disease and ulcerative colitis. Am J Gastroenterol 2007;102(2):313–23.
6. Yamazaki K, McGovern D, Ragoussis J, et al. Single nucleotide polymorphisms in TNFSF15 confer susceptibility to Crohn's disease. Hum Mol Genet 2005;14(22): 3499–506.
7. Jostins L, Ripke S, Weersma RK, et al. Host-microbe interactions have shaped the genetic architecture of inflammatory bowel disease. Nature 2012;491(7422): 119–24.
8. Liu JZ, van Sommeren S, Huang H, et al. Association analyses identify 38 susceptibility loci for inflammatory bowel disease and highlight shared genetic risk across populations. Nat Genet 2015;47(9):979–86.
9. Cleynen I, Boucher G, Jostins L, et al. Inherited determinants of Crohn's disease and ulcerative colitis phenotypes: a genetic association study. Lancet 2016; 387(10014):156–67.
10. Abraham C, Cho JH. Functional consequences of NOD2 (CARD15) mutations. Inflamm Bowel Dis 2006;12(7):641–50.
11. Economou M, Trikalinos TA, Loizou KT, et al. Differential effects of NOD2 variants on Crohn's disease risk and phenotype in diverse populations: a metaanalysis. Am J Gastroenterol 2004;99(12):2393–404.
12. Duerr RH, Taylor KD, Brant SR, et al. A genome-wide association study identifies IL23R as an inflammatory bowel disease gene. Science 2006;314(5804):1461–3.
13. Feagan BG, Sandborn WJ, Gasink C, et al. Ustekinumab as induction and maintenance therapy for Crohn's disease. N Engl J Med 2016;375(20):1946–60.
14. Stokkers PC, Reitsma PH, Tytgat GN, et al. HLA-DR and -DQ phenotypes in inflammatory bowel disease: a meta-analysis. Gut 1999;45(3):395–401.
15. Rioux JD, Xavier RJ, Taylor KD, et al. Genome-wide association study identifies new susceptibility loci for Crohn disease and implicates autophagy in disease pathogenesis. Nat Genet 2007;39(5):596–604.
16. Hampe J, Franke A, Rosenstiel P, et al. A genome-wide association scan of nonsynonymous SNPs identifies a susceptibility variant for Crohn disease in ATG16L1. Nat Genet 2007;39(2):207–11.
17. Cadwell K, Liu JY, Brown SL, et al. A key role for autophagy and the autophagy gene Atg16l1 in mouse and human intestinal Paneth cells. Nature 2008; 456(7219):259–63.
18. Kuballa P, Huett A, Rioux JD, et al. Impaired autophagy of an intracellular pathogen induced by a Crohn's disease associated ATG16L1 variant. PLoS One 2008;3(10):e3391.
19. Parkes M, Barrett JC, Prescott NJ, et al. Sequence variants in the autophagy gene IRGM and multiple other replicating loci contribute to Crohn's disease susceptibility. Nat Genet 2007;39(7):830–2.
20. McCarroll SA, Huett A, Kuballa P, et al. Deletion polymorphism upstream of IRGM associated with altered IRGM expression and Crohn's disease. Nat Genet 2008; 40(9):1107–12.

21. Xavier RJ, Huett A, Rioux JD. Autophagy as an important process in gut homeostasis and Crohn's disease pathogenesis. Gut 2008;57(6):717–20.
22. Barrett JC, Hansoul S, Nicolae DL, et al. Genome-wide association defines more than 30 distinct susceptibility loci for Crohn's disease. Nat Genet 2008;40(8): 955–62.
23. Tong Y, Yamaguchi H, Giaime E, et al. Loss of leucine-rich repeat kinase 2 causes impairment of protein degradation pathways, accumulation of alpha-synuclein, and apoptotic cell death in aged mice. Proc Natl Acad Sci U S A 2010; 107(21):9879–84.
24. Rioux JD, Silverberg MS, Daly MJ, et al. Genomewide search in Canadian families with inflammatory bowel disease reveals two novel susceptibility loci. Am J Hum Genet 2000;66(6):1863–70.
25. Okazaki T, Wang MH, Rawsthorne P, et al. Contributions of IBD5, IL23R, ATG16L1, and NOD2 to Crohn's disease risk in a population-based case-control study: evidence of gene-gene interactions. Inflamm Bowel Dis 2008;14(11): 1528–41.
26. Peyrin-Biroulet L, Deltenre P, de Suray N, et al. Efficacy and safety of tumor necrosis factor antagonists in Crohn's disease: meta-analysis of placebo-controlled trials. Clin Gastroenterol Hepatol 2008;6(6):644–53.
27. Uhlig HH, Schwerd T, Koletzko S, et al. The diagnostic approach to monogenic very early onset inflammatory bowel disease. Gastroenterology 2014;147(5): 990–1007.e3.
28. Glocker EO, Kotlarz D, Boztug K, et al. Inflammatory bowel disease and mutations affecting the interleukin-10 receptor. N Engl J Med 2009;361(21):2033–45.
29. de Ridder L, Weersma RK, Dijkstra G, et al. Genetic susceptibility has a more important role in pediatric-onset Crohn's disease than in adult-onset Crohn's disease. Inflamm Bowel Dis 2007;13(9):1083–92.
30. Seiderer J, Brand S, Herrmann KA, et al. Predictive value of the CARD15 variant 1007fs for the diagnosis of intestinal stenoses and the need for surgery in Crohn's disease in clinical practice: results of a prospective study. Inflamm Bowel Dis 2006;12(12):1114–21.
31. Cleynen I, Gonzalez JR, Figueroa C, et al. Genetic factors conferring an increased susceptibility to develop Crohn's disease also influence disease phenotype: results from the IBDchip European Project. Gut 2013;62(11):1556–65.
32. Adler J, Rangwalla SC, Dwamena BA, et al. The prognostic power of the NOD2 genotype for complicated Crohn's disease: a meta-analysis. Am J Gastroenterol 2011;106(4):699–712.
33. Sandborn WJ, Ghosh S, Panes J, et al. Tofacitinib, an oral Janus kinase inhibitor, in active ulcerative colitis. N Engl J Med 2012;367(7):616–24.
34. Sandborn WJ, Ghosh S, Panes J, et al. A phase 2 study of tofacitinib, an oral Janus kinase inhibitor, in patients with Crohn's disease. Clin Gastroenterol Hepatol 2014;12(9):1485–93.e2.
35. Brant SR, Picco MF, Achkar JP, et al. Defining complex contributions of NOD2/CARD15 gene mutations, age at onset, and tobacco use on Crohn's disease phenotypes. Inflamm Bowel Dis 2003;9(5):281–9.
36. Orchard TR, Chua CN, Ahmad T, et al. Uveitis and erythema nodosum in inflammatory bowel disease: clinical features and the role of HLA genes. Gastroenterology 2002;123(3):714–8.
37. Orchard TR, Thiyagaraja S, Welsh KI, et al. Clinical phenotype is related to HLA genotype in the peripheral arthropathies of inflammatory bowel disease. Gastroenterology 2000;118(2):274–8.

38. Orchard TR, Dhar A, Simmons JD, et al. MHC class I chain-like gene A (MICA) and its associations with inflammatory bowel disease and peripheral arthropathy. Clin Exp Immunol 2001;126(3):437–40.
39. Lyons JL, Rosenbaum JT. Uveitis associated with inflammatory bowel disease compared with uveitis associated with spondyloarthropathy. Arch Ophthalmol 1997;115(1):61–4.
40. Ellinghaus E, Ellinghaus D, Stuart PE, et al. Genome-wide association study identifies a psoriasis susceptibility locus at TRAF3IP2. Nat Genet 2010;42(11):991–5.
41. Wang MH, Fiocchi C, Zhu X, et al. Gene-gene and gene-environment interactions in ulcerative colitis. Hum Genet 2014;133(5):547–58.
42. Niess JH, Klaus J, Stephani J, et al. NOD2 polymorphism predicts response to treatment in Crohn's disease–first steps to a personalized therapy. Dig Dis Sci 2012;57(4):879–86.
43. Pierik M, Vermeire S, Steen KV, et al. Tumour necrosis factor-alpha receptor 1 and 2 polymorphisms in inflammatory bowel disease and their association with response to infliximab. Aliment Pharmacol Ther 2004;20(3):303–10.
44. Gutierrez A, Scharl M, Sempere L, et al. Genetic susceptibility to increased bacterial translocation influences the response to biological therapy in patients with Crohn's disease. Gut 2014;63(2):272–80.
45. Thomas D, Gazouli M, Karantanos T, et al. Association of rs1568885, rs1813443 and rs4411591 polymorphisms with anti-TNF medication response in Greek patients with Crohn's disease. World J Gastroenterol 2014;20(13):3609–14.
46. Jurgens M, Laubender RP, Hartl F, et al. Disease activity, ANCA, and IL23R genotype status determine early response to infliximab in patients with ulcerative colitis. Am J Gastroenterol 2010;105(8):1811–9.
47. Taylor KD, Plevy SE, Yang H, et al. ANCA pattern and LTA haplotype relationship to clinical responses to anti-TNF antibody treatment in Crohn's disease. Gastroenterology 2001;120(6):1347–55.
48. Louis E, Vermeire S, Rutgeerts P, et al. A positive response to infliximab in Crohn disease: association with a higher systemic inflammation before treatment but not with -308 TNF gene polymorphism. Scand J Gastroenterol 2002;37(7):818–24.
49. Mascheretti S, Hampe J, Kuhbacher T, et al. Pharmacogenetic investigation of the TNF/TNF-receptor system in patients with chronic active Crohn's disease treated with infliximab. Pharmacogenomics J 2002;2(2):127–36.
50. Song GG, Seo YH, Kim JH, et al. Association between TNF-alpha (-308 A/G, -238 A/G, -857 C/T) polymorphisms and responsiveness to TNF-alpha blockers in spondyloarthropathy, psoriasis and Crohn's disease: a meta-analysis. Pharmacogenomics 2015;16(12):1427–37.
51. Huang C, Haritunians T, Okou DT, et al. Characterization of genetic loci that affect susceptibility to inflammatory bowel diseases in African Americans. Gastroenterology 2015;149(6):1575–86.
52. Price WH. A high incidence of chronic inflammatory bowel disease in patients with Turner's syndrome. J Med Genet 1979;16(4):263–6.
53. Akolkar PN, Gulwani-Akolkar B, Heresbach D, et al. Differences in risk of Crohn's disease in offspring of mothers and fathers with inflammatory bowel disease. Am J Gastroenterol 1997;92(12):2241–4.
54. Beltran B, Nos P, Dasi F, et al. Mitochondrial dysfunction, persistent oxidative damage, and catalase inhibition in immune cells of naive and treated Crohn's disease. Inflamm Bowel Dis 2010;16(1):76–86.

55. Wang MH, Fiocchi C, Ripke S, et al. A novel approach to detect cumulative genetic effects and genetic interactions in Crohn's disease. Inflamm Bowel Dis 2013;19(9):1799–808.
56. Pinsk V, Lemberg DA, Grewal K, et al. Inflammatory bowel disease in the South Asian pediatric population of British Columbia. Am J Gastroenterol 2007; 102(5):1077–83.
57. Wang MH, Fiocchi C, Ripke S, et al. Model integrating genetic and environmental factors interactions can predict Crohn's disease risk. A Am J Gastroenterol 2014; 109(Supple 2):S503.
58. Polytarchou C, Koukos G, Iliopoulos D. Systems biology in inflammatory bowel diseases: ready for prime time. Curr Opin Gastroenterol 2014;30(4):339–46.

Epidemiology, Natural History, and Risk Stratification of Crohn's Disease

Satimai Aniwan, MD[a,b], Sang Hyoung Park, MD[a,c], Edward V. Loftus Jr, MD[a,*]

KEYWORDS

• Crohn's disease • Epidemiology • Risk factors • Natural history • Complications

KEY POINTS

- The incidence and prevalence of Crohn's disease in the Western world are continuously increasing, and are also rapidly increasing in newly industrialized countries, making Crohn's disease a truly global disease.
- Cigarette smoking, low dietary fiber intake, high dietary fat intake, improved childhood hygiene, and various medications are important environmental risk factors for Crohn's disease.
- Over time, the extent of Crohn's disease remains mostly stable, whereas disease behavior changes over time, with more patients developing stricturing or penetrating complications.
- Risk factors for a more unfavorable clinical course of Crohn's disease include younger age at diagnosis, extensive anatomic involvement, perianal disease, stricturing or penetrating behavior, deep ulcers, and prior surgical resection.

INTRODUCTION

Crohn's disease (CD) is a chronic condition that in some cases can result in significant morbidity and disability. The disease course can wax and wane over time, and there is a wide spectrum of severity. It is important to understand the epidemiology, risk

S. Aniwan and S.H. Park share co-first authorship.

Disclosure Statement: Dr E.V. Loftus Jr has consulted for AbbVie, Janssen, Takeda, UCB, Amgen, Pfizer, Eli Lilly, Salix, CVS Caremark, and Mesoblast; and has received research support from AbbVie, Janssen, Takeda, UCB, Genentech, Amgen, Pfizer, Receptos, Celgene, Gilead, Seres Therapeutics, and Robarts Clinical Trials.

[a] Division of Gastroenterology and Hepatology, Mayo Clinic, 200 First Street, South west, Rochester, MN 55905, USA; [b] Division of Gastroenterology, Thai Red Cross Society, King Chulalongkorn Memorial Hospital, Chulalongkorn University, Rama IV Road, Bangkok, 10330, Thailand; [c] Department of Gastroenterology, Asan Medical Center, University of Ulsan College of Medicine, 88, Olympic-ro 43-gil, Songpa-gu, Seoul 05505, Korea

* Corresponding author.

E-mail address: Loftus.Edward@mayo.edu

Gastroenterol Clin N Am 46 (2017) 463–480
http://dx.doi.org/10.1016/j.gtc.2017.05.003
gastro.theclinics.com

factors, and natural history of this incurable, lifelong disease for better management of patients and allocation of societal resources. By studying the association between demographics and initial clinical features of patients with CD and subsequent natural history, we may be able to stratify patients by their risks of clinical relapse, hospitalization, and surgery. Understanding the potential environmental risk factors and natural history of CD in a given patient guides the physician when counseling the patient and selecting a treatment strategy. Better risk stratification may improve the management of CD, thereby modifying disease outcomes. In this review, updated data regarding the incidence and prevalence of CD, important environmental risk factors, natural history of the disease, and important prognostic factors are discussed.

INCIDENCE AND PREVALENCE OF CROHN'S DISEASE

Inflammatory bowel disease (IBD) is a chronic and relapsing inflammatory disorder of the intestine, categorized into 2 identified subtypes: CD and ulcerative colitis (UC). UC was recognized as a medical condition approximately 60 years earlier than CD, and thus for years was thought to be more common than CD.[1] Because CD was formally recognized in 1932 as "regional enteritis,"[2] the incidence of CD has increased in the Western world, including North America, Europe, Australia, and New Zealand.[3] In particular, the incidence of CD has rapidly increased alongside human civilization and population growth during the last 50 years of the twentieth century.[4] Nowadays, the incidence of CD is highest in the Western region, ranging from 10 to 30 cases per 100,000 person-years.[3] Moreover, the prevalence of IBD is highest in the Western region, affecting up to 0.5% of the general population (**Fig. 1**).[3] Extrapolation of recent data from a population-based study in a well-defined region in the United States suggests that there are approximately 785,000 US residents with CD and 910,000 with UC, for a total of approximately 1.6 million US residents with IBD.[5] There may be geographic differences in CD incidence and prevalence across Western countries, as is the case in other immune-mediated diseases.[6] For example, studies of the European Crohn's and Colitis Organization's Epidemiology Committee (ECCO-EpiCom) inception cohort showed that the incidence of IBD is high in Western Europe, low in countries near the Mediterranean Sea, and varies from low to high throughout Eastern Europe.[7,8]

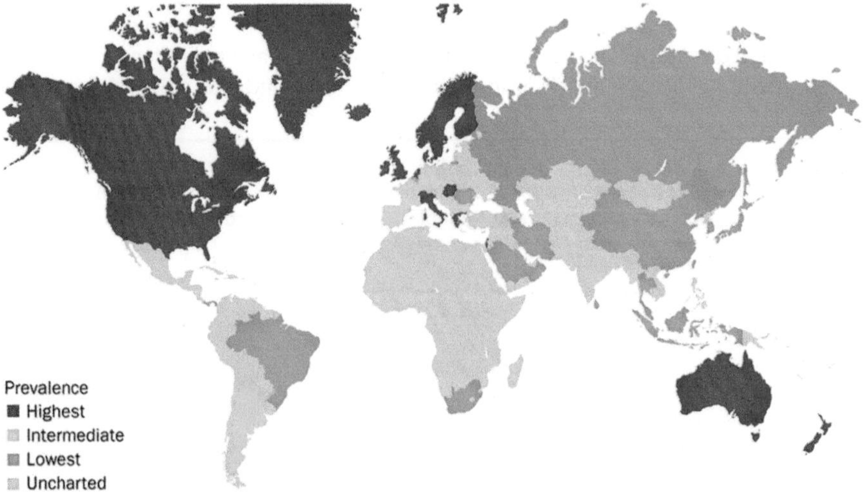

Fig. 1. The global prevalence of IBD in 2015. (*From* Kaplan GG. The global burden of IBD: from 2015 to 2025. Nat Rev Gastroenterol Hepatol 2015;12(12):722; with permission.)

IBD has traditionally been known as a disease of white people in the industrialized region of the Western world. However, industrialization has increased in other areas, such as Asia, since the late twentieth century. Alongside these changes, the incidence of UC, followed by that of CD, has increased in Asia at the turn of the twenty-first century, similar to that observed in Western countries during the twentieth century.[3,9] For example, in a population-based study from South Korea,[10] the annual incidence of CD was 0.05 cases per 100,000 person-years in 1986 to 1990, increasing up to 1.34 per 100,000 in 2001 to 2005. The prevalence of CD was 11.2 cases per 100,000 inhabitants in 2005, which was low compared with those in Western world, but rapidly increasing.[10] This trend was also observed in a multicenter epidemiologic study from Asia, the Asia-Pacific Crohn's and Colitis Epidemiologic Study (ACCESS), in which the pooled incidence of IBD in Asia was 1.4 cases per 100,000 person-years and increasing.[11] As in Western regions, there may be geographic differences in incidence between countries and within countries. In the ACCESS cohort, the highest incidence of IBD was in India, at 9.3 cases per 100,000 person-years, whereas the incidence of IBD within China ranged from 0.50 to 3.14 per 100,000 person-years for IBD and from 0.05 to 1.09 per 100,000 person-years for CD in different regions.[11] Differences in the degree of urbanization may affect the incidence of IBD within a country. Likewise, the incidence of IBD is also rapidly increasing in newly industrialized countries outside of Asia, such as in Central and South America.[4]

Several longitudinal analyses of population-based studies have reported that the incidence of IBD increased, then reached a plateau in the mid to late twentieth century, although there have been conflicting findings.[1,3] Globally, however, 75% of CD incidence studies and 60% of UC studies have demonstrated a statistically significant increase in incidence.[3] Recently, the incidence and prevalence of IBD in a population-based inception cohort from Olmsted County, Minnesota, was updated through 2011.[5] The incidence of CD was 6.9 cases per 100,000 person-years in 1970 to 1979 and 6.5 per 100,000 person-years in 1980 to 1990, increasing up to 9.0 per 100,000 person-years in 1990 to 1999, and 10.7 per 100,000 person-years in 2000 to 2010 (**Fig. 2**). A recently published article showed that the incidence of CD

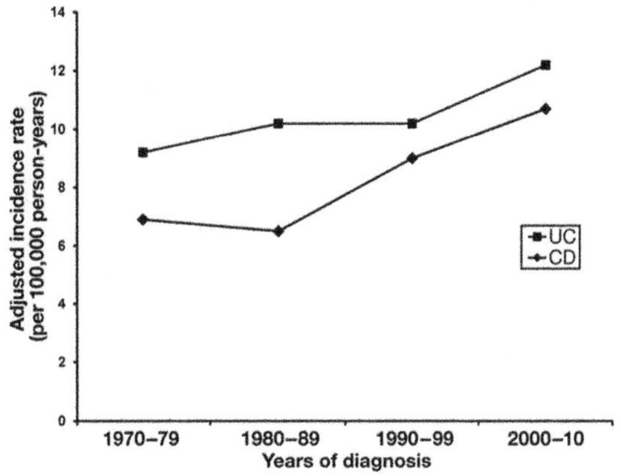

Fig. 2. Age-adjusted and sex-adjusted incidence rate of CD and UC in a population-based cohort of patients from Olmsted County between 1970 and 2010. (*From* Shivashankar R, Tremaine WJ, Harmsen WS, et al. Incidence and prevalence of Crohn's disease and ulcerative colitis in Olmsted County, Minnesota from 1970 through 2010. Clin Gastroenterol Hepatol 2017;15(6):859; with permission.)

increased in Denmark from 5.2 cases per 100,000 person-years to 9.1 per 100,000 person-years between 1980 and 2013.[12] The prevalence of IBD has increased over time even more dramatically than the incidence rate, because IBD is a chronic disease with a low mortality that is usually diagnosed in young individuals with relatively long life expectancy. This phenomenon has been known as "compounding prevalence."[1] For example, the prevalence of CD in Olmsted County was only 28 cases per 100,000 residents in 1965, increasing up to 105.7 per 100,000 residents in 1976, 132.7 per 100,000 residents in 1991, 174 per 100,000 residents in 2001, and 246.7 per 100,000 residents in 2011.[5,13–16] In contrast, some population-based studies from the Western world have reported a decreasing incidence of IBD. For example, a population-based study from Canada showed a decrease in both CD and UC incidence between 1996 and 2009.[17] Age-adjusted incidence rates for CD decreased from 27.4 cases per 100,000 person-years to 17.7 per 100,000 person-years during the study period. However, there may have been underestimation of cases, because diagnoses of IBD were not made based on clinical diagnoses and medical record review, but rather on a validated database scoring system (ie, administrative data such as *International Classification of Diseases, Ninth Revision* codes taken together with physician billing claims and, if hospitalized, discharge diagnoses).[18] Recently, Dahlhamer and colleagues[19] reported that the estimated prevalence of IBD in US adults was approximately 3 million persons using 2015 National Health Interview Survey (NHIS) data. This is a much higher figure than the previously reported estimate (approximately 1.6 million US residents based on the 2010 US White population).[5] The reason for this discrepancy is not entirely clear. However, the NHIS prevalence was based on patients' response to the question, "Have you ever been told by a doctor or other health professional that you had CD or UC?" Thus, there may be a possibility of overestimation, including other diagnosis such irritable bowel syndrome or infectious conditions.

Epidemiologic features of IBD can differ across age groups. Among elderly patients, the incidence of UC is higher than that of CD, and the incidence of CD in elderly patients (defined as >60–93 years of age according to the studies) varies across the Western region, ranging from 0 to 18.9 cases per 100,000 person-years.[20] This wide range of incidence may be because of the differences in the methods of data collection, data ascertainment, and definitions of diagnosis. In pediatric populations, the incidence of IBD continues to steadily increase.[21,22] A population-based study from Ontario, Canada, showed that the incidence of pediatric-onset IBD increased from 9.5 cases per 100,000 person-years in 1994 to 11.4 per 100,000 in 2005, and the prevalence increased from 42.1 per 100,000 persons in 1994 to 56.3 per 100,000 in 2005.[21] A pediatric population-based study from Iceland demonstrated that between 1951 and 2000 the incidence rate of CD increased from 0.2 cases per 100,000 person-years to 2.3 per 100,000, and the rate of UC increased from 1.1 per 100,000 to 2.4 per 100,000.[22]

IMPORTANT ENVIRONMENTAL RISK FACTORS

The putative roles of many environmental factors in the pathogenesis of IBD have been evaluated, but none of these factors exclusively explain the onset of IBD (**Fig. 3**).[23] Cigarette smoking has been the most consistently studied environmental risk factor. Smoking increases the risk of developing CD, in contrast to UC, in which current smoking is a protective factor and former smoking is a risk factor.[24] A meta-analysis of 9 studies including 10,610 patients demonstrated that current smoking is associated with the development of CD (odds ratio [OR] 1.76; 95% confidence

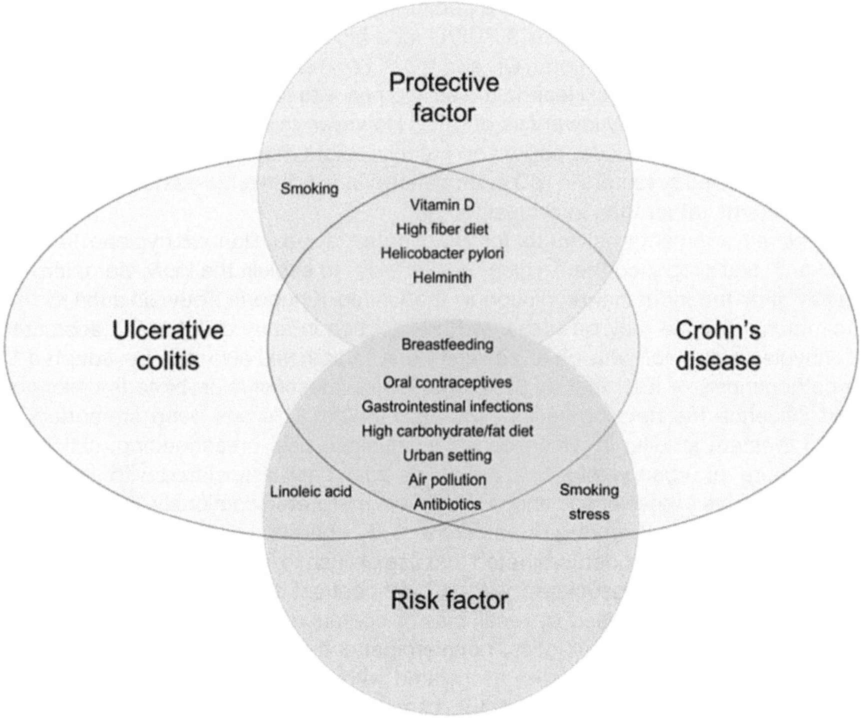

Fig. 3. The relationship between environmental factors and development of CD and UC. (*From* Ponder A, Long MD. A clinical review of recent findings in the epidemiology of inflammatory bowel disease. Clin Epidemiol 2013;5:244; with permission.)

interval [CI] 1.40–2.22), and former smoking is weakly associated with CD (OR 1.30; 95% CI 0.97–1.76).[25] Smoking might contribute to the development of CD by affecting the intestinal microbiota, as patients with CD who smoke demonstrate an intestinal dysbiosis.[26] However, studies from newly industrialized countries showed inconsistent data regarding the association between smoking and risk of CD. A study of risk factors from the ACCESS cohort demonstrated that smoking was not a risk factor for CD in 8 newly industrialized countries in Asia, whereas smoking quadrupled the risk of developing CD in Australia.[27] This result may mean that smoking differentially influences IBD risk according to races and regions, or that there is a delayed effect that has not yet manifested in these regions.[1] Alternatively, the exact rate of smoking could have been underestimated in Asian patients with IBD, because patients in these areas may be reluctant to disclose smoking history for cultural reasons.[28]

Dietary factors are known to be associated with IBD. The most common dietary pattern associated with an increased risk of IBD has been a diet low in fiber and high in animal fat.[29] In the prospective Nurses' Health Studies from the United States, women who had the highest quintile of long-term fiber intake had a 40% reduction in the risk of CD (OR 0.59, 95% CI 0.39–0.90).[30] The inverse association between dietary fiber intake and development of CD was observed especially with intake of fiber from fruits and vegetables, and not seen with intake of whole grains or cereals.[30] In contrast, a higher ratio of n-3:n-6 polyunsaturated fatty acids (PUFAs) was associated with a lower risk of UC, not CD.[31] In a pediatric population, high consumption of n-6 PUFAs and low consumption of n-3 PUFAs (or a high n-6:n-3 ratio) has been associated with an increased risk of both CD and UC.[32] Low levels of vitamin D may be a risk factor for IBD. In the Nurses' Health Studies, women with the predicted highest vitamin D levels had a significantly lower risk of CD.[33] However, the complex effect of individual variation in genetic susceptibility and gut microbiota may cause the heterogeneity in response to dietary factors in IBD pathogenesis, and future studies need to focus on dietary patterns rather than individual foods.

Another environmental risk factor for IBD of note may be childhood hygiene. In 1989, Strachan[34] first proposed the "hygiene hypothesis" to explain the increase of allergic disease after the industrial revolution in the United Kingdom. They postulated that autoimmune disease may be prevented by infection in early childhood, transmitted by unhygienic contact with older siblings. This hypothesis also can be adapted to the pathogenesis of IBD; that is, the disruption of intestinal microbiota in childhood could influence the development of IBD later in life. This has been supported by several Western studies in which early-life antibiotic use, breastfeeding, childhood pet exposure, or urban versus rural residence have been associated with risk of CD or UC.[35] However, these associations should be interpreted cautiously, because findings are not consistent among the different study cohorts. For example, Asian data from the ACCESS cohort demonstrated that use of flush toilets and antibiotics in childhood were negatively associated with UC, in contrast to Western studies.[27] This discrepancy could be caused by recall bias or confounding factors.[36]

Medications including antibiotics, nonsteroidal anti-inflammatory drugs (NSAIDs), and oral contraceptives have been associated with IBD risk. In a case-control study from Canada, 58% of pediatric-onset IBD cases had antibiotics prescribed in the first year of life compared with 39% of controls (OR 2.9; 95% CI 1.2–7.0), and 12% of adult-onset IBD cases had at least 3 antibiotic courses 2 to 5 years before diagnosis compared with 7% of controls (OR 1.5, 95% CI 1.3–1.8).[37,38] Antibiotic use may play a role in the disruption of gut microbiota, thereby increasing the risk of IBD. In the Nurses' Health Studies, frequent use of NSAIDs, but not aspirin, was associated with an increased risk of CD and UC, and this association was stronger with higher doses and longer duration of NSAID use.[39] Also, a meta-analysis revealed the association between the use of oral contraceptive agents and development of IBD, especially CD after adjusting for smoking (relative risk 1.46, 95% CI 1.26–1.70).[40]

NATURAL HISTORY OF CROHN'S DISEASE

Studies from population-based cohorts with long-term follow-up data for natural history of CD are summarized in **Table 1**.

Natural Course of Disease Location and Behavior

The Vienna classification was developed in 1998 to classify CD based on age at diagnosis, disease location, and disease behavior.[41] In 2005, the Vienna classification was modified, leading to the Montreal classification, which contains the same 3 categories with minor changes in each.[42] Modifications included an additional category for early age at diagnosis ($\leq$16 years), a modifier for proximal disease location (L1–3, $\pm$L4), and separating perianal disease from penetrating disease behavior (**Table 2**).

Across population-based studies, there are slight differences in the distribution of disease location at diagnosis of CD. These differences may be explained by geographic area and differences in investigative tools for evaluation. Overall, it could be estimated that the distribution of ileal, colonic, and ileocolonic location is of similar

Table 1
Population-based studies with follow-up data regarding the natural history of Crohn's disease

Country	Location	Number of Incident Cases of Crohn's Disease	Inclusion Period	Median Duration of Follow-up
United States	Olmsted County, Minnesota[68]	314	1940–2004	14 y
Denmark	Copenhagen County[44]	641	1962–1987 1991–1993 2003–2004	17 y 10 y 1 y
Hungary	Veszprem province[48]	506	1977–2009	11 y (interquartile range, 5.0–15.5 y)
United Kingdom	Cardiff, Wales[43]	341	1986–2003	7.7 y (range, 3.4–21.8 y)
France	Northern France (EPIMAD registry)[45]	8071	1988–2008	N/A
Norway	Inflammatory Bowel South-Eastern Norway (IBSEN study)[46]	200	1990–1993	5.3 y
Sweden	Stockholm County[53]	1389	1990–2001	N/A
European countries and Israel	European Collaborative Study Group On Inflammatory Bowel Disease (EC-IBD)[49]	358	1991–1993	10.3 y (range, 9.4–11 y)
Eastern and Western European countries	European Crohn's and Colitis Organization, Epidemiologic Committee (ECCO-EpiCom) cohort[63]	509	2010	1 y
Asian countries and Australia	Asia-Pacific Crohn's and Colitis Epidemiology (ACCESS) study[50]	181	2011	1 y

Table 2
The Vienna classification and the Montreal classification for Crohn's disease

Variable	Vienna Classification	Montreal Classification
Age at diagnosis (A)	A1: <40 y A2: ≥40 y	A1: ≤16 y A2: 17–40 y A3: >40 y
Disease location (L)	L1: ileal L2: colonic L3: ileocolonic L4: upper gastrointestinal tract	L1: ileal L2: colonic L3: ileocolonic L4: isolated upper gastrointestinal tract (added to L1–L3 when coexisting upper gastrointestinal disease)
Disease behavior (B)	B1: inflammatory B2: stricturing B3: penetrating	B1: inflammatory B2: stricturing B3: (internal) penetrating p- perianal disease modifier (added to B1–B3 when coexisting perianal disease)

proportion (**Fig. 4**). A temporal change in the proportion of disease location has been demonstrated in some of these studies. For example, in 3 cohorts from Cardiff, Wales, there was a trend toward more colonic disease at diagnosis after 1991. Colonic location at diagnosis was observed in 39% of patients in the first cohort (1986–1991), and this increased to 46% and 49% in the 1992 to 1997 and 1998 to 2003 cohorts, respectively.[43] Similarly, in a study from Copenhagen, Denmark, the prevalence of colonic disease rose from 30% in the first cohort (1962–1987) to 43% in the 1991 to 1993 cohort and 37% in the 2003 to 2004 cohorts.[44] In addition, those who presented with late-onset disease (age >40 years at diagnosis) were more likely to have colonic disease. In a French population-based registry, colonic disease occurred in 40% of those with late-onset disease (age 40–59 years at diagnosis) and in 65% with

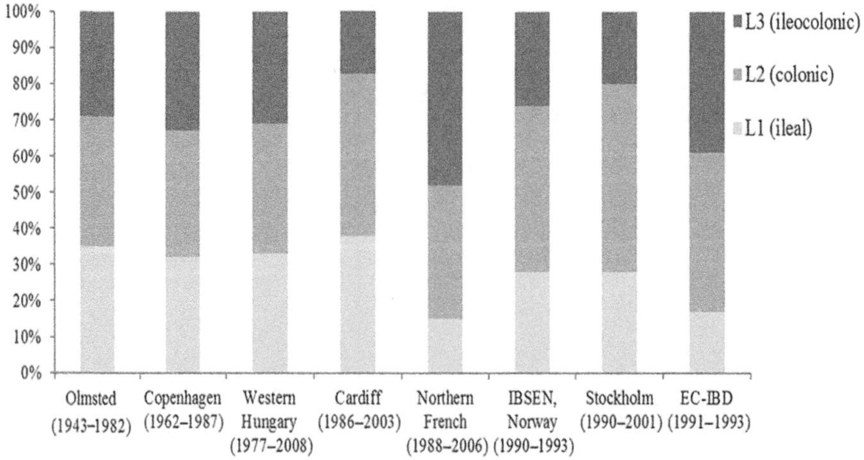

Fig. 4. Disease location at diagnosis of CD from population-based cohort studies.

elderly-onset disease (age ≥60 years at diagnosis) compared with only 20% among those with pediatric-onset disease (age <17 years at diagnosis).[45] Interestingly, CD location is less likely to change over time as reported by the Inflammatory Bowel South-Eastern Norway (IBSEN) study. After 5-year follow-up of 200 patients with incident CD, changes in disease location from either L1 or L2 to L3 occurred in only 13%.[46]

The most common disease behavior at diagnosis is inflammatory behavior. In population-based cohorts, 56% to 81% of patients with CD presented with inflammatory behavior, 5% to 24% had stricturing disease, and 4% to 23% presented with penetrating behavior (**Fig. 5**).[43,45,47–49] A trend of increase in the prevalence of inflammatory behavior was demonstrated in a recent study. In 3 cohorts from Western Hungary, there was a trend toward more inflammatory behavior at diagnosis; 42% in the 1977 to 1988 cohort, 53% in the 1989 to 1998 cohort, and 65% in the 1999 to 2008 cohort.[48] Importantly, changes in disease behavior over time have been described. After 5 years of follow-up in the Western Hungary cohort (1977–2008), 21% of 288 patients with inflammatory behavior at diagnosis developed either stricturing or penetrating behavior.[48] Among 249 patients with inflammatory disease behavior at diagnosis in the Olmsted County cohort diagnosed between 1970 and 2004, the cumulative risk of developing a stricturing or penetrating intestinal complication was 19% at 90 days, 22% at 1 year, and 51% at 20 years after diagnosis. Significant predictors of changes in disease behavior (from B1 to B2/B3) were the presence of ileal, ileocolonic, or upper gastrointestinal involvement (relative to colonic involvement).[47] Similarly, among 181 patients with CD in the ACCESS cohort diagnosed in 2011, 73% had no intestinal complication (B1) at diagnosis. The cumulative probability of changing from inflammatory to stricturing or penetrating disease behavior was 20% in the first year after diagnosis.[50]

Natural Course of Perianal Disease

The reported prevalence of perianal disease ranges from 11% to 25% in CD worldwide.[43,47,48] In the 1970 to 2004 Olmsted County cohort, the prevalence of perianal disease before or within 90 days of CD diagnosis was 16.7%. After a median follow-up duration of 8 years, an additional 11% developed perianal disease. Overall,

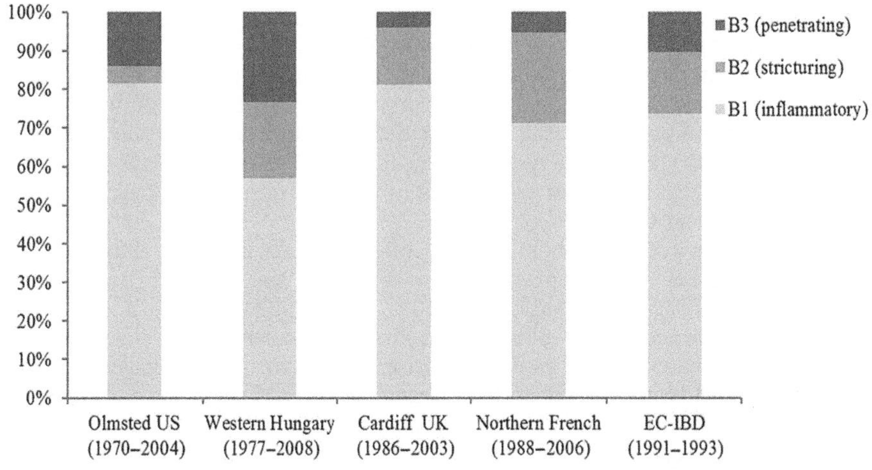

Fig. 5. Disease behavior at diagnosis of CD from population-based cohort studies.

28% of patients with CD experienced perianal disease in their disease course.[47] Regarding perianal fistula specifically, the overall prevalence in the 1970 to 1993 Olmsted County cohort was 20%. Almost half of patients (46%) had perianal fistula before or at diagnosis. The cumulative risk of developing perianal fistula was 21% at 10 years and 26% at 20 years after diagnosis.[51] One important predictor of developing perianal fistula is the presence of colonic disease. In a population-based study from Manitoba, the presence of colonic disease was associated with an increased risk of perineal fistula (OR 3.32, 95% CI 1.59–6.90), in contrast to ileal disease (OR 0.39, 95% CI 0.21–0.72).[52] Younger age at diagnosis may also be associated with the risk of developing perianal fistula. For example, in the cohort of patients with CD diagnosed in Stockholm County during 1990 to 2001, about 1 in 6 of the youngest patients in the cohort had perianal disease, whereas perianal fistulas were seen in fewer than 10% of the oldest patients.[53]

Natural Course of Disease Outcomes

Disease activity and relapse

A standard measure of disease activity in patients with CD has been the CD Activity Index. However, because of its complexity, requiring a 7-day symptom diary, it is not commonly used in clinical practice. The natural history of CD has been extensively studied; however, several studies used their own simple disease activity and relapse definition (**Table 3**). Only 2 population-based inception cohorts have described disease activity based on clinical and treatment response. A population-based study from Olmsted County, Minnesota, modeled the lifetime course of CD in various disease states using a Markov model; this particular model was unique in that the transition probabilities between disease states were derived by mapping disease states to the actual chronologic history of each patient. Over the lifetime disease course, a representative patient spent 24% in medical remission, 27% in mild disease, 1% in severe drug-responsive disease, 4% in severe drug-dependent disease, 2% in severe drug-refractory disease, 1% in surgery, and 41% in postsurgical remission. In addition, the proportion of patients in the medical remission state decreased and the proportion of patients in the postsurgical remission state increased, whereas the proportion of patients in other states remained stable over time.[54] In the 1962 to 1987 Copenhagen County cohort, the degree of clinical disease activity was prospectively collected each year after diagnosis. Within the first year after diagnosis, the proportions of patients with high activity, low activity, and clinical remission were 80%, 15%, and 5%, respectively. However, after the first year through 25 years, a decreasing proportion of high activity (30%), increasing proportion of remission (55%), and stable proportion of mild activity (15%) were observed. Half of patients (53%) had disease activity changing between remission and relapse over the 5-year period between years 3 and 8, but the degree of clinical activity at year 3 was mildly predictive of the overall clinical course over the next 5 years.[55]

Disease relapse occurs in most patients with CD. Data from the IBSEN cohort showed that 90% of 197 patients with a median of 10-year follow-up had disease relapse. The cumulative relapse rates were 53%, 85%, and 90% at 1, 5, and 10 years after diagnosis, respectively.[56] Similarly, the European collaborative study showed that 73% of 358 patients with a median follow-up of 10 years had disease recurrence. The cumulative all-type (medical and/or surgical) recurrence rates were 34%, 69%, and 77% at 1, 5, and 10 years after diagnosis, respectively. The cumulative surgical recurrence rates were 9%, 27%, and 34% at 1, 5, and 10 years after diagnosis, respectively.[49] Notably, these data predate the advent of biologic agents.

Table 3
Definition of disease activity and relapse from population-based studies of the natural history of Crohn's disease

Study	Inclusion Period	Definition of Disease Activity and Relapse
Copenhagen County, Denmark[55]	1962–1987	• *No activity:* ≤2 bowel movements/day without blood or pus, no abdominal pain, no systemic symptoms (fever, weight loss) • *Low activity:* 2–4 bowel movements with/without blood or pus, mild abdominal pain less than daily, no systemic symptoms • Moderate/high activity: >4 bowel movements/day with/without blood or pus, abdominal pain either severe or daily, with (high)/without (moderate) systemic symptoms
Olmsted County, Minnesota[54]	1970–1993	• *Remission:* no medication for Crohn's disease • *Mild:* treatment with sulfasalazine, 5-amino-salicylate, antibiotic, topical therapy • *Severe, drug responsive:* oral corticosteroids, immunosuppressive medications with documented improvement • *Severe, drug dependent:* oral corticosteroids, immunosuppressive medications lasting ≥6 mo with documented improvement • *Severe, drug refractory:* oral corticosteroids, immunosuppressive medications with no documented improvement within 2 mo for corticosteroids or 6 mo for immunosuppressive medication • *Surgery:* inpatient surgical procedures for Crohn's disease • *Postsurgical remission:* no medication for Crohn's disease after surgical procedure for Crohn's disease
Inflammatory Bowel South-Eastern Norway (IBSEN)[56]	1990–1994	• *Relapse:* an aggravation of symptoms leading to the need for more intensive medical/surgical treatment after achieving remission from the first attack at diagnosis
European Collaborative Study Group On Inflammatory Bowel Disease (EC-IBD)[49]	1991–1993	• *Nonsurgical recurrence:* an episode of increased disease activity requiring only medication change • *Surgical recurrence:* an episode of increased disease activity requiring surgical intervention (bowel resection, abscess drainage, fistula operation) with/without medication change
Copenhagen, Denmark[57]	2003–2004	• *Nonsurgical/medical recurrence:* an episode of increased disease activity leading to an increased dose of current medication or the addition of a new medication • *Surgical recurrence:* an episode of increased disease activity requiring surgical intervention (bowel resection, abscess drainage, perianal fistula operation) with/without medication change

Long-term data on disease activity and relapse from population-based cohorts in the current era of biologic agents and widespread use of immunomodulator drugs are limited. A recent Danish population-based cohort including 213 patients with CD diagnosed in 2003 to 2004 who were followed for a median of 7.7 years reported that the cumulative incidence of all-type recurrence was 40%, 63%, and 66% at 1, 5, and 7 years after diagnosis, respectively. The cumulative surgical recurrence rate was 6%, 18%, and 23% at 1, 5, and 7 years after diagnosis, respectively. Current smoking at the time of CD diagnosis was significantly associated with time to all-type recurrence (hazard ratio [HR] 1.65, 95% CI 1.11–2.44). Stricturing disease behavior was significantly associated with time to surgical recurrence (HR 3.45, 95% CI 1.47–8.09). Conversely, age ≥40 years at diagnosis was associated with decreased risk of all-type recurrence (HR 0.58, 95% CI 0.39–0.85), and disease locations of colonic, ileocolonic, and upper gastrointestinal were associated with decreased risks of surgical recurrence (relative to ileal location)[57] (**Table 4**).

Hospitalization

Among 221 patients with CD diagnosed between 1970 and 1997 in Olmsted County, 57% had at least 1 CD-related hospitalization. The crude hospitalization rate was 194 per 1000 person-years. During the first year after diagnosis, the crude hospitalization rate was more than twice the overall rate (474 per 1000 person-years).[58] A population-based study from Canada using the national-based hospital morbidity database reported a decrease in CD-related hospitalizations from 29.2 per 100,000 persons in 1994 to 1995 to 26.9 per 100,000 in 2000 to 2001. The readmission rate was approximately 20% per year and 35% over 7 years.[59] In the more recent Copenhagen cohort of 213 patients with CD diagnosed in 2003 to 2004 and followed until 2011, approximately half of patients (49%) had hospitalization in the first year after diagnosis. The hospitalization for CD declined from 7 days per person-year at the first year to 0.9 day per person-year at the fifth year. However, no significant predictors of the first hospitalization were identified in this study[57] (see **Table 4**).

Table 4
Summary of disease outcomes in population-based studies of Crohn's disease

Outcomes	Results	Comment	References
Disease activity and relapse	• Medical remission (one-fourth) • Disease relapses within 10 y (77%–90%) • Disease relapse requiring surgical treatment within 10 y (one-third)	• Heterogeneous definition of disease activity and relapse. • Long-term data beyond 10 y are not available in the era of biologic agents.	49,54–56
Hospitalization	• Two-thirds of patients require hospitalization • Half of hospitalizations occur in the first year then hospitalization rate (20% every year)	• Long-term data beyond 10 y are not available in the era of biologic agents.	57–59
Surgery	• Half of patients require surgery within 10 y	• Long-term data beyond 10 y are not available in the era of biologic agents.	48,56,60,61

Surgery

Surgery is common in patients with CD. Three different population-based cohort studies from Norway, Hungary, and Denmark reported the probability of surgical resection was 14% to 15%, 25% to 30%, and 38% to 52% at 1, 5, and 10 years after diagnosis, respectively.[48,56,60] In Olmsted County, an updated report indicated that 50% of patients with CD diagnosed between 1970 and 2004 underwent at least 1 major abdominal surgery after a median follow-up of 12 years. The cumulative risk for first major abdominal surgery was 38%, 48%, and 58% at 5, 10, and 20 years after diagnosis, respectively. The main indications for surgery were obstruction and medical treatment failure. Ileal or ileocecal resections were 72% of surgical procedures.[61] The predictors of first major abdominal surgery were disease location of upper gastrointestinal tract (HR 4.0, 95% CI 1.2–13.8), small bowel (HR 3.4, 95% CI 1.9–6.1), and ileocolon (HR 3.3, 95% CI 1.8–5.8), current smoking (HR 1.7; 95% CI 1.1–2.7), male gender (HR 1.6, 95% CI 1.02–2.4), penetrating disease behavior (HR 2.7, 95% CI 1.1–6.7), and initial use of corticosteroids (HR 1.6, 95% CI 1.03–2.5).[61] A decreased risk of surgery over 5 decades between post-1970 and 2011 was observed in a recent meta-analysis of population-based studies.[62] A recent cohort from 22 European countries (ECCO-EpiCom) including 509 patients with CD diagnosed in 2010 who were followed for 1 year reported that 15% of patients had surgery within the first year after diagnosis.[63] Similarly, the more recent Asia-Pacific ACCESS cohort from in 2011 demonstrated that within the first year of disease course, the cumulative probability of surgery was 8% in Asia and 12% in Australia.[50] The reduction in surgery rate may be attributed to the evolution of CD management (see **Table 4**).

RISK STRATIFICATION OF CROHN'S DISEASE

Clinical Risk Factors

The natural history of CD is characterized by changes in disease behavior over time, leading to the development of intestinal complications (eg, stricture, fistula, and abscess), requiring surgery, and setting the stage for disease recurrence. Some baseline clinical features associated with high risk of disease progression have been identified in population-based studies as mentioned previously and summarized in **Box 1**.

Endoscopic Risk Factors

In addition to clinical predictors, endoscopic features may identify patients with high risk of developing disease-related complications. In a retrospective cohort study from France, among 102 active patients with CD who underwent ileocolonoscopy between 1990 and 1996, 53 patients had extensive and deep ulcerations. During a median follow-up of 52 months, 58% of patients demonstrating extensive and deep ulceration required colectomy, compared with only 12% of patients without extensive deep ulcers. In multivariate analyses, the presence of extensive and deep ulcers at baseline colonoscopy was a significant predictor of colectomy (RR 5.4, 95% CI 2.6–11.2).[64] Conversely, mucosal healing after treatment was associated with corticosteroid-free remission and reduced risk of surgery. In the prebiologic era, it was shown in a Norwegian population-based cohort that mucosal healing at 1 year after diagnosis was associated with decreased endoscopic disease activity and decreased corticosteroid use at 5 years after diagnosis.[65] Thereafter, in the era of biologic agents, a referral-based prospective cohort from Belgium showed that among 183 patients with CD with a primary clinical response to infliximab, 68% had mucosal healing. During a median follow-up of 22 months, patients with mucosal healing had a

Box 1
Baseline predictors for poor disease outcomes of Crohn's disease

Clinical risk factors

Clinical predictors of disease recurrence (medical and/or surgical recurrence)[57,a]
- Current cigarette smoking
- Stricturing disease behavior (surgical relapse alone)

Clinical predictors of intestinal complications (change B1 to B2/B3) [47,b]
- Ileal location
- Ileocolonic location
- Upper gastrointestinal location

Clinical predictors of surgery[61,b]
- Small bowel location
- Ileocolonic location
- Upper gastrointestinal location
- Current cigarette smoking
- Male gender
- Penetrating disease behavior
- Initial use of corticosteroids

Endoscopic risk factors

Endoscopic predictors of corticosteroid-free remission[65]
- Deep ulceration[a]

Endoscopic predictors of surgery[66]
- Mucosal healing[c]

[a] Determined at diagnosis.
[b] Determined at 90 days after diagnosis.
[c] Determined at 1 year after diagnosis.

significantly lower risk of surgery relative to patients without mucosal healing (14% vs 38%; $P<.01$, respectively).[66]

Risk Stratification

According to the American Gastroenterological Association clinical decision support tool for CD evaluation and treatment, risk stratification has been developed to assess current and prior disease burden. Patients with young age (<30 years) at diagnosis, extensive anatomic involvement, perianal and/or severe rectal disease, stricturing and/or penetrating behavior, deep ulcers, and prior surgical resection are identified as moderate/high risk, whereas patients with age >30 years at diagnosis, limited anatomic involvement, nonstricturing and nonpenetrating behavior, no perianal disease, superficial ulcers, and no prior surgical resection are identified as low risk.[67]

SUMMARY

The incidence and prevalence of CD is increasing in both the Western world and in developing countries. Risk factors include cigarette smoking, a low-fiber/high-fat diet, and certain medications, such as antibiotics, NSAIDs and oral contraceptives. Approximately one-third of patients with CD had ileal, colonic, and ileocolonic location. More than 30% of the patients had a stricturing or penetrating complication at diagnosis, whereas one-fifth of the patients experienced intestinal complications within the first year after diagnosis. Hospitalization and surgery are common in patients with CD. Half of patients required hospitalization within the first year after diagnosis. Surgery occurred in 50% of patients with CD within 10 years after diagnosis. Risk factors for disease-related complications include young age at diagnosis, extensive anatomic involvement, perianal disease, stricturing or penetrating behavior, deep ulcers, and prior surgical resection. Identification of high-risk patients may improve the treatment paradigm and may improve disease outcomes.

REFERENCES

1. Kaplan GG. The global burden of IBD: from 2015 to 2025. Nat Rev Gastroenterol Hepatol 2015;12(12):720–7.
2. Crohn BB, Ginzburg L, Oppenheimer GD. Regional ileitis: a pathologic and clinical entity. J Am Med Assoc 1932;99(16):1323–9.
3. Molodecky NA, Soon IS, Rabi DM, et al. Increasing incidence and prevalence of the inflammatory bowel diseases with time, based on systematic review. Gastroenterology 2012;142(1):46–54.e42 [quiz: e30].
4. Kaplan GG, Ng SC. Understanding and preventing the global increase of inflammatory bowel disease. Gastroenterology 2016;152(2):313–21.e2.
5. Shivashankar R, Tremaine WJ, Harmsen WS, et al. Incidence and prevalence of Crohn's disease and ulcerative colitis in Olmsted County, Minnesota from 1970 through 2010. Clin Gastroenterol Hepatol 2017;15(6):857–63.
6. Bach JF. The effect of infections on susceptibility to autoimmune and allergic diseases. N Engl J Med 2002;347(12):911–20.
7. Burisch J, Pedersen N, Cukovic-Cavka S, et al. East-West gradient in the incidence of inflammatory bowel disease in Europe: the ECCO-EpiCom inception cohort. Gut 2014;63(4):588–97.
8. Vegh Z, Burisch J, Pedersen N, et al. Incidence and initial disease course of inflammatory bowel diseases in 2011 in Europe and Australia: results of the 2011 ECCO-EpiCom inception cohort. J Crohns Colitis 2014;8(11):1506–15.
9. Ng WK, Wong SH, Ng SC. Changing epidemiological trends of inflammatory bowel disease in Asia. Intest Res 2016;14(2):111–9.
10. Yang SK, Yun S, Kim JH, et al. Epidemiology of inflammatory bowel disease in the Songpa-Kangdong district, Seoul, Korea, 1986-2005: a KASID study. Inflamm Bowel Dis 2008;14(4):542–9.
11. Ng SC, Tang W, Ching JY, et al. Incidence and phenotype of inflammatory bowel disease based on results from the Asia-pacific Crohn's and colitis epidemiology study. Gastroenterology 2013;145(1):158–65.e152.
12. Lophaven SN, Lynge E, Burisch J. The incidence of inflammatory bowel disease in Denmark 1980-2013: a nationwide cohort study. Aliment Pharmacol Ther 2017;45(7):961–72.
13. Sedlack RE, Nobrega FT, Kurland LT, et al. Inflammatory colon disease in Rochester, Minnesota, 1935-1964. Gastroenterology 1972;62(5):935–41.
14. Sedlack RE, Whisnant J, Elveback LR, et al. Incidence of Crohn's disease in Olmsted County, Minnesota, 1935-1975. Am J Epidemiol 1980;112(6):759–63.
15. Loftus EV Jr, Silverstein MD, Sandborn WJ, et al. Crohn's disease in Olmsted County, Minnesota, 1940-1993: incidence, prevalence, and survival. Gastroenterology 1998;114(6):1161–8.
16. Loftus CG, Loftus EV Jr, Harmsen WS, et al. Update on the incidence and prevalence of Crohn's disease and ulcerative colitis in Olmsted County, Minnesota, 1940-2000. Inflamm Bowel Dis 2007;13(3):254–61.

17. Leddin D, Tamim H, Levy AR. Decreasing incidence of inflammatory bowel disease in eastern Canada: a population database study. BMC Gastroenterol 2014;14:140.
18. Rezaie A, Quan H, Fedorak RN, et al. Development and validation of an administrative case definition for inflammatory bowel diseases. Can J Gastroenterol 2012;26(10):711–7.
19. Dahlhamer JM, Zammitti EP, Ward BW, et al. Prevalence of inflammatory bowel disease among adults aged ≥18 years—United States, 2015. MMWR Morb Mortal Wkly Rep 2016;65(42):1166–9.
20. Stepaniuk P, Bernstein CN, Targownik LE, et al. Characterization of inflammatory bowel disease in elderly patients: a review of epidemiology, current practices and outcomes of current management strategies. Can J Gastroenterol Hepatol 2015;29(6):327–33.
21. Benchimol EI, Guttmann A, Griffiths AM, et al. Increasing incidence of paediatric inflammatory bowel disease in Ontario, Canada: evidence from health administrative data. Gut 2009;58(11):1490–7.
22. Agnarsson U, Bjornsson S, Johansson JH, et al. Inflammatory bowel disease in Icelandic children 1951-2010. Population-based study involving one nation over six decades. Scand J Gastroenterol 2013;48(12):1399–404.
23. Ponder A, Long MD. A clinical review of recent findings in the epidemiology of inflammatory bowel disease. Clin Epidemiol 2013;5:237–47.
24. Calkins BM. A meta-analysis of the role of smoking in inflammatory bowel disease. Dig Dis Sci 1989;34(12):1841–54.
25. Mahid SS, Minor KS, Soto RE, et al. Smoking and inflammatory bowel disease: a meta-analysis. Mayo Clin Proc 2006;81(11):1462–71.
26. Benjamin JL, Hedin CR, Koutsoumpas A, et al. Smokers with active Crohn's disease have a clinically relevant dysbiosis of the gastrointestinal microbiota. Inflamm Bowel Dis 2012;18(6):1092–100.
27. Ng SC, Tang W, Leong RW, et al. Environmental risk factors in inflammatory bowel disease: a population-based case-control study in Asia-Pacific. Gut 2015;64(7):1063–71.
28. Hwang SW, Seo H, Kim GU, et al. Underestimation of smoking rates in an East Asian population with Crohn's Disease. Gut Liver 2016;11(1):73–8.
29. Lewis JD, Abreu MT. Diet as a trigger or therapy for inflammatory bowel diseases. Gastroenterology 2016;152(2):398–414.e6.
30. Ananthakrishnan AN, Khalili H, Konijeti GG, et al. A prospective study of long-term intake of dietary fiber and risk of Crohn's disease and ulcerative colitis. Gastroenterology 2013;145(5):970–7.
31. Ananthakrishnan AN, Khalili H, Konijeti GG, et al. Long-term intake of dietary fat and risk of ulcerative colitis and Crohn's disease. Gut 2014;63(5):776–84.
32. Costea I, Mack DR, Lemaitre RN, et al. Interactions between the dietary polyunsaturated fatty acid ratio and genetic factors determine susceptibility to pediatric Crohn's disease. Gastroenterology 2014;146(4):929–31.
33. Ananthakrishnan AN, Khalili H, Higuchi LM, et al. Higher predicted vitamin D status is associated with reduced risk of Crohn's disease. Gastroenterology 2012;142(3):482–9.
34. Strachan DP. Hay fever, hygiene, and household size. BMJ 1989;299(6710):1259–60.
35. Ananthakrishnan AN. Epidemiology and risk factors for IBD. Nat Rev Gastroenterol Hepatol 2015;12(4):205–17.

36. Molodecky NA, Panaccione R, Ghosh S, et al. Challenges associated with identifying the environmental determinants of the inflammatory bowel diseases. Inflamm Bowel Dis 2011;17(8):1792–9.
37. Shaw SY, Blanchard JF, Bernstein CN. Association between the use of antibiotics in the first year of life and pediatric inflammatory bowel disease. Am J Gastroenterol 2010;105(12):2687–92.
38. Shaw SY, Blanchard JF, Bernstein CN. Association between the use of antibiotics and new diagnoses of Crohn's disease and ulcerative colitis. Am J Gastroenterol 2011;106(12):2133–42.
39. Ananthakrishnan AN, Higuchi LM, Huang ES, et al. Aspirin, nonsteroidal anti-inflammatory drug use, and risk for Crohn disease and ulcerative colitis: a cohort study. Ann Intern Med 2012;156(5):350–9.
40. Cornish JA, Tan E, Simillis C, et al. The risk of oral contraceptives in the etiology of inflammatory bowel disease: a meta-analysis. Am J Gastroenterol 2008;103(9): 2394–400.
41. Gasche C, Scholmerich J, Brynskov J, et al. A simple classification of Crohn's disease: report of the Working Party for the World Congresses of Gastroenterology, Vienna 1998. Inflamm Bowel Dis 2000;6(1):8–15.
42. Silverberg MS, Satsangi J, Ahmad T, et al. Toward an integrated clinical, molecular and serological classification of inflammatory bowel disease: report of a Working Party of the 2005 Montreal World Congress of Gastroenterology. Can J Gastroenterol 2005;19(Suppl A):5A–36A.
43. Ramadas AV, Gunesh S, Thomas GA, et al. Natural history of Crohn's disease in a population-based cohort from Cardiff (1986-2003): a study of changes in medical treatment and surgical resection rates. Gut 2010;59(9):1200–6.
44. Jess T, Riis L, Vind I, et al. Changes in clinical characteristics, course, and prognosis of inflammatory bowel disease during the last 5 decades: a population-based study from Copenhagen, Denmark. Inflamm Bowel Dis 2007;13(4):481–9.
45. Gower-Rousseau C, Vasseur F, Fumery M, et al. Epidemiology of inflammatory bowel diseases: new insights from a French population-based registry (EPIMAD). Dig Liver Dis 2013;45(2):89–94.
46. Henriksen M, Jahnsen J, Lygren I, et al. Clinical course in Crohn's disease: results of a five-year population-based follow-up study (the IBSEN study). Scand J Gastroenterol 2007;42(5):602–10.
47. Thia KT, Sandborn WJ, Harmsen WS, et al. Risk factors associated with progression to intestinal complications of Crohn's disease in a population-based cohort. Gastroenterology 2010;139(4):1147–55.
48. Lakatos PL, Golovics PA, David G, et al. Has there been a change in the natural history of Crohn's disease? Surgical rates and medical management in a population-based inception cohort from Western Hungary between 1977-2009. Am J Gastroenterol 2012;107(4):579–88.
49. Wolters FL, Russel MG, Sijbrandij J, et al. Phenotype at diagnosis predicts recurrence rates in Crohn's disease. Gut 2006;55(8):1124–30.
50. Ng SC, Zeng Z, Niewiadomski O, et al. Early course of inflammatory bowel disease in a population-based inception cohort study from 8 countries in Asia and Australia. Gastroenterology 2016;150(1):86–95.e83 [quiz: e13–84].
51. Schwartz DA, Loftus EV Jr, Tremaine WJ, et al. The natural history of fistulizing Crohn's disease in Olmsted County, Minnesota. Gastroenterology 2002;122(4): 875–80.

52. Tang LY, Rawsthorne P, Bernstein CN. Are perineal and luminal fistulas associated in Crohn's disease? A population-based study. Clin Gastroenterol Hepatol 2006;4(9):1130–4.
53. Lapidus A. Crohn's disease in Stockholm County during 1990-2001: an epidemiological update. World J Gastroenterol 2006;12(1):75–81.
54. Silverstein MD, Loftus EV, Sandborn WJ, et al. Clinical course and costs of care for Crohn's disease: Markov model analysis of a population-based cohort. Gastroenterology 1999;117(1):49–57.
55. Munkholm P, Langholz E, Davidsen M, et al. Disease-activity courses in a regional cohort of Crohn's-disease patients. Scand J Gastroenterol 1995;30(7):699–706.
56. Solberg IC, Vatn MH, Hoie O, et al. Clinical course in Crohn's disease: results of a Norwegian population-based ten-year follow-up study. Clin Gastroenterol Hepatol 2007;5(12):1430–8.
57. Vester-Andersen MK, Vind I, Prosberg MV, et al. Hospitalisation, surgical and medical recurrence rates in inflammatory bowel disease 2003-2011—a Danish population-based cohort study. J Crohns Colitis 2014;8(12):1675–83.
58. Ingle SB, Loftus EV, Harmsen WS, et al. Hospitalization rates for Crohn's disease patients in Olmsted County, Minnesota, in the pre-biologic era. Am J Gastroenterol 2007;102(Suppl 2):S487.
59. Bernstein CN, Nabalamba A. Hospitalization, surgery, and readmission rates of IBD in Canada: a population-based study. Am J Gastroenterol 2006;101(1):110–8.
60. Vester-Andersen MK, Prosberg MV, Jess T, et al. Disease course and surgery rates in inflammatory bowel disease: a population-based, 7-year follow-up study in the era of immunomodulating therapy. Am J Gastroenterol 2014;109(5):705–14.
61. Peyrin-Biroulet L, Harmsen WS, Tremaine WJ, et al. Surgery in a population-based cohort of Crohn's disease from Olmsted County, Minnesota (1970-2004). Am J Gastroenterol 2012;107(11):1693–701.
62. Frolkis AD, Dykeman J, Negron ME, et al. Risk of surgery for inflammatory bowel diseases has decreased over time: a systematic review and meta-analysis of population-based studies. Gastroenterology 2013;145(5):996–1006.
63. Burisch J, Pedersen N, Cukovic-Cavka S, et al. Initial disease course and treatment in an inflammatory bowel disease inception cohort in Europe: the ECCO-EpiCom cohort. Inflamm Bowel Dis 2014;20(1):36–46.
64. Allez M, Lemann M, Bonnet J, et al. Long term outcome of patients with active Crohn's disease exhibiting extensive and deep ulcerations at colonoscopy. Am J Gastroenterol 2002;97(4):947–53.
65. Froslie KF, Jahnsen J, Moum BA, et al. Mucosal healing in inflammatory bowel disease: results from a Norwegian population-based cohort. Gastroenterology 2007;133(2):412–22.
66. Schnitzler F, Fidder H, Ferrante M, et al. Mucosal healing predicts long-term outcome of maintenance therapy with infliximab in Crohn's disease. Inflamm Bowel Dis 2009;15(9):1295–301.
67. Sandborn WJ. Crohn's disease evaluation and treatment: clinical decision tool. Gastroenterology 2014;147(3):702–5.
68. Gollop JH, Phillips SF, Melton LJ 3rd, et al. Epidemiologic aspects of Crohn's disease: a population based study in Olmsted County, Minnesota, 1943-1982. Gut 1988;29(1):49–56.

The Microbiome in Crohn's Disease

Role in Pathogenesis and Role of Microbiome Replacement Therapies

Sahil Khanna, MBBS, MS*, Laura E. Raffals, MD

KEYWORDS

• Crohn's disease • Inflammatory bowel disease • Pathogenesis • Gut microbiota
• Microbiome • Fecal microbiota transplantation • Probiotics

KEY POINTS

- Patients with Crohn's disease have decreased microbial diversity, which plays an important role in the pathogenesis of Crohn's disease.
- Microbial restoration therapies are being studied for management of Crohn's disease and may be an adjunct to standard therapies in the future.
- It may be feasible to modify the gut microbiota community structure or function to treat patients with Crohn's disease with targeted therapies via individual agents, such as probiotics, bacterial consortia, or even dietary manipulation.
- Fecal microbiota transplantation should not be performed for Crohn's disease other than in research settings.
- A better understanding of host-microbe interactions in patients with Crohn's disease may help improve management of these patients.

INTRODUCTION

Crohn's disease, a subtype of inflammatory bowel disease (IBD), has been increasing in incidence over the last few decades.[1] Crohn's disease may involve any segment of the gastrointestinal tract and lead to complications, such as strictures and fistulas. The pathogenesis of Crohn's disease is multifactorial and involves the interplay of host genetics, host immune dysregulation, and environmental factors resulting in an aberrant immune response and subsequent intestinal inflammation.[2] The human gut microbiota, harboring more than 100 trillion microorganisms, serves as an important

Disclosure Statement: S. Khanna and L.E. Raffals have no relevant financial disclosures.
Division of Gastroenterology and Hepatology, Mayo Clinic, 200 First Street Southwest, Rochester, MN 55905, USA
* Corresponding author.
E-mail address: khanna.sahil@mayo.edu

Gastroenterol Clin N Am 46 (2017) 481–492
http://dx.doi.org/10.1016/j.gtc.2017.05.004
0889-8553/17/

component in the pathogenesis of Crohn's disease, by providing antigenic stimuli through altered microbial compositions that promote host-microbe imbalances leading to perturbed intestinal and immune homeostasis. An aggressive T-cell-mediated immune response to specific components of the intestinal microbiota in genetically susceptible hosts results in the inflammation of the bowel of Crohn's disease. Microbial dysbiosis is thought to be associated with either development or exacerbation of underlying Crohn's disease.[3]

CROHN'S DISEASE AND ALTERED MICROBIOME

Bacterial dysbiosis is likely a causative factor and an outcome in patients with Crohn's disease.[4] Although dysbiosis may develop as a result of bowel inflammation, dysbiosis may also have a role in perpetuating chronic inflammation. Studies of the gut microbiota in patients with Crohn's disease demonstrate an increase in pathogenic microorganisms, whereas populations of normal commensal phyla are diminished.[5,6] In one interesting study, pretreatment gut microbial samples from patients with new-onset Crohn's disease demonstrated an increased abundance of Enterobacteriaceae, Pasteurellacaea, Veillonellaceae, and Fusobacteriaceae, and decreased Erysipelotrichales, Bacteroidales, and Clostridiales.[7] Ileal and rectal mucosal samples demonstrated a reduction in Firmicutes, such as *Faecalibacterium prausnitzii*, and increased in Proteobacteria, such as *Escherichia coli*, and in *Veillonella*, *Haemophilus*, and *Fusibacteria*.[7] Similarly, previous studies have shown an increase in mucosa-associated *E coli* in Crohn's disease and several showing a reduction in *F prausnitzii*.[8–10] In another study, there were decreased populations of Bacteroidetes and Firmicutes in patients with Crohn's disease, whereas pathogenic organisms, such as *E coli*, *Campylobacter* species, and *Mycobacterium* species were increased.[11] Patients with Crohn's disease have a greater number of mucosal surface–associated bacteria with higher adherence and invasion compared with healthy control subjects.[12] Gut microbiome profiles from patients with isolated colonic Crohn's disease are more similar to that of healthy control subjects than microbiome profiles of patients with isolated ileal or ileocolonic Crohn's disease.[8–10,13] In one study, increased ileal mucosa-associated *E coli* and reduced ileal *F prausnitzii* was present in patients with ileal but not isolated colonic Crohn's disease.[13] However, studies have shown differences between the mucosa-associated microbiota in isolated colonic Crohn's disease and ulcerative colitis. Therefore, mucosa-associated microbiota changes in Crohn's disease are more marked than stool microbiome changes. The microbiota in isolated colonic Crohn's disease shows changes that tend to be less marked and less consistent than those found in Crohn's disease with ileal involvement. These findings could suggest future studies involving gut microbiome profiles in patients with Crohn's disease should incorporate mucosal microbiome sampling in addition to fecal sampling.

HOST MICROBIOME INTERACTIONS IN CROHN'S DISEASE

Evolution of Microbiome

Following birth, humans develop their gut microbiota through a variety of mechanisms. The mode of delivery (whether vaginal birth or birth by caesarean section), diet, and other environmental factors influence the microbial community as it evolves from a simple community containing a core set of resident bacteria to a more complex, diverse community. In early childhood the microbiota shifts in response to the environment including dietary influences, antibiotic exposure, and illness. Eventually, one's unique microbial community becomes a species-rich, complex community relatively stable and resistant to colonization by enteropathogens. In a healthy individual, the gut microbiota is resilient and can withstand transient changes and decreased microbial diversity stemming from a variety of disturbances. With age, the microbial community gradually changes and later in life is less diverse and resilient.[14]

Heredibility of the Microbial Community

The enteric microbiota is presumed to be influenced by one's genetic makeup; however, it is difficult to elucidate the specific contributions of environmental factors and genetics in individual gut microbial communities. Human studies have suggested heritability of microbiota composition; however, results have been inconsistent leaving room for further studies to understand to what degree host genetics matter.[15] The gut microbial communities of monozygotic twin pairs are more similar than mother-offspring pairs. However, in initial studies this concordance also seemed to be present in dizygotic twin pairs. In contrast, a recent twin study including 416 twin pairs found monozygotic twins had greater similarity in their gut microbiota than dizygotic twins highlighting the presumed genetic contribution to the gut microbiota.[16] The influence of host genetics is also relevant to the function of microbial community and subsequent interaction with the host immune system.[17,18] A UK study of 1126 twin pairs identified heritable taxa (some previously identified in other studies) and associations between some of these taxa and genes relevant to diet, metabolism, and immune defense.[19] Mouse studies have been more convincing of the genetic control of the gut microbiota. A study of inbred mice under controlled conditions found substantial influence of the host genetic makeup on the gut microbiota for many common taxa.[20]

The role of host genetics and the gut microbiota is of particular interest in IBD given the known genetic variants associated with IBD in genes known to regulate the immune response. A recent study by Imhann and colleagues[21] found significant differences in the gut microbiota of healthy individuals who carried a high genetic risk for IBD, including a decrease in the *Roseburia* spp known to be butyrate producers and decreased in patients with Crohn's disease compared with healthy individuals. There have been additional studies linking genetic variants and the microbiome. NOD2, the first discovered IBD susceptibility gene, is expressed in Paneth cells and initiates an immune response to bacterial lipopolysaccharides. If impaired it can affect the clearance of enteropathogens. Other IBD susceptibility genes, such as ATG16L1 and IL23R, also seem to have links to the host response to responses to microbes and are believed to contribute to intestinal dysbiosis found in Crohn's disease through disruption of the innate and adaptive immune response.[22]

Mucosal Immunity

Although host genetic factors influence the gut microbiota, the gut microbiota also influences the intestinal mucosal and systemic immune function. This is most evident in the immune dysfunction observed in germ-free mice.[23–25] The gut-associated lymphoid tissues, including isolated lymphoid follicles, spleen, lymph nodes, and Peyer patches, are poorly developed in germ-free mice. Germ-free mice colonized with commensal microbes increase IgA secretion and these mice also exhibit a $CD4^+$ T-cell deficiency that can be reversed with exposure to *Bacteroides fragilis* or oral capsular antigen PSA of *B fragilis*.[26] Other members of the microbiota (eg, *Lactobacilli* spp and peptidoglycan of gram-negative bacteria) also influence the development of the host mucosal immune system. *Bifidobacterium* spp and *Clostridium* spp are also important for gut health because they break down indigestible fiber to produce short-chain fatty acids (SCFAs) including butyrate, propionate, and acetate, which are vital to maintain the health and integrity of colonic epithelial cells.

The mucosal immune system has two major functions. This system must protect the host from enteric pathogens but remain tolerant to the resident microbiota overlying the intestinal epithelial layer. This necessary tolerance is achieved through a physical barrier (the mucus layer overlying the epithelium), and modulation of the immune response to commensal organisms.[27] Modulation of the immune response is influenced by exposure of microbes to the intestinal epithelial cells, specifically dendritic cells. For example, in in vitro experiments, dendritic cells stimulated by such isolates as *Lactobacilli* spp and *E coli* generate downstream signals to promote tolerance to these commensals.[28] Establishment of the microbiota with commensal organisms can further protect the host from pathogenic organisms through colonization resistance. The beneficial organisms compete for nutrients, resources, and locale pushing out pathogenic microbes. Ultimately there are many functions of the gut microbiota to protect the host and mitigate inflammation.

Understanding the role of the enteric microbiota in host immune function improves the understanding of the pathophysiology of disease states, such as IBD. Host genetic variants in IBD susceptibility genes (eg, NOD2, IL23R, ATG16L1, IBD5) lead to perturbations in the host immune response. These perturbations can result in defects in the mucosal barrier, loss of autophagy, and phagocytosis increasing susceptibility to enteropathogens. All of these downstream effects of genetic mutations can lead to changes in the gut microbiota composition and promote dysbiosis. Dysbiosis can further increase susceptibility to a proinflammatory response and further mucosal damage. This dysfunctional relationship between the gut microbes and the mucosal immune system results in a vicious cycle of microbial dysbiosis and immune activation ultimately resulting in a chronic intestinal inflammatory state.

MICROBIAL RESTORATION THERAPIES IN CROHN'S DISEASE

Because a perturbed microbiome is associated with Crohn's disease, it is conceivable that microbial restoration therapies could be useful in management of Crohn's disease. In patients with Crohn's disease, an understanding of the differences in composition of protective versus inflammatory bacteria and their down-stream metabolic functions may be useful to discover microbial therapeutic targets. It is well known that there is a limited role of antibiotics (treatment of abscesses and fistulae) in patients with Crohn's disease, suggesting that broad-spectrum nontargeted microbiome-destroying approaches are likely not useful. Also, the minimal clinical success with probiotics demonstrates that single or multiple nontargeted probiotic strains are likely not helpful in sustainable or even substantial alterations of the gut microbiome to lead to a meaningful clinical success. These findings may be caused by nonnative probiotic species, which may be unable to colonize the intestine and are rapidly cleared because of interactions with the native microbiome.

Fecal microbiota transplantation (FMT) is a potential emerging therapeutic option for diseases implicated in altered microbial compositions. The primary example is patients with recurrent *Clostridium difficile* infection (CDI) where FMT leads to greater than 90% cure rates as see in clinical series and clinical trials.[29] However, CDI is characterized by an induced defect in gut microbiota secondary to antibiotic exposure, which can be corrected by whole gut microbial transplantation. The high success rate is partly caused by lack of the underlying inciting factor (antibiotic exposure in most instances). Crohn's disease like other autoimmune diseases has a more complex pathogenesis involving host genetics and dysregulation of the host microbiome cross-talk.[2] The goals of FMT in Crohn's disease are to correct dysbiosis and restore a normal dialogue between the host immune system and the microbiota. However, the underlying genetic predisposition remains, which likely precludes a similar success as CDI for FMT in Crohn's disease.

Mouse Models

In a model of interleukin-10 knockout mice, ileocolonic resection (ICR) induced microbial functional and taxonomic shifts, decreased diversity, and depleted Bacteroidia and Clostridia.[30] After surgery, there was a significant loss of microbial diversity with predominance of Firmicutes and expansion of Proteobacteria. These mice had reduced colitis but worse ileitis with bacterial overgrowth, increased translocation, and reduction in tissue macrophages. After FMT, microbiome analysis revealed persistently decreased diversity in both ICR groups despite substantial diversity in the donor stool. The sham-transplanted group continued to have increased *Lactobacillus*, *Enterococcus*, *Streptococcus*, and *Staphylococcus* relative to control and FMT groups. In the FMT group, *Klebsiella* uniformly expanded in all animals after donor transplantation despite low relative abundance in donor stool. In addition to *Klebsiella*, an increase in *Bacteroides*, *Alistipes*, and *Parabacteroides* was seen in FMT animals. *Klebsiella* and *Bacteroides* accounted for most of the relative abundance. FMT prevented ileitis but restored colitis and allowed for a bloom of γ-proteobacteria. In the colon, ICR and sham transplant were associated with recruitment of tolerogenic dendritic cells, whereas FMT shifted these immune cell subsets to control profiles along with increasing cytokine levels.[30]

Human Studies

Microbial restoration therapies including FMT have been reported for patients with Crohn's disease and ulcerative colitis with equivocal evidence from underpowered, open-label case reports or studies with varied treatment protocols and delivery modalities. A systematic review of patients with Crohn's disease for FMT demonstrated a pooled estimate of clinical remission of 60.5% (95% confidence interval, 28.4%–85.6%) for Crohn's disease, which was higher than patients with ulcerative colitis of 22% (95% confidence interval, 10.4%–40.8%).[31] The subgroup analysis for Crohn's disease consisted of four studies and demonstrated moderate heterogeneity (Cochran Q, $P = .05$; $I^2 = 37\%$). This higher response rate was mainly driven by one study of nine patients.[32] In this study, metagenomic evaluation indicated evidence of FMT engraftment in seven of nine patients. There was an overall improvement in Crohn's disease activity indices and seven of nine patients were in remission at 2 weeks and five of nine patients who did not receive additional medical therapy were in remission at 6 and 12 weeks. No or modest improvement was seen in patients who did not engraft or whose microbiome was most similar to their donor.[32] A small case series demonstrated improvement in quality of life despite a lack of improvement in disease activity after FMT in Crohn's disease.[33] Most data for FMT is in patients with ulcerative colitis where randomized controlled trials have conflicting data but pooled data demonstrate a moderate benefit.[34] There are no results reported from placebo-controlled clinical trials of FMT for Crohn's disease.

Patients with concomitant CDI and Crohn's disease or ulcerative colitis frequently undergo FMT for management of CDI. These retrospective studies indicate that the response rates for FMT for CDI in patients with IBD are lower than patients without IBD.[35] Additionally, there has been a 25% reported risk of IBD flare after FMT. None of these studies have shown a benefit of a one-time FMT for the management of underlying IBD.

PREBIOTICS, PROBIOTICS, AND POSTBIOTICS IN CROHN'S DISEASE

As greater insight into the influence of the gut microbiota on the host immune response is gained, there is a need to explore ways to manipulate the microbiota or its function to modulate the host immune response and restore health. There have been many attempts to shape the gut microbial community with prebiotics and probiotics in patients with Crohn's disease with minimal efficacy. This apparent lack of efficacy may be in part caused by difficulties in administering known and consistent formulations of commensal organisms or poor tolerability of prebiotic doses needed to substantially change the enteric microbiota.

Prebiotics

Prebiotics promote the growth and colonization of beneficial organisms in the gut. Fiber is one of the oldest and most commonly used prebiotics. Some commensal organisms ferment indigestible fiber to produce SCFAs, which are a vital energy source for colonocytes. Reduction in SCFA producers has been noted in several IBD studies, including decreases in *Faecalibacterium*, *Phascolarctobacerium*, and *Roseburia* in Crohn's disease.[6,36] The study by Morgan and colleagues[36] also found a decrease in butanoate and propanoate metabolism genes in ileal Crohn's disease. Although a diet high in fiber has been associated with a decreased risk of Crohn's disease, there has not been evidence supporting its role in the treatment of Crohn's disease.[37]

Preliminary data suggest short-chain fructo-oligosaccharide has a rapid fermentation profile that may allow for normalization of ileal commensal microbes and enhanced luminal butyrate concentration in the ileum.[38] A small open-label study enrolled 10 patients with active ileocolonic Crohn's disease and administered 15 g of fructo-oligosaccharides (inulin) daily for 3 weeks.[39] Treatment resulted in a significant reduction in disease activity and an increase in fecal bifidobacteria concentrations. However, a sufficiently powered, randomized, double-blind, placebo-controlled study of fructo-oligosaccharides in active Crohn's disease did not find a clinical benefit despite evidence of affecting dendritic cell function.[40] At this time there is no convincing evidence to support the use of prebiotics for the treatment of active Crohn's disease. Further studies are needed to explore if prebiotics may have a role as adjuvant therapy or to help maintain remission.

Probiotics

Given the understanding of the relationship of dysbiosis and Crohn's disease, it seems logical that administration of probiotic strains could diversify the microbial community and help reshape the community to a more beneficial balance of microbes leading to improvement in disease activity. Most studies examining the role of probiotics in Crohn's disease have been designed to test efficacy for maintenance of remission. Studies have been small, often open-labeled, and varied in duration and end points. Probiotics examined have included *Lactobacilli GG*, *Lactobacilli johnsonii*, *E coli* Nissle 1917, and *Saccharomyces boulardii*. Some studies have included a combination of probiotics and prebiotics. One open-label, uncontrolled trial included 10 patients with active disease and administered a probiotic containing *Bifidobacterium breve*, *Bifidobacterium longum*, and *Lactobacillus casei*, and a prebiotic (psyllium).[41] Although seven patients reported improvement of symptoms, only two patients tapered off of corticosteroid therapy. Another larger study by Steed and colleagues[42] randomized 35 patients with Crohn's disease with active disease to *B longum*, and inulin/oligofructose growth substrate, or placebo. All patients continued on conventional therapy and were followed for 6 months. There were a significant number of patients lost to follow-up; however, of those patients who completed the study, 62% (8 of 13) in the treatment arm were in remission compared with 45% (5 of 11) in the placebo arm. Despite the limitations of this study from the high dropout rate, the study does raise the question of whether synbiotic consumption has some role in active Crohn's disease.[42]

The efficacy of probiotics for the induction of remission in Crohn's disease was explored in a Cochrane review in 2008. Only one small study (n = 11) met inclusion criteria and did not show a significant effect.[43] A recent meta-analysis and systemic review of probiotics in IBD also found probiotics were not effective in the induction and maintenance of remission in Crohn's disease.[44] These reviews further support the lack of data to support the efficacy of probiotics in Crohn's disease.

Postbiotics

Although there are no clear effective probiotic strains or therapeutically beneficial prebiotics for Crohn's disease, there is still hope that how best to formulate and administer microbial therapeutics will be discovered. This field will continue to advance as more is learned about the functional roles of the gut microbiota and its relationship with the host immune system. The identification of postbiotics is an emerging field in microbial therapeutics. Postbiotics are the bioactive molecules produced by a microbial community, which maintain the health of the gastrointestinal tract. Systems biology approaches incorporating advances in metagenomics and metabolomics may allow for identification of key metabolic pathways and bioactive postbiotics that have the potential to restore the healthy function of the gut microbial community.

MICROBIAL RESTORATION THERAPIES IN CROHN'S DISEASE: MORE QUESTIONS THAN ANSWERS

Microbial restoration therapies for Crohn's disease should be carried out only under research settings with an investigation drug use application from the Food and Drug Administration. Because microbial dysbiosis in Crohn's disease is likely a causative factor for and a result of underlying inflammation, microbial restoration therapies remain a major challenge in 2017. The exact nature of the perturbation of the microbiome is not completely understood and it has not been possible to differentiate the dysbiotic changes leading to onset of disease from those that are a result of inflammation. When underlying inflammation triggers Crohn's disease, the luminal microbiota change. This change in turn leads to abnormal host-microbiome interactions, which can aggravate underlying disease. Conceivably, the vicious circle of inflammation and dysbiosis may potentially be broken by controlling the underlying inflammation or by modulating the host microbiome by microbiome restoration therapies.

There are several considerations before microbiome restoration therapies should be used or tested for Crohn's disease. There are ongoing clinical trials of microbial restoration therapies for patients with IBD. Unlike CDI, where there seems to be no donor or recipient effect or no stool preparation effect on FMT success rates, Crohn's disease is more complicated. The efficacy and potentially safety of microbial restoration therapies in a patient with Crohn's disease is likely to be affected donor selection, Crohn's disease status, patient preparation, stool processing, and delivery method. Additionally, there is an urgent need to define end points and follow-up for these therapies in Crohn's disease (**Fig. 1**).

Considerations for donor screening for FMT for Crohn's disease are aimed at minimizing safety risks from FMT. These include a complete medical history for exclusion of microbiome-associated conditions, such as obesity, metabolic syndrome, anxiety,

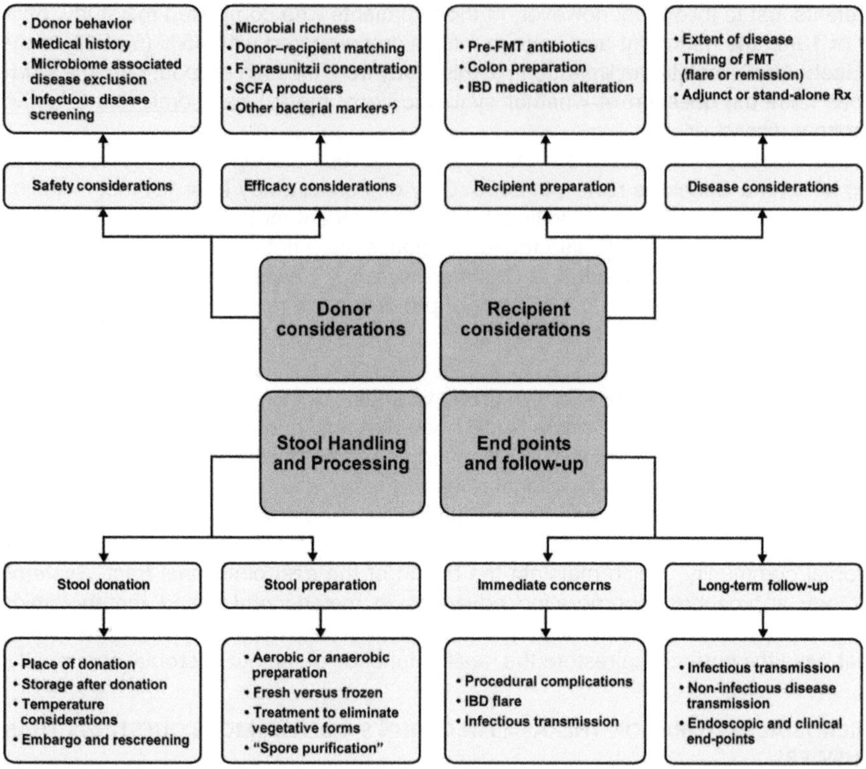

Fig. 1. Donor, recipient, disease, stool processing, and follow-up considerations for microbial restoration therapies for Crohn's disease.

depression, chronic diarrheal illnesses, recent hospitalization, and antibiotic exposure. Additionally, a careful screening of donor behavior (eg, tattoos, drug abuse), to avoid donors with risks for infectious diseases, along with comprehensive blood and stool testing for infectious diseases, should be performed.[45] Donor considerations specific to Crohn's disease possibly include an assessment of microbial richness, *F prausnitzii* concentration, and also an assessment of SCFA production. More research is needed to understand differences between related and unrelated donors, and there may be opportunities for donor-recipient matching or defined microbial consortia for FMT in Crohn's disease as the understanding of the host-microbiome in this patient population is expanded and ways to stably make meaningful changes in the host microbiome to potentially alter disease course are explored (see **Fig. 1**).

Recipient considerations for FMT in patients with Crohn's disease include decisions on benefit or lack of benefit of administration of gut-specific antibiotics (eg, oral vancomycin) before FMT, bowel preparation, and changes in Crohn's disease medications before FMT. Careful selection of disease extent and severity for FMT needs to be studied. Additionally, the timing and goal of FMT in these patients needs to be studied for maintenance of remission in patients already in remission or attempts to induce remission in patients with an ongoing disease flare. More research is needed to define if FMT should be used as a stand-alone treatment or as an adjunct to ongoing treatment (see **Fig. 1**).

Considerations around stool donation and processing include place of donation, stool processing temperatures, and choice of aerobic or anaerobic environment for processing and storage of stool. The optimal diluent used for stool processing and timing and optimal temperature for stability of the processed product still remains unknown. Also, some advocate an embargo of the stool product until donor rescreening is performed. The differential effects of fresh versus frozen stool are not seen in CDI but may play a role in Crohn's disease.[46] Additional concerns include treatment of stool to eliminate vegetative forms and pathogens and potentially use a purified spore form for FMT in these patients (see **Fig. 1**).

Patients with Crohn's disease who are enrolled in trials of FMT need close follow-up. Immediate concerns include procedural complications from colonoscopy, a risk of IBD flare, and a potential for infectious transmission especially because patients with Crohn's disease may be immunocompromised. Additional potential concerns include noninfectious disease transmission. Additionally, the timing and nature of microbial, endoscopic and clinical end points in clinical trials of FMT need to be defined (see **Fig. 1**).

MICROBIAL RESTORATION THERAPIES IN CROHN'S DISEASE: A CLOSER LOOK AT 2050

With ongoing research, it may be possible to manage patients with Crohn's disease with microbial restoration therapies in addition to conventional immunosuppression medications. Potential steps to tailor therapy for these patients include complete

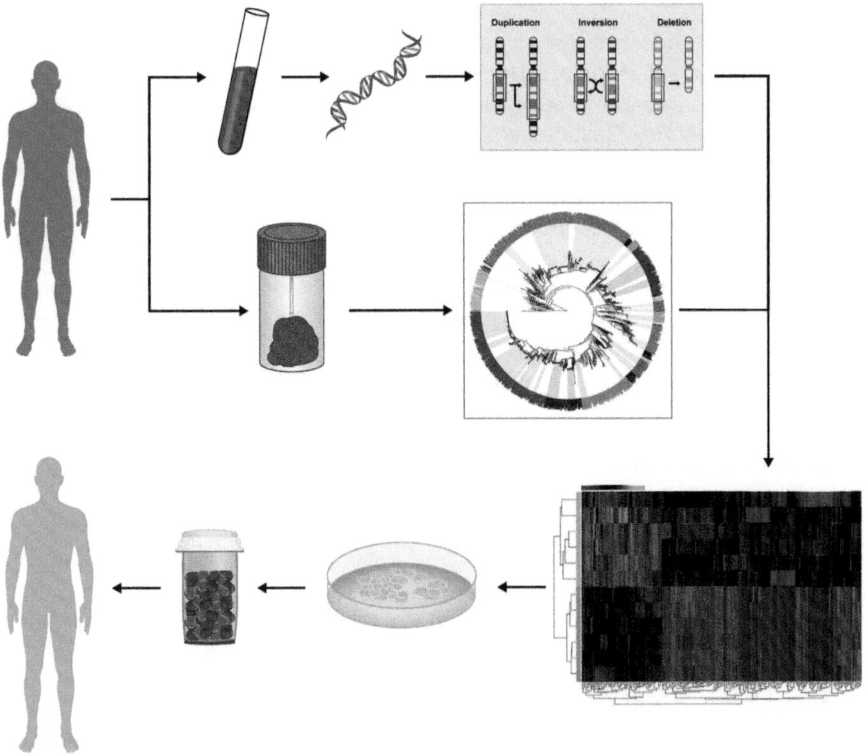

Fig. 2. An individualized approach for microbial restoration therapies in Crohn's disease by performing complete host gene and stool and mucosal microbiome sequencing, followed by computation of microbial dysbiosis and administer-defined microbial consortia or stool from specific donors.

host gene sequencing and microbiome sequencing of the stool and mucosa-associated microbiome. There would be technology and data available to decipher dysbiotic changes in host microbiome in context of host genetic makeup, and compute deficits or excess of microbial (bacterial, viral, or fungal) taxa; and treat these patients with defined scientifically grown microbial consortia or with donor stool from specific donors (**Fig. 2**).

SUMMARY

Patients with Crohn's disease have decreased microbial diversity, which plays an important role in the pathogenesis of Crohn's disease. A better understanding of host-microbe interactions in patients with Crohn's disease is needed. Microbial restoration therapies are being studied for management of Crohn's disease and may be an adjunct to standard therapies in the future. It may be feasible to modify the gut microbiota community structure or function to treat patients with Crohn's disease with targeted therapies via individual agents, such as probiotics, bacterial consortia, or even dietary manipulation. FMT should not be performed for Crohn's disease other than in research settings.

REFERENCES

1. Abraham C, Cho JH. Inflammatory bowel disease. N Engl J Med 2009;361(21):2066–78.
2. de Souza HS, Fiocchi C. Immunopathogenesis of IBD: current state of the art. Nat Rev Gastroenterol Hepatol 2016;13(1):13–27.
3. Colombel JF. Decade in review-IBD: IBD-genes, bacteria and new therapeutic strategies. Nat Rev Gastroenterol Hepatol 2014;11(11):652–4.
4. Kostic AD, Xavier RJ, Gevers D. The microbiome in inflammatory bowel disease: current status and the future ahead. Gastroenterology 2014;146(6):1489–99.
5. Sartor RB. Microbial influences in inflammatory bowel diseases. Gastroenterology 2008;134(2):577–94.
6. Frank DN, St Amand AL, Feldman RA, et al. Molecular-phylogenetic characterization of microbial community imbalances in human inflammatory bowel diseases. Proc Natl Acad Sci U S A 2007;104(34):13780–5.
7. Gevers D, Kugathasan S, Denson LA, et al. The treatment-naive microbiome in new-onset Crohn's disease. Cell Host Microbe 2014;15(3):382–92.
8. Willing BP, Dicksved J, Halfvarson J, et al. A pyrosequencing study in twins shows that gastrointestinal microbial profiles vary with inflammatory bowel disease phenotypes. Gastroenterology 2010;139(6):1844–54.e1.
9. Willing B, Halfvarson J, Dicksved J, et al. Twin studies reveal specific imbalances in the mucosa-associated microbiota of patients with ileal Crohn's disease. Inflamm Bowel Dis 2009;15(5):653–60.
10. Lopez-Siles M, Martinez-Medina M, Busquets D, et al. Mucosa-associated *Faecalibacterium prausnitzii* and *Escherichia coli* co-abundance can distinguish irritable bowel syndrome and inflammatory bowel disease phenotypes. Int J Med Microbiol 2014;304(3–4):464–75.
11. Chassaing B, Darfeuille-Michaud A. The commensal microbiota and enteropathogens in the pathogenesis of inflammatory bowel diseases. Gastroenterology 2011;140(6):1720–8.
12. Swidsinski A, Loening-Baucke V, Herber A. Mucosal flora in Crohn's disease and ulcerative colitis: an overview. J Physiol Pharmacol 2009;60(Suppl 6):61–71.

13. Baumgart M, Dogan B, Rishniw M, et al. Culture independent analysis of ileal mucosa reveals a selective increase in invasive *Escherichia coli* of novel phylogeny relative to depletion of *Clostridiales* in Crohn's disease involving the ileum. ISME J 2007;1(5):403–18.
14. Sartor RB, Wu GD. Roles for intestinal bacteria, viruses, and fungi in pathogenesis of inflammatory bowel diseases and therapeutic approaches. Gastroenterology 2017;152(2):327–39.e4.
15. Ley RE. The gene-microbe link. Nature 2015;518(7540):S7.
16. Goodrich JK, Waters JL, Poole AC, et al. Human genetics shape the gut microbiome. Cell 2014;159(4):789–99.
17. Turnbaugh PJ, Hamady M, Yatsunenko T, et al. A core gut microbiome in obese and lean twins. Nature 2009;457(7228):480–4.
18. Turnbaugh PJ, Backhed F, Fulton L, et al. Diet-induced obesity is linked to marked but reversible alterations in the mouse distal gut microbiome. Cell Host Microbe 2008;3(4):213–23.
19. Goodrich JK, Davenport ER, Beaumont M, et al. Genetic determinants of the gut microbiome in UK twins. Cell Host Microbe 2016;19(5):731–43.
20. Org E, Parks BW, Joo JW, et al. Genetic and environmental control of host-gut microbiota interactions. Genome Res 2015;25(10):1558–69.
21. Imhann F, Vich Vila A, Bonder MJ, et al. Interplay of host genetics and gut microbiota underlying the onset and clinical presentation of inflammatory bowel disease. Gut 2016. [Epub ahead of print].
22. Chu H, Khosravi A, Kusumawardhani IP, et al. Gene-microbiota interactions contribute to the pathogenesis of inflammatory bowel disease. Science 2016; 352(6289):1116–20.
23. Bouskra D, Brezillon C, Berard M, et al. Lymphoid tissue genesis induced by commensals through NOD1 regulates intestinal homeostasis. Nature 2008; 456(7221):507–10.
24. Macpherson AJ, Harris NL. Interactions between commensal intestinal bacteria and the immune system. Nat Rev Immunol 2004;4(6):478–85.
25. Ishikawa H, Tanaka K, Maeda Y, et al. Effect of intestinal microbiota on the induction of regulatory CD25+ CD4+ T cells. Clin Exp Immunol 2008;153(1):127–35.
26. Mazmanian SK, Liu CH, Tzianabos AO, et al. An immunomodulatory molecule of symbiotic bacteria directs maturation of the host immune system. Cell 2005; 122(1):107–18.
27. Sekirov I, Russell SL, Antunes LC, et al. Gut microbiota in health and disease. Physiol Rev 2010;90(3):859–904.
28. Zeuthen LH, Fink LN, Frokiaer H. Epithelial cells prime the immune response to an array of gut-derived commensals towards a tolerogenic phenotype through distinct actions of thymic stromal lymphopoietin and transforming growth factor-beta. Immunology 2008;123(2):197–208.
29. van Nood E, Dijkgraaf MG, Keller JJ. Duodenal infusion of feces for recurrent *Clostridium difficile*. N Engl J Med 2013;368(22):2145.
30. Perry T, Jovel J, Patterson J, et al. Fecal microbial transplant after ileocolic resection reduces ileitis but restores colitis in IL-10-/- mice. Inflamm Bowel Dis 2015; 21(7):1479–90.
31. Colman RJ, Rubin DT. Fecal microbiota transplantation as therapy for inflammatory bowel disease: a systematic review and meta-analysis. J Crohns Colitis 2014;8(12):1569–81.

32. Suskind DL, Brittnacher MJ, Wahbeh G, et al. Fecal microbial transplant effect on clinical outcomes and fecal microbiome in active Crohn's disease. Inflamm Bowel Dis 2015;21(3):556–63.
33. Wei Y, Zhu W, Gong J, et al. Fecal microbiota transplantation improves the quality of life in patients with inflammatory bowel disease. Gastroenterol Res Pract 2015; 2015:517597.
34. Moayyedi P. Fecal transplantation: any real hope for inflammatory bowel disease? Curr Opin Gastroenterol 2016;32(4):282–6.
35. Khoruts A, Rank KM, Newman KM, et al. Inflammatory bowel disease affects the outcome of fecal microbiota transplantation for recurrent *Clostridium difficile* infection. Clin Gastroenterol Hepatol 2016;14(10):1433–8.
36. Morgan XC, Tickle TL, Sokol H, et al. Dysfunction of the intestinal microbiome in inflammatory bowel disease and treatment. Genome Biol 2012;13(9):R79.
37. Hou JK, Abraham B, El-Serag H. Dietary intake and risk of developing inflammatory bowel disease: a systematic review of the literature. Am J Gastroenterol 2011;106(4):563–73.
38. Barnes JL, Hartmann B, Holst JJ, et al. Intestinal adaptation is stimulated by partial enteral nutrition supplemented with the prebiotic short-chain fructooligosaccharide in a neonatal intestinal failure piglet model. JPEN J Parenter Enteral Nutr 2012;36(5):524–37.
39. Lindsay JO, Whelan K, Stagg AJ, et al. Clinical, microbiological, and immunological effects of fructo-oligosaccharide in patients with Crohn's disease. Gut 2006; 55(3):348–55.
40. Benjamin JL, Hedin CR, Koutsoumpas A, et al. Randomised, double-blind, placebo-controlled trial of fructo-oligosaccharides in active Crohn's disease. Gut 2011;60(7):923–9.
41. Fujimori S, Tatsuguchi A, Gudis K, et al. High dose probiotic and prebiotic cotherapy for remission induction of active Crohn's disease. J Gastroenterol Hepatol 2007;22(8):1199–204.
42. Steed H, Macfarlane GT, Blackett KL, et al. Clinical trial: the microbiological and immunological effects of synbiotic consumption: a randomized double-blind placebo-controlled study in active Crohn's disease. Aliment Pharmacol Ther 2010; 32(7):872–83.
43. Butterworth AD, Thomas AG, Akobeng AK. Probiotics for induction of remission in Crohn's disease. Cochrane Database Syst Rev 2008;(3):CD006634.
44. Dong J, Teng G, Wei T, et al. Methodological quality assessment of meta-analyses and systematic reviews of probiotics in inflammatory bowel disease and pouchitis. PLoS One 2016;11(12):e0168785.
45. Tariq R, Weatherly R, Kammer P, et al. Donor screening experience for fecal microbiota transplantation in patients with recurrent *C. difficile* infection. J Clin Gastroenterol 2016. [Epub ahead of print].
46. Lee CH, Steiner T, Petrof EO, et al. Frozen vs fresh fecal microbiota transplantation and clinical resolution of diarrhea in patients with recurrent *Clostridium difficile* infection: a randomized clinical trial. JAMA 2016;315(2):142–9.

Endoscopic and Radiographic Assessment of Crohn's Disease

Badr Al-Bawardy, MD[a,*], Stephanie L. Hansel, MD, MS[a], Jeff L. Fidler, MD[b], John M. Barlow, MD[b], David H. Bruining, MD[a]

KEYWORDS

- Crohn's disease • Mucosal healing • Endoscopy • Computed tomography • MRI • Ultrasound • Enterography

KEY POINTS

- Crohn's disease (CD) is a transmural chronic inflammatory disorder that can affect any part of the gastrointestinal tract.
- Assessments of disease activity and response to therapy are essential to the management of CD.
- Clinical symptoms correlate poorly with CD activity and long-term outcomes.
- Endoscopic and radiographic responses have been associated with favorable clinical outcomes.
- There are multiple endoscopic and radiologic scoring systems that provide objective measurements of disease activity and response to therapy in CD.

BACKGROUND

Management algorithms for Crohn's disease (CD) patients continue to rapidly evolve. A key concept that is driving the search for objective disease assessment tools is the notion that symptoms often do not correlate with disease activity. A powerful study by Modigliani and colleagues[1] demonstrated no significant correlation between endoscopic disease activity measured with the CD endoscopic index of severity (CDEIS) and clinical symptoms measured with the CD activity index (CDAI). This has been followed by more recent work noting the lack of agreement between CDAI and C-reactive protein (CRP), fecal calprotectin, and endoscopic interrogations with the simple

Disclosure Statement: No disclosures (B. Al-Bawardy, S.L. Hansel, J.L. Fidler, J.M. Barlow). Consultant to Medtronics (D.H. Bruining).
[a] Division of Gastroenterology and Hepatology, Mayo Clinic, 200 First Street Southwest, Rochester, MN 55905, USA; [b] Department of Radiology, Mayo Clinic, 200 First Street Southwest, Rochester, MN 55905, USA
* Corresponding author.
E-mail address: albawardy.badr@mayo.edu

Gastroenterol Clin N Am 46 (2017) 493–513
http://dx.doi.org/10.1016/j.gtc.2017.05.005
gastro.theclinics.com

endoscopic score for CD (SES-CD) scoring system.[2] In both the ACCENT 1 (A Crohn's Disease Clinical Trial Evaluating Infliximab in a New Long-Term Treatment Regimen) and the SONIC (Study of Biologic and Immunomodulator Naive Patients in Crohn's Disease) trials, nearly 18% of patients with symptoms and CDAIs suggesting active CD disease did not have mucosal ulcerations on baseline ileocolonoscopy (IC).[3,4] In short, symptoms alone cannot reliably predict disease activity and should not be used to guide management decisions.

Endoscopic and radiographic assessments, however, can provide accurate and objective CD activity assessments. These modalities complement each other. IC is the gold standard for establishing an inflammatory bowel disease (IBD) diagnosis with tissue acquisition. It also provides detailed and prognostic mucosal assessments, and allows performance of therapeutic stricture dilation. Capsule endoscopy (CE) can evaluate the mucosa of the entire gastrointestinal tract. Computed tomography enterography (CTE), magnetic resonance enterography (MRE), and ultrasound (US) can provide transmural disease assessments in regions inaccessible to standard endoscopic techniques, diagnose penetrating disease complications, detect and screen for unsuspected strictures before CE, and detect extraintestinal IBD manifestations. Clinical research now demonstrates that mucosal healing on endoscopy or radiologic response to medical therapy is associated with better long-term outcomes.[5,6] These endoscopic and radiologic tools continue to evolve with the creation of objective scoring systems that are discussed in this review article.

ENDOSCOPY

CD can involve any segment of the gastrointestinal tract from the mouth to the anus. Hence, endoscopic modalities for the evaluation of CD include IC, esophagogastroduodenoscopy (EGD), CE, and balloon-assisted enteroscopy (BAE). Endoscopic applications in CD include the initial diagnosis, assessment of disease extent and severity, response to therapy, evaluation for postoperative recurrence, colorectal neoplasia surveillance, and therapeutic intervention such as stricture dilation. For establishing the initial CD diagnosis, IC is the gold standard, often demonstrating mucosal erythema, edema, mucosal friability, aphthous ulcerations, serpiginous ulcerations, skip lesions, and strictures (**Fig. 1**). Histologic findings of chronic inflammation include crypt architectural distortion and noncaseating granulomas. EGD is the preferred test for evaluating upper gut CD involvement, which can affect up to 16% of adult CD patients.[7] BAE is used to obtain tissue confirmation of CD when TI and colonic skipping is present, and to perform therapeutic interventions such as stricture dilation and retrieval of retained capsule endoscope.

CE is a minimally invasive modality for small bowel examination in CD. Potential indications include assessing for proximal small bowel disease and monitoring response to medical therapy. The yield of CE in suspected and established CD has varied in the literature, ranging from 50% to 70%.[8] CE is reported to have a higher sensitivity for proximal small bowel CD mucosal lesions than CTE or MRE.[9] The utilization of CE has been limited by the risk of capsule retention that can approach 2.6% in some patient populations.[10] Therefore, patency capsule administration should be considered in CD patients with a history of obstructive symptoms, strictures, prior small bowel resection or anastomosis, or in the absence of recent CTE or MRE imaging.[11]

A critical role of endoscopy is to assess response to therapy and achievement of mucosal healing. Mucosal healing in CD is defined as the absence of ulcerations. In contrast to clinical symptoms, mucosal healing in IBD has been associated with favorable long-term outcomes, including clinical remission, lower rates of surgery,

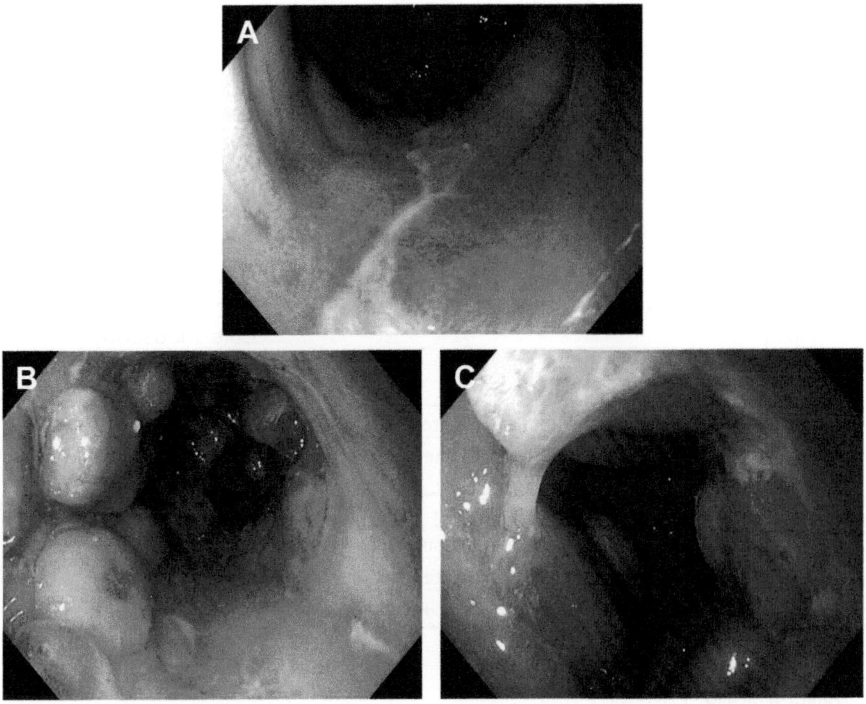

Fig. 1. Colonoscopy images of a 38-year-old man with ileocolonic CD demonstrating colonic linear ulceration (*A*), cobblestoning with associated stricture in the descending colon (*B, C*).

decreased hospitalizations, and improved quality of life.[6,12–14] Partial mucosal healing (decreased inflammation but with persistent ulcerations) is also associated with favorable outcomes such as decreased rates of surgery.[15] Deep remission, defined as mucosal healing plus a CDAI less than 150, has also been proposed as a CD treatment target. Fewer data are available regarding outcomes of achieving deep remission. Multiple endoscopic scoring tools have been developed to allow more objective reporting of disease activity.

ENDOSCOPIC SCORING SYSTEMS

Crohn's Disease Endoscopic Index of Severity

In 1989, the Crohn's disease endoscopic index of severity (CDEIS) was the first endoscopic score to be developed and validated.[16] The score depends on variables (superficial ulcers, deep ulcers, percentage of disease surface, and ulcerated surface in each segment on a 10 cm visual analog scale) in 5 intestinal segments (terminal ileum, ascending colon, transverse colon, descending colon, and sigmoid colon or rectum) (**Table 1**). The score also incorporates the presence of ulcerated stenosis and nonulcerated stenosis in any of the intestinal segments for total scores that range from 0 to 44. The inter-rater and intrarater reliability of the CDEIS has been shown to be substantial, with the intraclass correlation coefficients (ICCs) of 0.71 (0.63–0.76) and 0.89 (0.86–0.93), respectively.[17]

Various CDEIS scoring thresholds have been used. It has been proposed that a decrease of the CDEIS by greater than 4 to 5 points can be used as a definition of endoscopic response (sensitivity of 70% and specificity of 68%–84%), whereas a CDEIS less than 6 to 7 can be used as the definition of endoscopic remission

Table 1
Crohn's disease endoscopic index of severity

	Rectum	Sigmoid and Left Colon	Transverse Colon	Right Colon	Ileum	Total	
Deep ulceration (12 if present in the segment, 0 if absent)	0	0	0	0	0	0	1
Superficial ulceration (6 if present in the segment, 0 if absent)	0	0	0	0	0	0	2
Surface involved by the disease (cm)	0	0	0	0	0	0	3
Ulcerated surface measured (cm)	0	0	0	0	0	0	4
	Total 1 + total 2 + total 3 + total 4				=	0	A
	Number (n) of segments totally or partially explored				=	0	n
	Total A divided by n				=	0	B
	3 if ulcerated stenosis anywhere, 0 if not				+	0	C
	3 if non ulcerated stenosis anywhere, 0 if not				+	0	D
	Total score = B + C + D				=	0	CDEIS

Score range: 0–44.
Severe disease: CDEIS ≥ 12.
Moderate disease: CDEIS 9–12.
Mild disease: CDEIS = 3–9.
Remission: CDEIS = 0–3.
Data from Mary JY, Modigliani R. Development and validation of an endoscopic index of the severity for Crohn's disease: a prospective multicentre study. Groupe d'Etudes Therapeutiques des Affections Inflammatoires du Tube Digestif (GETAID). Gut 1989;30(7):983–9; and Peyrin-Biroulet L, Panes J, Sandborn WJ, et al. Defining disease severity in inflammatory bowel diseases: current and future directions. Clin Gastroenterol Hepatol 2016;14(3):348–54.

(sensitivity of 86%–92% and a specificity of 82%–88%).[18] However, this has varied in the literature, in which severe disease has been defined as a score equal to or greater than 12, moderate disease 9 to 12, mild disease 3 to 9, and remission 0 to 3.[19] Recently, the International Organization for the Study of Inflammatory Bowel Disease (IOIBD) suggested that a greater than 50% decrease in CDEIS be considered the definition of endoscopic response.[18] This recommendation stemmed from post hoc analysis of 172 subjects in the SONIC trial. In this analysis, greater than 50% reduction in CDEIS at 26 weeks predicted corticosteroid-free clinical remission at 50 weeks with a sensitivity of 73% (95% CI, 65%–82%) and specificity of 46% (95% CI, 35%–58%).[20]

The widespread utilization of CDEIS in clinical practice remains limited. This is due to the complex and cumbersome nature of recording the variables in multiple segments. Moreover, it can potentially underestimate severity if only 1 segment is involved. Finally, the inter-rater and intrarater reliability was reported among IBD experts and it is unclear if these results can be reproduced in other settings.

Simple Endoscopic Score for Crohn's Disease

The simple endoscopic score for Crohn's disease (SES-CD), developed as a simplified version of the CDEIS, was proposed and validated in 2004.[21] Similar to the CDEIS, the score incorporates 4 variables (size of ulcers, proportion of ulcerated surface, proportion of surface affected, and presence of stenosis) in 5 intestinal segments (**Table 2**). For the validation stage, the SES-CD was found to have a high correlation with the CDEIS (correlation coefficient of 0.88).[21] The SES-CD scores range from 0 to 56. Severe disease is defined as a score equal to or greater than 16, moderate disease 7 to 15, mild disease 3 to 6, and inactive disease equal to or less than 2.[19] Post hoc analysis of 172 subjects from the SONIC trial also demonstrated that greater than 50% reduction in SES-CD at 26 weeks predicted corticosteroid free clinical remission at 50 weeks with a sensitivity of 74% (66%–83%) and a specificity of 48% (36%–60%).[20] SES-CD has been shown to have high inter-rater and intrarater reliability with ICC of 0.83 (0.75–0.88) and 0.91 (0.89–0.95), respectively.[17] The IOIBD, using a Delphi process, proposed a greater than 50% decrease in SES-CD as the definition for response and an SES-CD of 0 to 2 as the definition of remission.[18]

The SES-CD has its strengths and limitations. It has been embraced in clinical practice more than the CDEIS due to its simplified design. Limitations include the possibility of underestimation of disease burden because it assumes segments that are not examined to be lesion free. Further research is warranted to better define values that can predict improved long-term outcomes.

Rutgeerts Score

The risk of CD clinical recurrence after resection is variable and depends on the resected intestinal segment, patient, and disease-related factors. The 1-year rate of clinical CD recurrence is as high as 38%, whereas the endoscopic recurrence rate can approach 85% to 93%.[22] In 1990, Rutgeerts and colleagues[23] developed a score for the postoperative endoscopic severity of CD recurrence at the neoterminal ileum and ileocolonic anastomosis. The ileum is graded from i0 to i4 in order of increasing severity (**Table 3**). The Rutgeerts score 1 year after resection has been shown to correlate with the risk of clinical recurrence at 3 years.[23] In a study of 89 subjects, the majority (80%) of i0 and i1 subjects had lesions that had not changed at 3 years. On the other hand, 92% of subjects with i3 and i4 lesions had recurrent disease at 3 years. Hence, subjects with i2-i4 lesions are often classified as having postoperative recurrence of CD, whereas patients with i0 and i1 lesions are described as having endoscopic remission.[18]

Table 2
Simple endoscopic severity for Crohn's disease

Variable	0	1	2	3
Size of ulcers (cm)	None	Aphthous ulcers (0.1–0.5)	Large ulcers (0.5–2)	Very large ulcers (>2)
Ulcerated surface	None	<10%	10%–30%	>30%
Affected surface	Unaffected	<50%	50%–75%	>75%
Presence of narrowing	None	Single can be passed	Multiple can be passed	Cannot be passed

Score range: 0–56.
Severe disease: SES-CD ≥16.
Moderate disease: SES-CD = 7–15.
Mild disease: SES-CD = 3–6.
Inactive disease: SES-CD ≤2.
Data from Daperno M, D'Haens G, Van Assche G, et al. Development and validation of a new, simplified endoscopic activity score for Crohn's disease: the SES-CD. Gastrointest Endosc 2004;60(4):505–12; and Peyrin-Biroulet L, et al. Defining disease severity in inflammatory bowel diseases: current and future directions. Clin Gastroenterol Hepatol 2016;14(3):348–54.

Table 3
Rutgeerts score

Endoscopic Score	Definition
i0	No aphthous ulcers
i1	≤5 aphthous ulcers
i2	>5 aphthous ulcers with normal intervening mucosa or skip areas of larger lesions or lesions confined to the ileocolonic anastomosis
i3	Diffuse aphthous ileitis with diffusely inflamed mucosa
i4	Diffuse inflammation with already larger ulcers, nodules, and/or narrowing

Postoperative recurrence: Rutgeerts score equals i2–i4.

Data from Rutgeerts P, Geboes K, Vantrappen G, et al. Predictability of the postoperative course of Crohn's disease. Gastroenterology 1990;99(4):956–63; and Vuitton, L, Marteau P, Sandborn WJ, et al. IOIBD technical review on endoscopic indices for Crohn's disease clinical trials. Gut 2016;65(9):1447–55.

Despite global popularity, the Rutgeerts score has several limitations that should be acknowledged. It has not been formally validated and it has only moderate interobserver agreement.[24] The score also depends on reaching and traversing the ileocolonic anastomosis, which is not always possible in CD patients.

Capsule Endoscopy Scoring Systems

The Lewis score was first proposed in 2008.[25] It is calculated by dividing the small bowel into 3 equal parts, or tertiles, based on small bowel transit time. For each tertile, villous appearance (edema), ulceration (number, size, and extent), and presence of stenosis are recorded (**Fig. 2**). Subscores are calculated for each tertile based on extent and distribution of edema and the number, size and, distribution of ulcerations. The cumulative or final score is calculated by adding the worst affected tertile subscore to the stenosis score (**Table 4**). Absent or clinically insignificant inflammation is denoted with a score less than 135, mild inflammation with a score of 135 to 790, and moderate-severe inflammation with a scores equal to or greater than 790. The Lewis score has strong interobserver agreement and can potentially be used to assess response to medical therapy.[26]

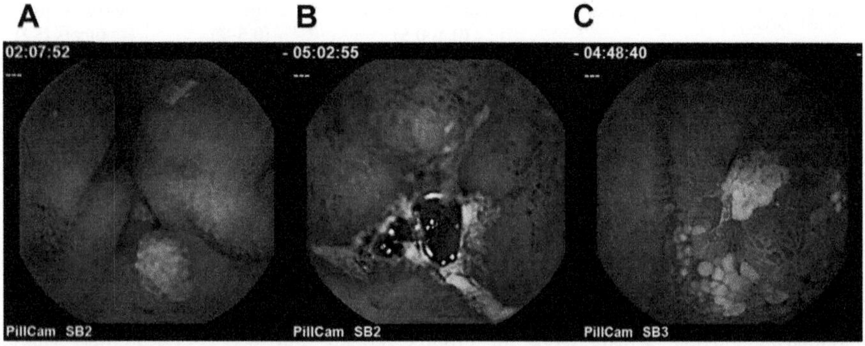

Fig. 2. CE images of a CD patient showing aphthae (*A*), edema, erythema and ulceration (*B*), and ulceration with associated stenosis (*C*).

Table 4
Capsule endoscopy Lewis score

Parameter	Descriptor or Number (Numerical Score)	Longitudinal Extent[a] (Numerical Score)	Descriptor (Numerical Score)
Villous appearance[a] (worst-affected tertile)	Normal (0) Edematous (1)	Short-segment (8) Long-segment (12) Whole tertile (20)	Single (1) Patchy (14) Diffuse (17)
Ulcers[b,c] (worst-affected tertile)	None (0) Single (3) Few (5) Multiple (10)	Short-segment (5) Long-segment (10) Whole tertile (15)	<¼ (9) ¼–½ (12) >½ (18)
Stenosis (whole study)	None (0) Single (14) Multiple (20)	Ulcerated (24) Nonulcerated (2)	Traversed (7) Not traversed (10)

Score total: worst-affected tertile villous appearance and ulcers plus stenosis score.
Clinically insignificant inflammation: Lewis score <135.
Mild inflammation: Lewis score = 135–790.
Moderate to severe inflammation: Lewis scores ≥790.
[a] Short-segment <10%; long-segment 11%–50%; whole tertile >50%.
[b] Ulcer number: single = 1, few = 2–7, multiple ≥8.
[c] Ulcer descriptor (size): proportion of the capsule picture filled by the largest ulcer.
Data from Gralnek IM, Defranchis R, Seidman E, et al. Development of a capsule endoscopy scoring index for small bowel mucosal inflammatory change. Aliment Pharmacol Ther 2008;27(2):146–54; and Cotter J, Dias de Castro F, Magalhaes J, et al. Validation of the Lewis score for the evaluation of small-bowel Crohn's disease activity. Endoscopy 2015;47(4):330–5.

The capsule endoscopy Crohn's disease activity index (CECDAI), or Niv score, was also proposed in 2008 and subsequently validated in a prospective multicenter study.[27,28] The CECDAI evaluates 3 parameters that include inflammation, extent of disease, and presences of strictures. The inflammatory score ranges from 0 (no inflammation) to 5 (large ulcers >2 cm). The extent of disease score ranges from 0 (no disease) to 3 (diffuse disease), and presence of stricture scores range from 0 (none) to 3 (obstruction) (**Table 5**). This scoring system divides the small bowel into 2 segments (proximal and distal) based on transit time. Based on a formula, a segmental score, as well as a total score, can be calculated. The score ranges from 0 to 36 and there are currently no cut-off values to define disease activity or severity other than that a score less than 4 is equivalent to endoscopic remission. Further prospective studies are needed to elucidate the definition of mucosal healing with CE and response to therapy using CE scores.

RADIOLOGIC IMAGING MODALITIES

Multiple radiologic modalities exist for the evaluation of CD. This includes CTE, MRE, and US. These imaging modalities have replaced small bowel follow-through examinations at most academic centers. Imaging complements endoscopy because it permits detection of active small bowel transmural inflammation, postoperative recurrence, penetrating and extraintestinal complications of CD, evaluates small bowel segments not reachable by conventional endoscopy, and monitors response to therapy.

Robust data support the use of CTE and MRE in CD patients. The sensitivities and specificities of CTE and MRE for detecting active inflammation in CD are

Table 5
Capsule endoscopy Crohn's disease activity index

Parameter	Score and Descriptor
A. Inflammation	0: None 1: Mild to moderate (edema, hyperemia, or denudation) 2: Severe (edema, hyperemia, or denudation) 3: Bleeding, exudate, erosion, aphthae, ulcer <0.5 cm 4: Pseudopolyp, ulcer 0.5–2 cm 5: Ulcer >2 cm
B. Extent of Disease	0: None 1: Single-segment (focal disease) 2: 2–3 Segments (patchy disease) 3: >3 Segments (diffuse disease)
C. Stricture	0: None 1: Single, traversed 2: Multiple, traversed 3: Obstruction

CECDAI: proximal segment (A × B + C) + distal segment (A × B + C).
Score range: 0–36.
Clinical or endoscopic remission: CECDAI <4.
Data from Gal E, Geller A, Fraser G, et al. Assessment and validation of the new capsule endoscopy Crohn's disease activity index (CECDAI). Dig Dis Sci 2008;53(7):1933–7; and Niv Y, Ilani S, Levi Z, et al. Validation of the capsule endoscopy Crohn's disease activity index (CECDAI or Niv score): a multicenter prospective study. Endoscopy 2012;44(1):21–6.

comparable and exceed 90%.[29,30] An advantage of CTE and MRE is the ability to identify isolated transmural disease not detected by IC.[31] The complementary role of imaging in the diagnosis of CD is nicely demonstrated in a series of 153 subjects who underwent endoscopic terminal ileal (TI) intubation.[32] In this series, 53.7% of subjects who had normal endoscopic TI examinations had demonstrated active CD via imaging due to TI skipping or transmural disease.[32] In a large cohort, CTE has also been shown to identify penetrating disease and extraintestinal CD manifestations as a new finding in up to two-thirds of patients.[33] In addition, CTE has been reported to alter management plans in nearly 50% of CD patients.[34] MRI of the pelvis is the imaging test of choice for evaluating perianal CD because it has a sensitivity of 86% and specificity of 69%, and when combined with other modalities, such as endoscopic US and examination under anesthesia, the sensitivity approaches 100%.[35,36]

Abdominal US is an intriguing test for evaluating small bowel CD at select IBD centers. The potential advantages of US include portability, low cost, avoidance of ionizing radiation, and (in some protocols) the avoidance of intravenous or oral contrast agents. The overall per patient sensitivity and specificity of US for the diagnosis of CD is 85% and 98%, respectively.[29] The accuracy of US is influenced by disease location because the highest accuracy is observed in the TI and left colon.[29] In a direct comparison to MRE, US was less accurate at defining disease extent and detecting enteroenteric fistulas.[37] Performance of US in detecting proximal small bowel CD and postoperative recurrence improved with administration of oral contrast, such as small intestinal contrast US (SICU).[38–40] The role of US in the diagnosis and management of CD is evolving but its use has been limited by operator expertise and patients' body habitus (eg, difficulty with elevated body mass index).

MAGNETIC RESONANCE SCORING SYSTEMS

Magnetic Resonance Index of Activity Score

The magnetic resonance index of activity (MaRIA) score was first reported in 2009 (**Fig. 3**). In the initial derivation study of 50 subjects who had IC performed as the reference standard, the MRE findings of wall thickness, postcontrast wall signal intensity, relative contrast enhancement (RCE), pseudopolyps, lymph node enlargement, presence of edema, and ulcerations correlated with disease activity.[41] The presence of increased wall thickness (P = .007), RCE (P = .01), edema (P = .02), and ulcers on MRE (P = .003) highly correlated with the CDEIS.[41] The MaRIA score is calculated using wall thickness, RCE, edema, and ulceration (**Table 6**) with the equation: $1.5 \times$ wall thickness $+ 0.02 \times$ RCE $+ 5 \times$ edema $+ 10 \times$ ulceration.

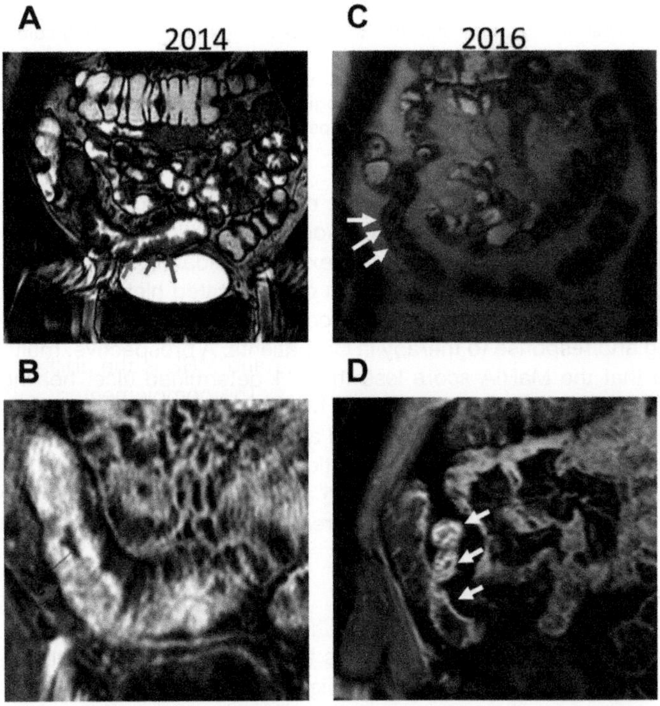

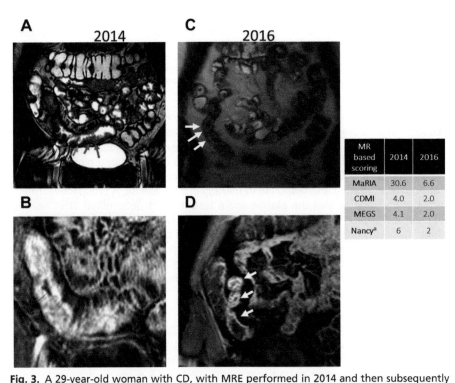

MR based scoring	2014	2016
MaRIA	30.6	6.6
CDMI	4.0	2.0
MEGS	4.1	2.0
Nancy[a]	6	2

Fig. 3. A 29-year-old woman with CD, with MRE performed in 2014 and then subsequently in 2016 (after treatment with adalimumab 40 mg subcutaneously every 2 weeks). (*A*) 2014 coronal fast-imaging using steady-state acquisition sequence demonstrating distal ileum, including terminal ileum with moderate wall thickening (*red arrows*) and ulcerations (*blue arrow*). (*B*) 2014 coronal postcontrast LAVA sequence demonstrating distal ileum, including terminal ileum with moderate wall thickening (10.4 mm) and mucosal hyperenhancement (*red arrow*) consistent with active CD. (*C*) 2016 coronal T2 half-fourier acquisition single-shot turbo spin-echo sequence demonstrating thickening (4.4 mm) of a segment of ileum (*white arrows*), less than previous MRE in 2014. (*D*) 2016 coronal T1 volumetric interpolated breath-hold fat-saturated postgadolinium sequence demonstrating bowel wall hyperenhancement (*white arrows*) much less pronounced than previous MRE in 2014. [a] Ileum segment. (*From* Deepak P, Fletcher JG, Fidler JL, et al. Computed tomography and magnetic resonance enterography in Crohn's disease: assessment of radiologic criteria and endpoints for clinical practice and trials. Inflamm Bowel Dis 2016;22:2285; with permission.)

Table 6
Magnetic resonance index of activity score

MRE Feature	Description
Bowel wall thickness	Measured in millimeters
RCE	Calculation of pregadolinium and postgadolinium contrast wall signal intensity in the bowel wall and the standard deviation of precontrast and postcontrast signal intensity noise measured outside the body
Edema	Hyperintensity on T2-weighted sequences of the colon wall relative to the signal of psoas muscle
Ulcers	Deep depressions in the mucosal surface of a thickened segment

Abbreviation: RCE, relative contrast enhancement.
MaRIA = 1.5 × wall thickness + 0.02 × RCE + 5 × edema + 10 × ulceration.
The global MaRIA score is calculated as the sum of the MaRIA in the ileum, ascending colon, transverse colon, descending colon, sigmoid, and rectum.
Adapted from Deepak P, Fletcher JG, Fidler JL, et al. Computed tomography and magnetic resonance enterography in Crohn's disease: assessment of radiologic criteria and endpoints for clinical practice and trials. Inflamm Bowel Dis 2016;22:2280–8; with permission.

The MaRIA score was shown to have significant correlation (r = 0.82) with the CDEIS.[41] The score also showed high accuracy for the detection of active CD (receiver operating characteristic [ROC] = 0.89). An external validation study of subjects who had an IC as the reference standard also demonstrated high correlation with the CDEIS (r = 0.80).[42] In addition, the MaRIA score has been shown to be predictive of ulcer healing and response to therapy in CD patients. A prospective, multicenter study showed that the MaRIA score less than 11 determined ulcer healing with sensitivity of 94% and accuracy of 90%, and a MaRIA score less than 7 determined mucosal healing with a sensitivity of 85% and accuracy of 83%.[43] The implementation of the MaRIA score in clinical practice has been limited by its time-consuming nature. It is also does not take into account the length of disease involvement. Modifications may allow more widespread use of the MaRIA score in the near future.

Crohn's Disease MRI Index Score (London)

The Crohn's disease MRI index (CDMI) score was first derived and validated in 2012.[44] It is a qualitative MRI scoring system designed for nonperforating small bowel CD. The derivation cohort was composed of 16 subjects who underwent MRE within 2 weeks of small bowel resection. The surgical specimen was graded for transmural acute inflammation (score 0–13). MRI parameters of mural thickness (coefficient: 1.34, 95% CI 0.36–2.32, P = .007) and T2 signal intensity (coefficient: 0.90, 95% CI −0.24–2.04, P = .06) were the best predictors for the acute inflammation score. The equation to calculate the CDMI is: 1.79 + 1.34 mural thickness + 0.94 mural T2 signal intensity (**Table 7**). This score was validated in a cohort of 26 subjects, demonstrating a correlation between the CDMI and the endoscopic acute inflammatory score from TI biopsies. A CDMI cutoff value of 4.1 predicted the presence of histopathologic acute inflammation with a sensitivity of 81% and area under the curve (AUC) of 0.76.[44] The advantage of using the CDMI score is that it is simpler and more time-efficient to calculate compared with MaRIA. However, it has similar limitations to the MaRIA in that it does not take into account disease extent.

Table 7
Crohn's disease MRI index

Score	0	1	2	3
Mural thickness[a]	1–3 mm	>3–5 mm	>5–7 mm	>7 mm
Mural T2 signal[b]	Equivalent to normal bowel wall	Minor increase in signal-bowel wall appears dark gray on fat-saturated images	Moderate increase in signal-bowel wall appears light gray on fat-saturated images	Marked increase in signal-bowel wall contains areas of white high signal approaching that of luminal content
Perimural T2 signal	Equivalent to normal mesentery	Increase in mesenteric signal but no fluid	Small fluid rim (≤2 mm)	Larger fluid rim (>2 mm)
Mural enhancement pattern	Not applicable	Homogeneous	Mucosal	Layered
Enhancement[c]	Equivalent to normal bowel wall	Minor enhancement: bowel wall signal greater than normal small bowel but significantly less than nearby vascular structures	Moderate enhancement: bowel wall signal increased but somewhat less than nearby vascular structures	Marked enhancement: bowel wall signal approaches that of nearby vascular structures
Lymph nodes	Absent	Cluster <1 cm	1 node >1 cm	3 nodes >1 cm
Lymph node enhancement[c]	Less than nearby vascular structure	Equivalent or greater to nearby vascular structure	Lymph node enhancement[c]	Less than nearby vascular structure
Comb sign	Absent	Present		

CDMI = 1.79 + 1.34 mural thickness + 0.94 mural T2 score.
[a] Measured using electronic calipers.
[b] Compared with normal small bowel.
[c] Compared with nearest vessel.
Adapted from Deepak P, Fletcher JG, Fidler JL, et al. Computed tomography and magnetic resonance enterography in Crohn's disease: assessment of radiologic criteria and endpoints for clinical practice and trials. Inflamm Bowel Dis 2016;22:2280–8; with permission.

Magnetic Resonance Enterography Global Score

The magnetic resonance enterography global score (MEGS) was first introduced in 2014 and is derived from the CDMI.[45] The derivation cohort of MEGS consisted of 71 CD subjects who underwent MRE, fecal calprotectin, and CRP. The score was derived from the following variables: mural thickness, mural T2 signal, mesenteric edema, T1 enhancement, mural enhancement pattern, and haustral folds (colon only). The variables are scored in each of the 9 intestinal segments: jejunum, ileum, terminal ileum, cecum, ascending colon, transverse colon, descending colon, sigmoid, and rectum (**Table 8**). The score also accounts for disease length in each segment and extramural features such as lymphadenopathy, comb sign (dilated vasa recta), and the presence of

Table 8
Magnetic resonance enterography global score

Score	0	1	2	3
Mural thickness small bowel[a]	<3 mm	>3–5 mm	>5–7 mm	>7 mm
Mural T2 signal[b]	Equivalent to normal bowel wall	Minor increase in signal, bowel wall appears dark gray on fat saturated images	Moderate increase in signal, bowel wall appears light gray on fat saturated images	Marked increase in signal, bowel wall contains areas of white high signal approaching that of luminal content
Perimural T2 signal (mesenteric edema)	Equivalent to normal mesentery	Increase in mesenteric signal but no fluid	Small fluid rim (≤2 mm)	Larger fluid rim (>2 mm)
T1 enhancement[c]	Equivalent to normal bowel wall	Minor enhancement: bowel wall signal greater than normal small bowel but significantly less than nearby vascular structures	Moderate enhancement: bowel wall signal increased but somewhat less than nearby vascular structures	Marked enhancement: bowel wall signal approaches that of nearby vascular structures
Mural enhancement pattern	Not applicable or homogeneous	Mucosal	Layered	—
Haustral loss (colon only)	None	<1/3 segment	1/3–2/3 segment	>2/3 segment
Multiplication factor per segment Length of disease segment	—	0–5 cm × 1	5–15 cm × 1.5	>15 cm × 2

Additional score for extramural features				
Score	0	5	—	—
Lymph nodes (≥1 cm measured in shortest diameter)	Absent	Present	—	—
Comb sign (linear densities on the mesenteric side of affected bowel segments)	Absent	Present	—	—
Abscess	Absent	Present	—	—
Fistulae	Absent	Present	—	—

MEGS = 1.8.wall thickness + 0.08.mural T2 signal + 0.19.length − 0.192.

[a] Measured using electronic calipers.

[b] Compared with normal small bowel.

[c] Compared with nearest vessel.

Adapted from Deepak P, Fletcher JG, Fidler JL, et al. Computed tomography and magnetic resonance enterography in Crohn's disease: assessment of radiologic criteria and endpoints for clinical practice and trials. Inflamm Bowel Dis 2016;22:2280–8; with permission.

fistula or abscess. Using Logistic regression, wall thickness ($P = .005$), mural T2 signal ($P = .027$), and length of disease ($P = .017$) were predictive of active disease (fecal calprotectin >100 μg/g). The equation to calculate MEGS is: 1.8.wall thickness + 0.08.mural T2 signal + 0.19.length − 0.192.

On subsequent imaging studies, the MEGS scoring system has performed well. A positive correlation between a MEGS score and fecal calprotectin ($r = 0.46$, $P<.001$) and CRP ($r = 0.388$, $P = .002$) has been reported.[45] MEGS also demonstrated a sensitivity of 65% and specificity of 78% for predicting active intestinal disease. This scoring system was further validated in a cohort of 36 CD subjects undergoing anti–tumor necrosis factor (anti-TNF) treatment.[46] A significant decrease in MEGS was noted in clinical responders versus nonresponders to anti-TNF therapy with a sensitivity of 58% and specificity of 70%. One of the strengths of MEGS is the ability to account for disease length, proximal small bowel disease, and extramural features. By comparison, in the derivation study, CDMI score had weaker positive correlation with fecal calprotectin ($r = 0.39$, $P = .001$) and no correlation with CRP ($r = 0.144$, $P = .259$) compared with MEGS.[45]

Nancy Score

The Nancy score was first described in 2010 in 40 CD subjects undergoing colonoscopy and MRI assessment (211 segments analyzed).[47] In this derivation cohort, subjects underwent MR colonography with diffusion-weighted imaging (DWI) without oral or rectal contrast and a colonoscopy within 48 hours. DWI is an imaging technique that derives image contrast from motion of water molecules between tissues. The MR-DWI colonography scans were correlated to the SES-CD in 6 intestinal segments: rectum, sigmoid, left colon, transverse colon, right colon, and ileum. The sum of 6 variables (DWI hyperintensity, rapid gadolinium enhancement, differentiation between the mucosa-submucosa complex and the muscularis propria, bowel wall thickening, edema, and presence of ulceration) is calculated in each segment to give the segmental score. The segmental scores are added to give the total score (range: 0–36) (**Table 9**). A segmental score greater than 2 was associated with colonic inflammation with a sensitivity of 58.3% and specificity of 84.5% (area under the receiver operating characteristic: 0.779, $P = .0001$).[47] In addition, there was correlation of the segmental score ($r = 0.565$, $P<.0001$) and the total score ($r = 0.539$, $P = .001$) with the SES-CD. Future studies are needed for validation.[48]

Clermont-Ferrand Index (Clermont Score)

The Clermont-Ferrand index score was introduced in 2013 as an MRE scoring system that incorporates DWI and the quantitative apparent diffusion coefficient (ADC). A decrease in ADC is associated with restricted diffusion and active inflammation. The score was first described prospectively in a cohort of 31 CD subjects and compared with the MaRIA score.[49] This initial study demonstrated a high correlation between DWI hyperintensity and disease activity as measured by MRE ($P = .001$). An ADC cutoff of 1.6×10^{-3} mm^2/s had a sensitivity of 82.4% and specificity of 100% for active disease. The equation to calculate the Clermont score is: 1.646 × bowel thickness − 1.321 × ADC + 5.613 × edema + 8.306 × ulceration + 5.039. The Clermont score was prospectively validated in a cohort of 130 subjects (848 segments evaluated).[50] This work confirmed that an ADC cutoff value of 1.9×10^{-3} mm^2/s has a sensitivity of 85.9% to 96.9% and specificity of 81.6% to 98.1% in distinguishing active from inactive ileocolonic CD. The Clermont score also showed high correlation to the MaRIA score, predominantly for ileal and not colonic disease.

Table 9
Nancy score

Radiological Item of the Magnetic Resonance Score	MR Sequence	Definition
DWI hyperintensity	DWI	Presence of hyperintensity in the colonic wall segment in the DWI sequence.
Rapid gadolinium enhancement after intravenous contrast medium administration	Gradient-echo T1-weighted, arterial phase	Gadolinium enhancement in the arterial phase (20–25 s after gadolinium infusion)
Differentiation between the mucosa-submucosa complex and the muscularis propria	Single-shot fast-spin echo short-time echo without fat saturation	Distinction in the colonic wall between 2 layers: (1) mucosa-submucosa complex hyperintensity, (2) muscularis propria hypointensity
Bowel wall thickening	Gradient-echo T1-weighted, delayed phase	Thickness of the colonic wall exceeding 5 mm
Parietal edema	Single-shot fast-spin echo, short-time echo, without fat saturation	Thickness of the colonic wall exceeding 5 mm and hyperintensity of the mucosa-submucosa complex
Ulceration	2-Dimensional steady-state, free-precession imaging	Loss of substance in the mucosa-submucosa complex

Six different radiological signs are recorded per segment (MR-score-S) in 5 colonic segments and the ileum, with total MR-score (MR-score-T) calculated by adding the segmental scores (MR-score-S), with values ranging from 0 to 36.

Adapted from Deepak P, Fletcher JG, Fidler JL, et al. Computed tomography and magnetic resonance enterography in Crohn's disease: assessment of radiologic criteria and endpoints for clinical practice and trials. Inflamm Bowel Dis 2016;22:2280–8; with permission.

Similar to the other scoring systems, unique advantages and limitations exist. One proposed advantage of DWI-based scoring systems, such as the Clermont score, is the ability to avoid use of intravenous contrast agents. A limitation of the Clermont score is the lack of data regarding the performance of the score in proximal small bowel segments. In addition, it has not been validated with the use of endoscopic findings. There is also uncertainty in the reproducibility of ADC values. Finally, as in the MaRIA score, the Clermont score can be time-consuming to generate in the clinical setting. **Table 10** illustrates the derivation and validation of the various radiologic scores.

MRI Perianal Fistula Scoring System

Van Assche and colleagues[51] first proposed and validated an MRI perianal fistula scoring system in 2003 (**Fig. 4**). The derivation and validation cohort was composed of 18 subjects with perianal disease who underwent treatment with infliximab. The score incorporated fistula number, location, extension, hyperintensity on T2-weighted images, presence of fluid collections, and rectal wall involvement. The score ranges from 0 to 30. In the development phase, the score was measured at baseline and after infliximab treatment (week 6 and week 10) with good interobserver agreement ($P<.001$). After 6 and 10 weeks of treatment, the decrease in the MRI score was significantly more pronounced in clinical responders versus nonresponders

Table 10
Derivation and validation of radiologic scores

	Derivation (Subjects, Segments)	Validation (Subjects, Segments)	Therapeutic Response Assessment (Subjects or Segments)	Gold Standard
MaRIA	50, 213	48, 258	Yes	IC (CDEIS)
CDMI	16, 44	26, 26	No	Surgical specimen (AIS)
MEGS	71, 639	36, 801	Yes	Extension of CDMI and correlated to clinical indices (HBI, fecal calprotectin, CRP, and CD activity score)
Nancy	40, 211	—	No	IC (SES-CD)
Clermont	31, —	130, 848	No	MaRIA (≥7 active = active disease)

Abbreviations: AIS, surgical specimen; CD, Crohn's disease; CDEIS, Crohn's disease endoscopic index of severity; CDMI, Crohn's disease MRI index; CRP, C-reactive protein; HBI, Harvey Bradshaw Index; MaRIA, magnetic resonance Index of activity; MEGS, magnetic resonance enterography global score; SES-CD, simple endoscopic severity for Crohn's disease; IC, ileocolonoscopy.

Adapted from Deepak P, Fletcher JG, Fidler JL, et al. Computed tomography and magnetic resonance enterography in Crohn's disease: assessment of radiologic criteria and endpoints for clinical practice and trials. Inflamm Bowel Dis 2016;22:2283; with permission.

($P = .03$). A follow-up study of 59 CD subjects with median follow-up of 9.8 (1.4–46.1) months after initiation of infliximab showed a significant decrease in this score that correlated with clinical improvement in 54.7% of subjects.[52] Despite its potential use as an objective disease assessment tool, widespread clinical implementation has been sparse.

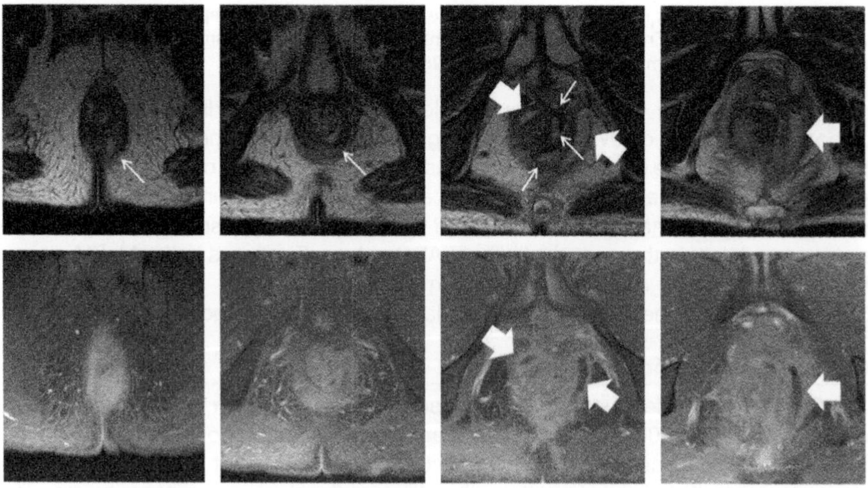

Fig. 4. Axial T2 weighted images (*top row*) from inferior to superior (*left to right*) and corresponding contrast-enhanced images demonstrate a complex perianal fistula arising at the 5 o'clock position of the anal canal and multiple abscesses. Multiple high T2 signal intensity tracts (*arrows*) are seen in the intersphincteric space with a horseshoe configuration. There are associated fluid collections (*block arrows*) with extension to the left ischioanal fossa. Findings are consistent with a Van Assche score of 19.

CROHN'S DISEASE ULTRASOUND SCORING SYSTEMS

Two CD US scoring systems have been proposed. In 2009, Rigazio and colleagues[53] proposed a semiquantitative bowel US scoring system for the prediction of surgery. In a cohort of 147 subjects (49 cases who underwent surgery within 30 days of US, 98 matched controls), bowel wall thickness (>4.5 mm), US pattern (disrupted stratification), presence of fistulae or abscesses, and presence of stenosis were independently associated with risk of surgery. The score is calculated with the following formula: $(2.5 \times \text{US pattern}) + (1.5 \times \text{bowel thickness}) + (3 \times \text{presence of fistulae/abscesses}) + (1.5 \times \text{presence of stenosis})$. Each of the 4 variables is given a score of 0 or 1. A total score greater than 3 predicted the risk for surgery with an odds ratio of 23.4 (95% CI 9.55–57.32) and AUC of 0.902 (95% CI 0.842–0.945).[53]

In 2012, Calabrese and colleagues[54] developed a numerical index to quantify bowel damage using SICU termed the sonographic lesion index for CD (SLIC). A total of 110 ileal and ileocolonic CD subjects were included in the derivation study and followed for 1 year after index SICU. The score is derived from multiple continuous and discrete variables, including wall thickness, lumen diameter, length of lesion, and number of lesion sites. It is calculated via a complex mathematic model with a total score range of 0 to 200. Median SLIC was higher in subjects with CRP greater than 5 mg/dL (P = .003) and CDAI greater than 150 (P<.005).[54] The total score was subdivided into 5 classes (A–E) from lowest to highest. Subjects with score ranges in the D and E class were more likely to undergo surgery at 1 year compared with the other classes (P<.0001). A subsequent study of subjects with ileal and ileocolonic CD demonstrated improvement in SLIC after anti-TNF induction therapy in clinical responders compared with nonresponders.[55]

LÉMANN INDEX

The Lémann index was formulated as a novel tool to assess digestive damage in patients with CD.[56] It was created by a multicenter, international collaboration involving 24 centers in 15 countries. The digestive tract is divided into 4 organs: upper digestive tract, small bowel, colon-rectum, and anus. Each organ is further divided into segments and scored based on surgical history, stricturing lesions, and penetrating lesions. Segmental scores can be used to generate organ indexes and, eventually, the global index named the Lémann Index. It is hoped that further modifications can simplify this system to allow more widespread use in clinical practice.

LIMITATIONS AND FUTURE DIRECTIONS

Mucosal healing, defined as absence of mucosal ulcerations, has been dependably shown to be associated with favorable clinical outcomes in IBD patients. This includes long-term clinical remission, lower rates of surgery, fewer hospitalizations, and improved quality of life.[6,12–14] Hence, proactive endoscopic disease assessment to reach the goal of mucosal healing may be critical to alter the natural history of this disease process. Endoscopic scoring tools may have a role in assessing the degree of improvement that is associated with positive clinical outcomes. However, the threshold values for endoscopic scores that are associated with improved long-term clinical outcomes have not been validated. Only post hoc analysis from the SONIC trial has demonstrated that greater than 50% reduction in CDEIS and SES-CD at 26 weeks predicted corticosteroid-free clinical remission at 50 weeks.[20] Further studies for validation of endoscopic scoring targets are needed.

Cross-sectional imaging allows for objective noninvasive assessment of disease activity and response to therapy in CD. As with endoscopic activity scores, many radiologic scoring tools are limited by the lack of validated scoring thresholds to establish disease activity and mucosal healing. The MaRIA score is an exception in which it has been shown that a score less than 7 predicts endoscopic mucosal healing with a sensitivity of 85% and accuracy of 83%.[43] In a retrospective study of 150 CD subjects, CTE or MRE lesion improvement was defined by decreased enhancement or length of disease without worsening of other parameters of active inflammation.[5] In this cohort, complete radiologic responders were defined as having improvement of all lesions, nonresponders had worsening lesions, and partial responders had all other scenarios. Complete radiologic responders had significantly decreased risk of subsequent corticosteroid use, hospitalizations, and CD surgery.[5] This work needs to be further explored in prospective studies.

SUMMARY

Endoscopic and radiologic modalities are critical for disease assessments in patients with CD. Indications include disease diagnosis; assessment of disease activity, extent, and severity; detecting complications; and monitoring response to medical therapy. Given the need for objective tools, multitudes of scoring systems have been developed. These systems will continue to evolve as clinicians seek simplified, reproducible, and objective endoscopic and radiologic methods to assess patients with CD.

REFERENCES

1. Modigliani R, Mary JY, Simon JF, et al. Clinical, biological, and endoscopic picture of attacks of Crohn's disease. Evolution on prednisolone. Groupe d'Etude Therapeutique des Affections Inflammatoires Digestives. Gastroenterology 1990;98(4):811–8.
2. Jones J, Loftus EV Jr, Panaccione R, et al. Relationships between disease activity and serum and fecal biomarkers in patients with Crohn's disease. Clin Gastroenterol Hepatol 2008;6(11):1218–24.
3. Hanauer SB, Feagan BG, Lichtenstein GR, et al. Maintenance infliximab for Crohn's disease: the ACCENT I randomised trial. Lancet 2002;359(9317):1541–9.
4. Colombel JF, Sandborn WJ, Reinisch W, et al. Infliximab, azathioprine, or combination therapy for Crohn's disease. N Engl J Med 2010;362(15):1383–95.
5. Deepak P, Fletcher JG, Fidler JL, et al. Radiological response is associated with better long-term outcomes and is a potential treatment target in patients with small bowel Crohn's Disease. Am J Gastroenterol 2016;111(7):997–1006.
6. Reinink AR, Lee TC, Higgins PD. Endoscopic mucosal healing predicts favorable clinical outcomes in inflammatory bowel disease: a meta-analysis. Inflamm Bowel Dis 2016;22(8):1859–69.
7. Annunziata ML, Caviglia R, Papparella LG, et al. Upper gastrointestinal involvement of Crohn's disease: a prospective study on the role of upper endoscopy in the diagnostic work-up. Dig Dis Sci 2012;57(6):1618–23.
8. Dionisio PM, Gurudu SR, Leighton JA, et al. Capsule endoscopy has a significantly higher diagnostic yield in patients with suspected and established small-bowel Crohn's disease: a meta-analysis. Am J Gastroenterol 2010;105(6): 1240–8 [quiz: 1249].
9. Jensen MD, Nathan T, Rafaelsen SR, et al. Diagnostic accuracy of capsule endoscopy for small bowel Crohn's disease is superior to that of MR enterography or CT enterography. Clin Gastroenterol Hepatol 2011;9(2):124–9.

10. Liao Z, Gao R, Xu C, et al. Indications and detection, completion, and retention rates of small-bowel capsule endoscopy: a systematic review. Gastrointest Endosc 2010;71(2):280–6.
11. Pennazio M, Spada C, Eliakim R, et al. Small-bowel capsule endoscopy and device-assisted enteroscopy for diagnosis and treatment of small-bowel disorders: European Society of Gastrointestinal Endoscopy (ESGE) Clinical Guideline. Endoscopy 2015;47(4):352–76.
12. Shah SC, Colombel JF, Sands BE, et al. Systematic review with meta-analysis: mucosal healing is associated with improved long-term outcomes in Crohn's disease. Aliment Pharmacol Ther 2016;43(3):317–33.
13. Neurath MF, Travis SP. Mucosal healing in inflammatory bowel diseases: a systematic review. Gut 2012;61(11):1619–35.
14. Casellas F, Barreiro de Acosta M, Iglesias M, et al. Mucosal healing restores normal health and quality of life in patients with inflammatory bowel disease. Eur J Gastroenterol Hepatol 2012;24(7):762–9.
15. Schnitzler F, Fidder H, Ferrante M, et al. Mucosal healing predicts long-term outcome of maintenance therapy with infliximab in Crohn's disease. Inflamm Bowel Dis 2009;15(9):1295–301.
16. Mary JY, Modigliani R. Development and validation of an endoscopic index of the severity for Crohn's disease: a prospective multicentre study. Groupe d'Etudes Therapeutiques des Affections Inflammatoires du Tube Digestif (GETAID). Gut 1989;30(7):983–9.
17. Khanna R, Zou G, D'Haens G, et al. Reliability among central readers in the evaluation of endoscopic findings from patients with Crohn's disease. Gut 2016;65(7): 1119–25.
18. Vuitton L, Marteau P, Sandborn WJ, et al. IOIBD technical review on endoscopic indices for Crohn's disease clinical trials. Gut 2016;65(9):1447–55.
19. Peyrin-Biroulet L, Panes J, Sandborn WJ, et al. Defining disease severity in inflammatory bowel diseases: current and future directions. Clin Gastroenterol Hepatol 2016;14(3):348–54.
20. Ferrante M, Colombel JF, Sandborn WJ, et al. Validation of endoscopic activity scores in patients with Crohn's disease based on a post hoc analysis of data from SONIC. Gastroenterology 2013;145(5):978–86.
21. Daperno M, D'Haens G, Van Assche G, et al. Development and validation of a new, simplified endoscopic activity score for Crohn's disease: the SES-CD. Gastrointest Endosc 2004;60(4):505–12.
22. Buisson A, Chevaux JB, Allen PB, et al. Review article: the natural history of postoperative Crohn's disease recurrence. Aliment Pharmacol Ther 2012;35(6): 625–33.
23. Rutgeerts P, Geboes K, Vantrappen G, et al. Predictability of the postoperative course of Crohn's disease. Gastroenterology 1990;99(4):956–63.
24. Marteau P, Laharie D, Colombel JF, et al. Interobserver variation study of the Rutgeerts score to assess endoscopic recurrence after surgery for Crohn's disease. J Crohns Colitis 2016;10(9):1001–5.
25. Gralnek IM, Defranchis R, Seidman E, et al. Development of a capsule endoscopy scoring index for small bowel mucosal inflammatory change. Aliment Pharmacol Ther 2008;27(2):146–54.
26. Cotter J, Dias de Castro F, Magalhaes J, et al. Validation of the Lewis score for the evaluation of small-bowel Crohn's disease activity. Endoscopy 2015;47(4):330–5.

27. Gal E, Geller A, Fraser G, et al. Assessment and validation of the new capsule endoscopy Crohn's disease activity index (CECDAI). Dig Dis Sci 2008;53(7): 1933–7.
28. Niv Y, Ilani S, Levi Z, et al. Validation of the Capsule Endoscopy Crohn's Disease Activity Index (CECDAI or Niv score): a multicenter prospective study. Endoscopy 2012;44(1):21–6.
29. Panes J, Bouzas R, Chaparro M, et al. Systematic review: the use of ultrasonography, computed tomography and magnetic resonance imaging for the diagnosis, assessment of activity and abdominal complications of Crohn's disease. Aliment Pharmacol Ther 2011;34(2):125–45.
30. Siddiki H, Fletcher JG, Hara AK, et al. Validation of a lower radiation computed tomography enterography imaging protocol to detect Crohn's disease in the small bowel. Inflamm Bowel Dis 2011;17(3):778–86.
31. Siddiki HA, Fidler JL, Fletcher JG, et al. Prospective comparison of state-of-the-art MR enterography and CT enterography in small-bowel Crohn's disease. AJR Am J Roentgenol 2009;193(1):113–21.
32. Samuel S, Bruining DH, Loftus EV Jr, et al. Endoscopic skipping of the distal terminal ileum in Crohn's disease can lead to negative results from ileocolonoscopy. Clin Gastroenterol Hepatol 2012;10(11):1253–9.
33. Bruining DH, Siddiki HA, Fletcher JG, et al. Prevalence of penetrating disease and extraintestinal manifestations of Crohn's disease detected with CT enterography. Inflamm Bowel Dis 2008;14(12):1701–6.
34. Bruining DH, Siddiki HA, Fletcher JG, et al. Benefit of computed tomography enterography in Crohn's disease: effects on patient management and physician level of confidence. Inflamm Bowel Dis 2012;18(2):219–25.
35. Siddiqui MR, Ashrafian H, Tozer P, et al. A diagnostic accuracy meta-analysis of endoanal ultrasound and MRI for perianal fistula assessment. Dis Colon Rectum 2012;55(5):576–85.
36. Schwartz DA, Wiersema MJ, Dudiak KM, et al. A comparison of endoscopic ultrasound, magnetic resonance imaging, and exam under anesthesia for evaluation of Crohn's perianal fistulas. Gastroenterology 2001;121(5):1064–72.
37. Castiglione F, Mainenti PP, De Palma GD, et al. Noninvasive diagnosis of small bowel Crohn's disease: direct comparison of bowel sonography and magnetic resonance enterography. Inflamm Bowel Dis 2013;19(5):991–8.
38. Calabrese E, La Seta F, Buccellato A, et al. Crohn's disease: a comparative prospective study of transabdominal ultrasonography, small intestine contrast ultrasonography, and small bowel enema. Inflamm Bowel Dis 2005;11(2):139–45.
39. Castiglione F, Bucci L, Pesce G, et al. Oral contrast-enhanced sonography for the diagnosis and grading of postsurgical recurrence of Crohn's disease. Inflamm Bowel Dis 2008;14(9):1240–5.
40. Calabrese E, Petruzziello C, Onali S, et al. Severity of postoperative recurrence in Crohn's disease: correlation between endoscopic and sonographic findings. Inflamm Bowel Dis 2009;15(11):1635–42.
41. Rimola J, Rodriguez S, Garcia-Bosch O, et al. Magnetic resonance for assessment of disease activity and severity in ileocolonic Crohn's disease. Gut 2009; 58(8):1113–20.
42. Rimola J, Ordas I, Rodriguez S, et al. Magnetic resonance imaging for evaluation of Crohn's disease: validation of parameters of severity and quantitative index of activity. Inflamm Bowel Dis 2011;17(8):1759–68.

43. Ordas I, Rimola J, Rodriguez S, et al. Accuracy of magnetic resonance enterography in assessing response to therapy and mucosal healing in patients with Crohn's disease. Gastroenterology 2014;146(2):374–82.
44. Steward MJ, Punwani S, Proctor I, et al. Non-perforating small bowel Crohn's disease assessed by MRI enterography: derivation and histopathological validation of an MR-based activity index. Eur J Radiol 2012;81(9):2080–8.
45. Makanyanga JC, Pendse D, Dikaios N, et al. Evaluation of Crohn's disease activity: initial validation of a magnetic resonance enterography global score (MEGS) against faecal calprotectin. Eur Radiol 2014;24(2):277–87.
46. Prezzi D, Bhatnagar G, Vega R, et al. Monitoring Crohn's disease during anti-TNF-alpha therapy: validation of the magnetic resonance enterography global score (MEGS) against a combined clinical reference standard. Eur Radiol 2016;26(7): 2107–17.
47. Oussalah A, Laurent V, Bruot O, et al. Diffusion-weighted magnetic resonance without bowel preparation for detecting colonic inflammation in inflammatory bowel disease. Gut 2010;59(8):1056–65.
48. Peyrin-Biroulet L, Laurent V. Is diffusion-weighted Magnetic Resonance Imaging for assessing Crohn's disease ready for prime time? Experience with the Nancy Score. Inflamm Bowel Dis 2015;21(10):E25.
49. Buisson A, Joubert A, Montoriol PF, et al. Diffusion-weighted magnetic resonance imaging for detecting and assessing ileal inflammation in Crohn's disease. Aliment Pharmacol Ther 2013;37(5):537–45.
50. Hordonneau C, Buisson A, Scanzi J, et al. Diffusion-weighted magnetic resonance imaging in ileocolonic Crohn's disease: validation of quantitative index of activity. Am J Gastroenterol 2014;109(1):89–98.
51. Van Assche G, Vanbeckevoort D, Bielen D, et al. Magnetic resonance imaging of the effects of infliximab on perianal fistulizing Crohn's disease. Am J Gastroenterol 2003;98(2):332–9.
52. Karmiris K, Bielen D, Vanbeckevoort D, et al. Long-term monitoring of infliximab therapy for perianal fistulizing Crohn's disease by using magnetic resonance imaging. Clin Gastroenterol Hepatol 2011;9(2):130–6.
53. Rigazio C, Ercole E, Laudi C, et al. Abdominal bowel ultrasound can predict the risk of surgery in Crohn's disease: proposal of an ultrasonographic score. Scand J Gastroenterol 2009;44(5):585–93.
54. Calabrese E, Zorzi F, Zuzzi S, et al. Development of a numerical index quantitating small bowel damage as detected by ultrasonography in Crohn's disease. J Crohns Colitis 2012;6(8):852–60.
55. Zorzi F, Stasi E, Bevivino G, et al. A sonographic lesion index for Crohn's disease helps monitor changes in transmural bowel damage during therapy. Clin Gastroenterol Hepatol 2014;12(12):2071–7.
56. Pariente B, Mary JY, Danese S, et al. Development of the Lemann index to assess digestive tract damage in patients with Crohn's disease. Gastroenterology 2015; 148(1):52–63.e3.

Intestinal and Nonintestinal Cancer Risks for Patients with Crohn's Disease

Sushil K. Garg, MBBS[a], Fernando S. Velayos, MD[b],
John B. Kisiel, MD[c,*]

KEYWORDS

- Inflammatory bowel diseases • Colorectal neoplasms • Skin neoplasms/secondary
- Lymphoma • Monoclonal antibodies/adverse effects
- 6-mercaptopurine/adverse effects

KEY POINTS

- Population-based studies show that patients with Crohn's disease (CD) are at increased risk of cancers of the colorectum, small bowel, skin, lymph nodes, and uterine cervix.
- Intestinal cancers seem to be more common among patients with long-standing and poorly controlled CD; cancers outside the intestines seem to be increased by immunosuppressive therapies.
- Cancers of the colorectum, skin, and uterine cervix are preventable; patients should be counseled on cancer risks and receive tailored cancer surveillance.

INTRODUCTION

Crohn's disease (CD) is a form of chronic inflammatory bowel disease (IBD) with an incidence in North American of 20 cases per 100,000 person-years[1] and a prevalence of approximately 200 to 300 cases per 100,000 adults.[2] In CD, inflammation occurs transmurally, extending from the mucosa to the muscularis layer and serosa. The most commonly affected intestinal segments are the terminal ileum and colon. At the time of diagnosis, 40% of patients exhibit disease with an ileocolic distribution, 30% suffer from an isolated ileal disease, and 30% have disease affecting only the colon. Approximately 5% to 10% of patients exhibit associated lesions of the upper

Disclosure Statement: Drs S.K. Garg and F.S. Velayos have no relevant financial disclosures; Dr J. B. Kisiel is supported by the Maxine and Jack Zarrow Family Foundation of Tulsa Oklahoma.
[a] Department of Internal Medicine, University of Minnesota, Minneapolis, MN, USA; [b] Division of Gastroenterology, University of California San Francisco, San Francisco, CA, USA; [c] Division of Gastroenterology and Hepatology, Mayo Clinic, 200 First Street, Southwest, Rochester, MN 55905, USA
* Corresponding author.
E-mail address: kisiel.john@mayo.edu

http://dx.doi.org/10.1016/j.gtc.2017.05.006

gastrointestinal tract, and 20% to 30% show perianal disease. Onset of disease typically occurs in the second or third decade of life; thus, patients can be exposed to decades of chronic inflammation in the intestines and other sites of CD-related extraintestinal disease.

Chronic immune-mediated inflammatory diseases such as CD are strongly associated with cancer.[3] Accordingly, patients with CD have increased rates of intestinal and nonintestinal cancers.[4] The risk of cancer in CD patients can be related to cellular damage sustained during chronic inflammatory disease itself, or owing to life style factors like smoking, or owing to medications, which may blunt innate immune system cancer surveillance. Measuring the magnitude of cancer risks for patients with CD has evolved in recent years. Historically, the scientific literature on this topic has been dominated by case-control studies conducted in referral centers. More recently, large observational studies in administrative databases and population-level cohorts are thought to provide more realistic estimates of neoplastic complication rates with greater levels of precision. We, therefore, aimed to review the magnitude of risk for the development of intestinal and nonintestinal cancer in CD patients, discuss modifiable and nonmodifiable covariates, and inform these estimates largely from data published within the last 10 years. The focus of this review is to evaluate the epidemiologic characteristics, pathogenesis, and surveillance to prevent most commonly reported cancers in patients with CD.

COLORECTAL CANCER IN CROHN'S DISEASE

Epidemiology

Colorectal cancer (CRC) is ranked as the third most common cancer in the world.[5] Each year, approximately 900,000 new cases of CRC are identified and 500,000 deaths occur worldwide. From 2009 to 2013, the number of new cases of colon and rectal cancer was 41.0 per 100,000 and the number of deaths was 15.1 per 100,000 per year.[6] Adenocarcinoma of the colorectum is a major cause of morbidity and mortality in IBD. CRC accounts for about 10% to 15% of deaths in patients with IBD,[7] and causes 1 in 12 deaths of patients with CD.[4] The prognosis of sporadic CRC and IBD-related CRC are thought to be similar, both having an overall 5-year survival of 50%.[8] However, the median age at diagnosis of IBD-related CRC, at 60 years of age, seems to be lower than that of sporadic CRC, at 70 years of age.[9]

It has long been understood that patients with IBD of the colon are at increased risk for CRC; however, our understanding of the magnitude of that risk is evolving. In recent years, high-quality population-based studies have shown that patients with IBD have about a 2- to 3-fold increase in CRC risk compared with the general population. CD seems to increase the risk of colonic but not rectal cancers.[10] Important and emerging trends in CRC risk among CD patients are shown in **Table 1**. There may be a decreased risk in more recent years, as shown by many recent large studies.[9,11–14] Caution must be taken when comparing these results because not all reports stratify CD patients by disease distribution; risk seems to remain considerably higher for patients with known colonic CD.[15] It is likely that recent advances are due to the impact of modern biologic therapy for CD, aggressive and appropriate surgical CD management, and the role of surveillance colonoscopy for CRC. These practices have been influenced by a greater understanding of the pathogenesis of CD-associated CRC.

Pathogenesis of Colorectal Cancer in Crohn's Disease

The pathogenesis of ulcerative colitis-induced CRC has been studied extensively. Most of the literature on colitis-induced CRC is from ulcerative colitis. Like sporadic

Table 1
Colorectal cancer risk in Crohn's disease

Outcome	Risk Estimate (95% CI)	Comparison Group	Study Design	Publication Year, Reference
CRC in CD	OR 1.9 (1.4–2.5)	Healthy controls	Metaanalysis, population-based cohorts	Jess et al,[10] 2005
CRC in CD	SIR 1.6 (1.2–2.0)	Healthy controls	US administrative database cohort	Herrinton et al,[12] 2012
CRC in CD	RR 0.85 (0.67–1.07)	Healthy controls	Danish nationwide cohort	Jess et al,[9] 2012
CRC in CD	SIR 1.6 (1.2–2.0)	Healthy controls	Metaanalysis, population-based cohorts	Lutgens et al,[11] 2013
CRC in CD	RR 0.86 (0.85–0.87)	Healthy controls	US administrative database cohort	Garg & Loftus,[13] 2016
CRC in CD	SIR 0.89 (0.15–2.95)	Healthy controls	Norwegian inception cohort	Hovde et al,[14] 2016
CRC in colonic CD	SIR 2.97 (1.08–6.46)	Healthy controls	Dutch population-based cohort	van den Heuvel et al,[15] 2016
Colon cancer in CD	SIR 2.5 (1.7–3.5)	Healthy controls	Metaanalysis, population-based cohorts	Jess et al,[10] 2005
Rectal cancer, in CD	SIR 1.4 (0.8–2.6)	Healthy controls	Metaanalysis, population-based cohorts	Jess et al,[10] 2005

Abbreviations: CD, Crohn's disease; CRC, colorectal cancer; OR, odds ratio; RR, relative risk; SIR, standardized incidence ratio.

CRC, IBD-CRC is believed to arise through the progressive accumulation of genetic abnormalities that cause abnormal cell growth and tumor architecture, which progress along an adenoma–carcinoma sequence.[16] The types of genetic abnormalities seem to be similar between sporadic and IBD-associated colorectal neoplasms, but may occur at different rates and in a different sequence, as summarized in **Fig. 1**, and are reviewed extensively elsewhere.[17,18] In clinical practice, colorectal neoplasms in patients with IBD are heterogeneous and multiple tumorigenesis pathways may be occurring in the same individual. Among CRC and its precursors, there are several morphologic categories. Endoscopically visible dysplastic precursors most often present as a mass or lesion. These may be discretely polypoid and amenable to endoscopic therapy or may be carpetlike, spreading, or ulcerated, and unresectable by endoscopic techniques. Neoplasms may also be endoscopically unapparent and thus are found only on random biopsy; termed "flat dysplasia," these neoplasms are also strongly linked to a subsequent diagnosis of CRC.[19] Last, there is no evidence to suggest that sporadic and IBD colorectal neoplasms are mutually exclusive.

Ultimately, the development of CRC in chronic colitis is thought to be accelerated by the inflammatory activity of the disease itself. This is reflected not only in case control studies showing a strong association of colorectal neoplasms with active histologic inflammation,[20,21] but also in careful examination of the other known clinical risk factors for CRC in CD, which likely reflect a large cumulative burden of inflammatory activity over an individual's lifetime (**Table 2**).

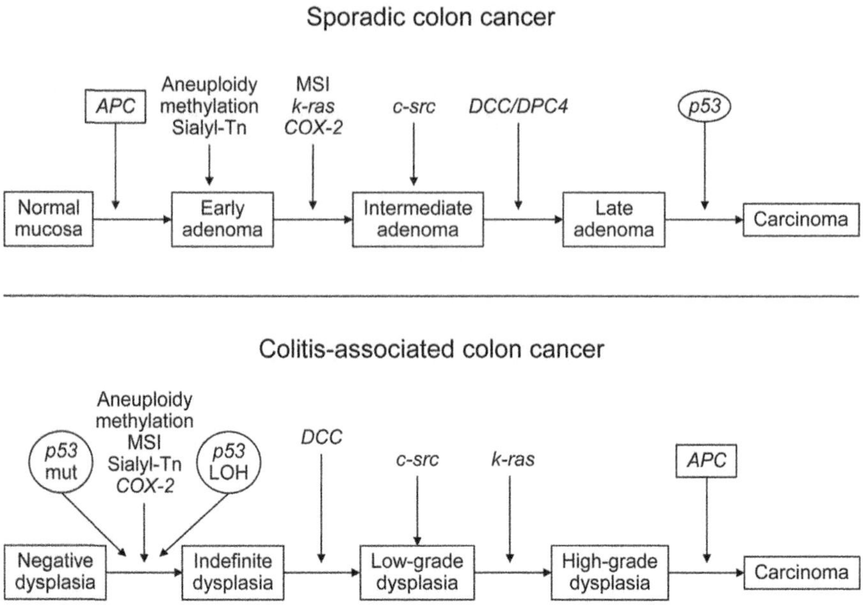

Fig. 1. Comparison of genetic and epigenetic changes in sporadic and colitis-associated CRC. CRC, colorectal cancer; LOH, loss of heterozygosity; Mut, mutation. (*From* Xie J, Itzkowitz SH. Cancer in inflammatory bowel disease. World J Gastroenterol 2008;14(3):378–89; with permission.)

Surveillance of Colorectal Cancer in Patients with Crohn's Disease

Because CRC risk seems to increase with increasing extent of colonic involvement and the duration of the disease history, current US society guidelines recommend regular surveillance colonoscopies beginning 8 to 10 years after CD involving one-third of the colon or less is diagnosed[22,23]; the surveillance interval is every 1 to 3 years, and should be tailored on the basis of additional risk factors. In patients with CD and primary sclerosing cholangitis, surveillance should be started immediately upon primary sclerosing cholangitis diagnosis and should be performed annually.[22] In addition to these guidelines on surveillance intervals, there are emerging data on surveillance examination techniques. Dye-spray enhanced surveillance colonoscopy, or "chromoendoscopy," seems to offer increased yield over standard definition white light colonoscopy and is, therefore, strongly recommended by expert consensus.[24] Use of chromoendoscopy should be considered for at-risk CD patients if the expertise required for this technique is available.

SMALL BOWEL ADENOCARCINOMA

Epidemiology

Small bowel adenocarcinomas (SBA) contribute to only 2% of all gastrointestinal cancers, with an overall low risk in the general population.[25] However, the risk of SBA in CD patients is 20 to 30 times higher than in patients without CD[10]; this corresponds with an incidence of approximately 0.3 (95% CI, 0.1–0.5) cases per 1000 patient-years.[26] In 8 studies, metaanalyzed by Canavan and colleagues,[27] the relative risk (RR) of SBA in CD is 31.2 (95% CI, 15.9–60.9). Subgroup analysis based on geographic region showed RR of 19.4 (95% CI, 7.4–50.8), 63.3 (95% CI,

Table 2
Risk factors for colorectal cancer in patients with Crohn's disease

	Risk Estimate (95% CI)	Comparison Group	Study Design	Publication Year, Reference
Disease duration since diagnosis	CRC Incidence	General population	Metaanalysis of community- and referral-based cohorts	Canavan et al,[27] 2006
10 y	2.9% (1.5%–5.3%)			
20 y	5.6% (3.1%–10.4%)			
30 y	8.3% (4.5%–15.1%)			
Age at CD diagnosis ≤25 y	RR 21.4 (11.39–40.44)	Age at CD diagnosis >25 y	Metaanalysis of population and referral based cohorts	Von Roon et al,[63] 2007
Colonic CD	SIR 4.3 (2.0–9.4)	Ileal or ileocolonic CD	Metaanalysis of population-based cohorts	Jess et al,[10] 2005
Colonic CD	RR 4.5 (1.3–14.9)	Ileal CD	Metaanalysis of population- and referral-based cohorts	Canavan et al,[27] 2006
PSC in CD	OR 6.78 (1.65–27.9)	CD without PSC	Referral center case-control	Lindstrom et al,[64] 2011
First-degree relative with CRC	RR 2.5 (1.4–4.4)	CD patients without CRC family history	Population-based cohort	Askling et al,[65] 2001
First-degree relative with CRC, diagnosed before age 50	RR 9.2 (3.7–23)	CD patients without CRC family history	Population-based cohort	Askling et al,[65] 2001

Abbreviations: CD, Crohn's disease; CRC, colorectal cancer; OR, odds ratio; PSC, primary sclerosing cholangitis; RR, relative risk; SIR, standardized incidence ratio.

23.7–168.5), and 44.2 (95% CI, 8.9–199.7) for Scandinavia, the United Kingdom, and North America, respectively. This study did not find a difference in RR of SBA based on setting of study (referral vs population based). There was also no change in risk of SBA in CD patients over time. A study of the Nationwide Inpatient Sample in the United States[13] showed no change in the incidence of SBA in CD patients over time; however, the incidence continues be high despite improvement in diagnostic modalities.

Risk Factors

Risk factors for SBA in CD include long-standing disease,[28–31] a previous history of stricture repair,[32–35] and excluded/bypassed bowel segments.[36–38] Protective factors are not very well-studied, but are thought to be prolonged used of aspirin[39,40] and small bowel resection.[40]

Pathogenesis

The pathogenesis of SBA in patients with CD is unclear because of the rarity of the disease. Patients with long-standing disease (>8 years) develop SBA in the inflamed portion of the bowel, which suggests that the pathogenesis of SBA in CD is likely inflammation driven.

Prevention and Treatment

No systematic screening for SBA has been proposed in patients with ileal CD owing to the small number of total cases reported. However, in high-risk patients, such as those with long-standing CD associated with strictures who have not undergone small bowel resection, regular imaging with computed tomography or magnetic resonance enterography and/or ileocolonoscopy with targeted biopsies should be performed and sudden change in symptoms, including onset of systemic symptoms, small bowel obstruction, and progression of disease on imaging, should raise the suspicion of malignancy. Enterographic features of SBAs include annular/constricting lesions or those with eccentric or circumferential wall thickening and irregular borders.[41] MRI may also identify spread to regional lymph nodes or distant metastases.

LYMPHOPROLIFERATIVE DISORDERS

Epidemiology

The incidence of lymphoproliferative disorders (LD) has increased markedly worldwide, especially in western countries.[42] Non-Hodgkin lymphoma (NHL) represents 4.3% of all new cancer cases seen in the United States alone. From 2009 to 2013, the number of new cases of NHL was up to 19.5 per 100,000 patients per year. The number of deaths was 6.0 per 100,000 patients per year.[6] NHL is much more common than Hodgkin lymphoma. During the same period, the number of new cases of Hodgkin lymphoma was 2.6 per 100,000 patients per year, and the number of deaths was 0.4 per 100,000 patients per year.[6] Hodgkin lymphoma is more common among young adults and among men than women.

Assessment of the baseline risk of lymphoma and other LD in CD patients has been complicated by the need to differentiate between the risks of lymphoma attributable to CD itself versus the increased risk owing to exposure to treatment for CD. It is well-known that patients who are on immunosuppressive therapy, including treatment for CD, are at increased risk of lymphoma, especially NHL; further, risk of lymphoma increases with the intensity of immunosuppression. **Table 3** highlights that much of the lymphoma risk in CD is attributable to the use of thiopurine therapy. Among IBD patients who discontinue thiopurines, the risk of developing lymphoma was similar to that among patients who had never taken them.[43]

Because thiopurines are now often used in combination with anti-tumor necrosis factor-α (anti-TNF) therapies,[44,45] it has been challenging to determine if the increased rates of LD in thiopurine users could also be attributable to anti-TNF use in more recent years. Data from both a metaanalysis[46] and a large prospective Crohn's Therapy, Resource, Evaluation, and Assessment Tool (TREAT) registry[47] do not demonstrate a strong association between anti-TNF therapy and lymphoma.

Diagnosis of Lymphoproliferative Disorders

Currently there is no screening or effective method for the early diagnosis of LD in patients receiving treatment for CD. Symptoms of LD should be suspected in patients with unexplained headache, fever, weight loss, and presence of hepatomegaly or splenomegaly. Given that there are no specific monitoring recommendations,

Table 3
Lymphoma risk in Crohn's disease

Outcome	Risk Estimate (95% CI)	Comparison Group	Study Design	Publication Year, Reference
Lymphoma in IBD	SIR 1.3 (1.0–1.6)	General population	Swedish population-based cohort	Askling et al,[66] 2005
NHL in CD	SIR 1.55 (1.2–2.0)	General population	Swedish population-based cohort	Askling et al,[66] 2005
Lymphoma in IBD	RR 1.39 (0.50–3.40)	General population	UK administrative database	Lewis et al,[67] 2001
Lymphoma in men with CD	IRR 3.63 (1.53–8.62)	General population	Canadian population database	Bernstein et al,[68] 2001
Lymphoma in TP-treated CD	HR 5.28 (2.01–13.9)	CD treated without TP	French prospective cohort	Kotlyar et al,[43] 2015
NHL in anti-TNF–treated CD	SIR 1.7 (0.5–7.1)	NHL in TP-treated CD	Metaanalysis of RCTs, cohorts, or case series	Siegel et al,[46] 2009
Lymphoma in IFX-treated CD	SIR 2.01 (0.87, 3.95)	General population (SEER)	Prospective registry	Lichtenstein et al,[47] 2014

Abbreviations: CD, Crohn's disease; CRC, colorectal cancer; IBD, inflammatory bowel disease; IRR, incident rate ratio; NHL, non-Hodgkin lymphoma; OR, odds ratio; RCT, randomized controlled trial; RR, relative risk; SEER, Surveillance Epidemiology End Results Database; SIR, standardized incidence ratio; TNF, tumor necrosis factor; TP, thiopurines; UK, United Kingdom.

physicians should clearly communicate the increased risk of lymphomas associated with these therapies. It should also be emphasized that undertreated CD is many times more likely to cause permanently disabling complications. Because this discussion can be impeded by the strong emotional reaction to the rare but frightening possibility of lymphoma and because patients often do not fully understand risk terminology, decision tools and communication aids may be helpful.[48]

NONMELANOMA SKIN CANCER

Epidemiology

Nonmelanoma skin cancer (NMSC) is the most common cutaneous malignancy in the general population[49]; these include squamous cell carcinoma and basal cell skin cancer. Because of underlying immune system dysregulation and immunosuppressive medication use, CD patients are thought to be at increased NMSC risk (**Table 4**). The CESAME study was the first large prospective study to assess the possible impact of thiopurines on the risk of NMSC in IBD patients.[50] This study showed that patients with IBD who are taking thiopurines are at almost 5-time higher risk of lymphoma (HR, 5.28; 95% CI, 2.01–13.9) compared with patients who were never exposed to these drugs. This study also showed that male sex, advanced age, and longer duration of IBD were associated with increased risk of LD. The risk of developing lymphoma in IBD patients after discontinuation of thiopurines was similar to that among patients who had never taken them.

Table 4
Risk of NMSC in Crohn's disease with and without thiopurines

Outcome	Risk Estimate (95% CI)	Comparison Group	Study Design	Publication Year, Reference
NMSC in IBD	IRR 1.64 (1.54–1.74)	Matched, non-IBD controls	Retrospective administrative database	Long et al,[69] 2010
NMSC in first year after CD diagnosis	RR 2.1 (1.8–2.3)	General population	Danish population-based cohort	Kappelman et al,[55] 2014
NMSC in IBD	HR 2.28 (1.50–3.45)	IBD patient with no thiopurines use	Metaanalysis referral-based and population-based	Ariyaratnam & Subramanian,[70] 2014

Abbreviations: HR, hazard ratio; IBD, inflammatory bowel disease; IRR, incident rate ratio; NMSC, nonmelanoma skin cancer; RCTs, randomized controlled trials; RR, risk ratio.

Anti-TNF therapy does not seem to independently increase the risk of NMSC above that attributable to thiopurines. A pooled prospective analysis of randomized controlled trials for the treatment of active CD with adalimumab done by Osterman and colleagues[51] found that adalimumab monotherapy was not associated with an increased risk of NMSC or other malignancies when compared with the general population; however, there was an increased risk with coadministration of adalimumab with immunomodulator therapy.[51] Similarly, Lichtenstein and colleagues,[47] used the TREAT registry data to show higher incidence of squamous cell carcinoma in patients receiving other treatments only (0.08 per 100 patient-years) than in infliximab-treated patients (0.05 per 100 patient-years).[47] The risk of NMSC is greater in patients receiving combination therapy and this risk may be possibly, mostly attributable to the use of thiopurines.

Risk Factors, Pathogenesis, and Prevention of Nonmelanoma Skin Cancer in Crohn's Disease

Patient with fair skin, atypical moles, advanced age, outdoor occupation, and a family or personal history of skin cancer are high risk of NMSC. Ultraviolet (UV) B radiation causes direct damage to DNA and RNA, leading to generation of mutagenic photoproducts, which in turns leads to NMSC.[52] Azathioprine causes the accumulation of 6-thioguanine in the patients' DNA, which in turns leads to the formation of excessive reactive oxygen species lead to DNA mutations and oxidative stress, which is linked to oncogenesis.[52]

Patients should be counseled about sunscreen use and avoidance of tanning beds or other sources of UV light. Patient should be advised to use broad-spectrum sunscreen that protects against both UV A and B light. Additionally, annual screening skin examination by a dermatologist should be considered in patients who are receiving immunomodulators and/or biologics.[42]

MELANOMA

Epidemiology

Melanoma is the fifth most common cancer among men in the United States.[53] There has been shown to be an increased risk of melanoma in patients with CD. A study done by Long and colleagues[54] and published in 2012 showed that patients with CD were at significantly increased risk for melanoma (adjusted HR, 1.28; 95% CI, 1.00–1.64) compared with controls. The same study found that patients with CD who were receiving biologics were at increased risk of melanoma (HR, 1.94; 95% CI, 1.03–3.68) compared with patients who did not. There was no increased risk of melanoma with use of 5-aminosalicylic acid and thiopurines. Other studies have shown this relationship as well. A study done by Kappelman and colleagues[55] in 2014 showed increased risk of melanoma (standardized incidence ratio [SIR], 1.4; 95% CI, 1.0–1.9) in CD patients. Last, a metaanalysis performed by Singh and colleagues[53] in 2014, which included 7 studies, confirmed an increased risk of melanoma in CD (RR, 1.80; 95% CI, 1.17–2.75). Interestingly, this study did not find an increased risk among patients taking biologics or in studies performed after 1998, the year in which infliximab was approved in the United States to treat CD.

Pathogenesis, Risk Factors, and Prevention of Melanoma in Crohn's Disease

Potential mechanisms of this increased risk of melanoma in IBD patients include underlying immune dysfunction resulting in altered tumor surveillance,[53] increased susceptibility to infection with oncogenic viruses such as melanoma-associated retroviruses, direct pharmacologic effects of medications on DNA metabolism, and immunosuppression from medications.[53]

Risk factors for melanoma include fair skin, advancing age, male sex, immunosuppression, presence of atypical and multiple nevi, a personal history of NMSC, family history of melanoma, excessive UV light exposure, and intense sun exposure.[56] As reviewed, patients with IBD who are treated with anti-TNF therapy may be at additional risk, but studies on this topic have reached differing conclusions.

Patients with CD should be counseled about increased risk of melanoma. These patients should avoid excessive sun exposure and should use sunscreen. An annual screening skin examination by a dermatologist should be considered in patients who are receiving immunomodulators and/or biologics.[53]

CERVICAL CANCER AND CERVICAL DYSPLASIA IN CROHN'S DISEASE

Epidemiology

Cervical cancer is the second most common cancer in women worldwide.[42] The risk of cervical neoplasia in IBD, however, has been controversial. A recent population-based study conducted in Denmark involving 8717 women with Crohn's disease observed increased risks of low-grade squamous intraepithelial lesion (incident rate ratio [IRR], 1.26; 95% CI, 1.07–1.48), high-grade squamous intraepithelial lesion (IRR, 1.28; 95% CI, 1.13–1.45), and cervical cancer (IRR, 1.53; 95% CI, 1.04–2.27) in these patients, despite normal screening frequency.[57] Patients with CD aged 0 to 25 years (IRR, 1.30; 95% CI, 1.11–1.51) and 26 to 39 years (IRR, 1.30; 95% CI, 1.06–1.58) at diagnosis were at significantly increased risk of high-grade squamous intraepithelial lesion, and those aged 0 to 25 at diagnosis of CD were at increased risk of cervical cancer (IRR, 2.70; 95% CI, 1.47–4.96). Further analysis showed that medical therapy with mesalamine, azathioprine, and corticosteroids did not impact cervical neoplasia risk in CD. Although patients with CD who had ever used anti–TNF-α therapy were at a significantly increased risk of high-grade squamous intraepithelial lesion (IRR, 1.85, 95% CI, 1.12–3.04) compared with nonusers, there was no increased risk of cervical cancer. One important limitation of this study was that it did not have information on patients' smoking history, a modifiable risk factor for squamous cervical cancer.[58]

Another study by Singh and colleagues[59] showed a significantly increased risk of cervical abnormalities in women with CD who were exposed to 10 or more prescriptions of oral contraceptives (OR, 1.66; 95% CI, 1.08–2.54) or had a combined exposure to corticosteroids and immunosuppressants (OR, 1.41; 95% CI, 1.09–1.81).[59] A study conducted by Jess and colleagues[60] also showed an increased risk of carcinoma in situ and cervical dysplasia in patients with CD (SIR, 1.65; 95% CI, 1.10–2.37). Subgroup analysis showed that patients with young age of diagnosis (CD at age 0–19 years; SIR, 2.52; 95% CI, 1.26–4.51), smokers (SIR, 2.15; 95% CI, 1.27–3.40), and those patients treated with 5-aminosalicylic acid (SIR, 1.69; 95% CI, 1.08–2.51) or thiopurines (SIR, 2.47; 95% CI, 1.54–3.73) were at greatest risk for cervical dysplasia. A recent metaanalysis demonstrated increased risk of high-grade cervical dysplasia and cervical cancer among patients with IBD who were on immunosuppressive medications (OR, 1.34; 95% CI, 1.23–1.46) compared with the general population.[61]

Risk Factors, Surveillance, and Prevention of Cervical Neoplasia in Crohn's Disease

Traditional risk factors for the development of cervical cancer are well-known and they include prolonged oral contraceptive use, a high number of sexual partners, early age at first intercourse (before age 20), tobacco smoking, coinfection with other sexually transmitted diseases, low socioeconomic class, and high parity.[52] In studies involving patients with CD, young age of diagnosis of CD, and use of immunosuppressants were identified as additional CD-specific risk factors.

There are no specific cervical cancer screening guidelines for patients with IBD. The American College of Obstetrics and Gynecology recommends that women who are immunocompromised should undergo cervical cancer screening annually starting at age 21.[52] Routine use of quadrivalent or 9-valent human papilloma virus (HPV) vaccine in men and women between the ages of 9 and 26 years is also recommended. Women who receive the HPV vaccine should still undergo regular cervical cancer screening because the vaccine does not cover all high-risk HPV phenotypes.

FISTULA-ASSOCIATED PERIANAL CANCER

Up to 38% of patients with CD can have perianal CD associated with fistulae and fissures. A study published by Shwaartz and colleagues[62] examined 2382 patients with fistulizing perianal CD and found a prevalence of 0.79% for cancer in a fistula tract. One-half of these cases were squamous cell carcinoma and one-half were diagnosed with adenocarcinoma. Most of these patients had long-standing CD and chronic fistulas. Mean time from fistula diagnosis to cancer diagnosis was 6 years. Because symptoms of cancer are usually like those of perianal disease without cancer, a high index of suspicion is required in patients with difficult to control perianal CD. Examination under anesthesia with biopsies of the fistula tract may be necessary to establish an early diagnosis.

SUMMARY

Patients with CD are at increased risk for malignancy owing to both underlying disease and CD therapies. The benefits of therapy outweigh risks and long-term complications of under-treated disease may be debilitating. Although there are no surveillance measures for SBA or LD in CD, many cancers in CD may be preventable.

- CRC
  - Patient with CD involving one-third or more of the colon should start surveillance colonoscopies 8 to 10 years after diagnosis.

- Interval between surveillance colonoscopies should be every 1 to 3 years based on additional risk factors, such as inflammation severity, pseudopolyps, strictures, and family history of CRC.
- Patients with CD and primary sclerosing cholangitis should start surveillance colonoscopies immediately after diagnosis and should undergo surveillance colonoscopies every year.
- Use of chromoendoscopy should be considered for at risk CD patients if the expertise required for this technique is available.

- Skin cancer
  - Avoid excessive sun exposure and use a high-strength sun block if they are being treated with thiopurines; strict avoidance of tanning beds.
  - Annual dermatologic examination if treated with thiopurines or anti-TNF agents.
- Cervical cancer
  - Patients with CD should receive HPV vaccination between the ages of 9 and 26 years.
  - Screening for cervical cancer should start at the age of 21 years.
  - Patients with CD if immunosuppressed should have annual Pap smear.

ACKNOWLEDGMENTS

The authors would like to express thanks to Patricia J. Erwin, MLS, for her support for literature search.

REFERENCES

1. Loftus EV Jr. Clinical epidemiology of inflammatory bowel disease: incidence, prevalence, and environmental influences. Gastroenterology 2004;126(6):1504–17.
2. Kappelman MD, Rifas-Shiman SL, Kleinman K, et al. The prevalence and geographic distribution of Crohn's disease and ulcerative colitis in the United States. Clin Gastroenterol Hepatol 2007;5(12):1424–9.
3. Franks AL, Slansky JE. Multiple associations between a broad spectrum of autoimmune diseases, chronic inflammatory diseases and cancer. Anticancer Res 2012;32(4):1119–36.
4. Jess T, Winther KV, Munkholm P, et al. Intestinal and extra-intestinal cancer in Crohn's disease: follow-up of a population-based cohort in Copenhagen County, Denmark. Aliment Pharmacol Ther 2004;19(3):287–93.
5. Ferlay J, Soerjomataram I, Dikshit R, et al. Cancer incidence and mortality worldwide: sources, methods and major patterns in GLOBOCAN 2012. Int J Cancer 2015;136(5):E359–86.
6. Howlader N, NA, Krapcho M, et al, editors. SEER cancer statistics review, 1975-2013. Bethesda (MD): National Cancer Institute; 2016. Available at: http://seer.cancer.gov/csr/1975_2013/. based on November 2015 SEER data submission, posted to the SEER web site.
7. Dyson JK, Rutter MD. Colorectal cancer in inflammatory bowel disease: what is the real magnitude of the risk? World J Gastroenterol 2012;18(29):3839–48.
8. Rhodes JM, Campbell BJ. Inflammation and colorectal cancer: IBD-associated and sporadic cancer compared. Trends Mol Med 2002;8(1):10–6.
9. Jess T, Simonsen J, Jorgensen KT, et al. Decreasing risk of colorectal cancer in patients with inflammatory bowel disease over 30 years. Gastroenterology 2012;143(2):375–81.e1 [quiz: e13–4].

10. Jess T, Gamborg M, Matzen P, et al. Increased risk of intestinal cancer in Crohn's disease: a meta-analysis of population-based cohort studies. Am J Gastroenterol 2005;100(12):2724–9.
11. Lutgens MW, van Oijen MG, van der Heijden GJ, et al. Declining risk of colorectal cancer in inflammatory bowel disease: an updated meta-analysis of population-based cohort studies. Inflamm Bowel Dis 2013;19(4):789–99.
12. Herrinton LJ, Liu L, Levin TR, et al. Incidence and mortality of colorectal adenocarcinoma in persons with inflammatory bowel disease from 1998 to 2010. Gastroenterology 2012;143(2):382–9.
13. Garg SK, Loftus EV Jr. Risk of cancer in inflammatory bowel disease: going up, going down, or still the same? Curr Opin Gastroenterol 2016;32(4):274–81.
14. Hovde O, Hoivik ML, Henriksen M, et al. Malignancies in patients with inflammatory bowel disease: results from 20 years of follow-up in the IBSEN study. J Crohns Colitis 2017;11(5):571–7.
15. van den Heuvel TR, Wintjens DS, Jeuring SF, et al. Inflammatory bowel disease, cancer and medication: cancer risk in the Dutch population-based IBDSL cohort. Int J Cancer 2016;139(6):1270–80.
16. Fearon ER, Vogelstein B. A genetic model for colorectal tumorigenesis. Cell 1990; 61(5):759–67.
17. Xie J, Itzkowitz SH. Cancer in inflammatory bowel disease. World J Gastroenterol 2008;14(3):378–89.
18. Kisiel JB, Ahlquist DA. Stool DNA testing for cancer surveillance in inflammatory bowel disease: an early view. Therap Adv Gastroenterol 2013;6(5):371–80.
19. Thomas T, Abrams KA, Robinson RJ, et al. Meta-analysis: cancer risk of low-grade dysplasia in chronic ulcerative colitis. Aliment Pharmacol Ther 2007; 25(6):657–68.
20. Rutter M, Saunders B, Wilkinson K, et al. Severity of inflammation is a risk factor for colorectal neoplasia in ulcerative colitis. Gastroenterology 2004;126(2):451–9.
21. Gupta RB, Harpaz N, Itzkowitz S, et al. Histologic inflammation is a risk factor for progression to colorectal neoplasia in ulcerative colitis: a cohort study. Gastroenterology 2007;133(4):1099–105 [quiz: 1340–1].
22. Farraye FA, Odze RD, Eaden J, et al. AGA technical review on the diagnosis and management of colorectal neoplasia in inflammatory bowel disease. Gastroenterology 2010;138(2):746–74, 774.e1–4; [quiz: e12–3].
23. Fornaro R, Caratto M, Caratto E, et al. Colorectal cancer in patients with inflammatory bowel disease: the need for a real surveillance program. Clin Colorectal Cancer 2016;15(3):204–12.
24. Laine L, Kaltenbach T, Barkun A, et al. SCENIC international consensus statement on surveillance and management of dysplasia in inflammatory bowel disease. Gastroenterology 2015;148(3):639–51.e28.
25. Aparicio T, Zaanan A, Svrcek M, et al. Small bowel adenocarcinoma: epidemiology, risk factors, diagnosis and treatment. Dig Liver Dis 2014;46(2):97–104.
26. Laukoetter MG, Mennigen R, Hannig CM, et al. Intestinal cancer risk in Crohn's disease: a meta-analysis. J Gastrointest Surg 2011;15(4):576–83.
27. Canavan C, Abrams KR, Mayberry J. Meta-analysis: colorectal and small bowel cancer risk in patients with Crohn's disease. Aliment Pharmacol Ther 2006;23(8): 1097–104.
28. Mizushima T, Ohno Y, Nakajima K, et al. Malignancy in Crohn's disease: incidence and clinical characteristics in Japan. Digestion 2010;81(4):265–70.
29. Mellemkjaer L, Johansen C, Gridley G, et al. Crohn's disease and cancer risk (Denmark). Cancer Causes Control 2000;11(2):145–50.

30. Kvist N, Jacobsen O, Norgaard P, et al. Malignancy in Crohn's disease. Scand J Gastroenterol 1986;21(1):82–6.
31. Kamiya T, Ando T, Ishiguro K, et al. Intestinal cancers occurring in patients with Crohn's disease. J Gastroenterol Hepatol 2012;27(Suppl 3):103–7.
32. Partridge SK, Hodin RA. Small bowel adenocarcinoma at a strictureplasty site in a patient with Crohn's disease: report of a case. Dis Colon Rectum 2004;47(5): 778–81.
33. Menon AM, Mirza AH, Moolla S, et al. Adenocarcinoma of the small bowel arising from a previous strictureplasty for Crohn's disease: report of a case. Dis Colon Rectum 2007;50(2):257–9.
34. Jaskowiak NT, Michelassi F. Adenocarcinoma at a strictureplasty site in Crohn's disease: report of a case. Dis Colon Rectum 2001;44(2):284–7.
35. Barwood N, Platell C. Case report: adenocarcinoma arising in a Crohn's stricture of the jejunum. J Gastroenterol Hepatol 1999;14(11):1132–4.
36. Senay E, Sachar DB, Keohane M, et al. Small bowel carcinoma in Crohn's disease. Distinguishing features and risk factors. Cancer 1989;63(2):360–3.
37. Schuman BM. Adenocarcinoma arising in an excluded loop of ileum. N Engl J Med 1970;283(3):136–7.
38. Greenstein AJ, Janowitz HD. Cancer in Crohn's disease. The danger of a bypassed loop. Am J Gastroenterol 1975;64(2):122–4.
39. Solem CA, Harmsen WS, Zinsmeister AR, et al. Small intestinal adenocarcinoma in Crohn's disease: a case-control study. Inflamm Bowel Dis 2004;10(1):32–5.
40. Piton G, Cosnes J, Monnet E, et al. Risk factors associated with small bowel adenocarcinoma in Crohn's disease: a case-control study. Am J Gastroenterol 2008;103(7):1730–6.
41. Amzallag-Bellenger E, Oudjit A, Ruiz A, et al. Effectiveness of MR enterography for the assessment of small-bowel diseases beyond Crohn disease. Radiographics 2012;32(5):1423–44.
42. Magro F, Peyrin-Biroulet L, Sokol H, et al. Extra-intestinal malignancies in inflammatory bowel disease: results of the 3rd ECCO Pathogenesis Scientific Workshop (III). J Crohns Colitis 2014;8(1):31–44.
43. Kotlyar DS, Lewis JD, Beaugerie L, et al. Risk of lymphoma in patients with inflammatory bowel disease treated with azathioprine and 6-mercaptopurine: a meta-analysis. Clin Gastroenterol Hepatol 2015;13(5):847–58.e4 [quiz: e48–50].
44. Colombel JF, Sandborn WJ, Reinisch W, et al. Infliximab, azathioprine, or combination therapy for Crohn's disease. N Engl J Med 2010;362(15):1383–95.
45. Panaccione R, Ghosh S, Middleton S, et al. Combination therapy with infliximab and azathioprine is superior to monotherapy with either agent in ulcerative colitis. Gastroenterology 2014;146(2):392–400.e3.
46. Siegel CA, Marden SM, Persing SM, et al. Risk of lymphoma associated with combination anti-tumor necrosis factor and immunomodulator therapy for the treatment of Crohn's disease: a meta-analysis. Clin Gastroenterol Hepatol 2009; 7(8):874–81.
47. Lichtenstein GR, Feagan BG, Cohen RD, et al. Drug therapies and the risk of malignancy in Crohn's disease: results from the TREAT Registry. Am J Gastroenterol 2014;109(2):212–23.
48. Siegel CA. Lost in translation: helping patients understand the risks of inflammatory bowel disease therapy. Inflamm Bowel Dis 2010;16(12):2168–72.
49. Rogers HW, Weinstock MA, Feldman SR, et al. Incidence estimate of nonmelanoma skin cancer (keratinocyte carcinomas) in the U.S. population, 2012. JAMA Dermatol 2015;151(10):1081–6.

50. Beaugerie L, Brousse N, Bouvier AM, et al. Lymphoproliferative disorders in patients receiving thiopurines for inflammatory bowel disease: a prospective observational cohort study. Lancet 2009;374(9701):1617–25.
51. Osterman MT, Sandborn WJ, Colombel JF, et al. Increased risk of malignancy with adalimumab combination therapy, compared with monotherapy, for Crohn's disease. Gastroenterology 2014;146(4):941–9.
52. Sifuentes H, Kane S. Monitoring for extra-intestinal cancers in IBD. Curr Gastroenterol Rep 2015;17(11):42.
53. Singh S, Nagpal SJ, Murad MH, et al. Inflammatory bowel disease is associated with an increased risk of melanoma: a systematic review and meta-analysis. Clin Gastroenterol Hepatol 2014;12(2):210–8.
54. Long MD, Martin CF, Pipkin CA, et al. Risk of melanoma and nonmelanoma skin cancer among patients with inflammatory bowel disease. Gastroenterology 2012; 143(2):390–9.e1.
55. Kappelman MD, Farkas DK, Long MD, et al. Risk of cancer in patients with inflammatory bowel diseases: a nationwide population-based cohort study with 30 years of follow-up evaluation. Clin Gastroenterol Hepatol 2014;12(2):265–73.e1.
56. Azoury SC, Lange JR. Epidemiology, risk factors, prevention, and early detection of melanoma. Surg Clin North Am 2014;94(5):945–62, vii.
57. Rungoe C, Simonsen J, Riis L, et al. Inflammatory bowel disease and cervical neoplasia: a population-based nationwide cohort study. Clin Gastroenterol Hepatol 2015;13(4):693–700.e1.
58. International Collaboration of Epidemiological Studies of Cervical Cancer. Comparison of risk factors for invasive squamous cell carcinoma and adenocarcinoma of the cervix: collaborative reanalysis of individual data on 8,097 women with squamous cell carcinoma and 1,374 women with adenocarcinoma from 12 epidemiological studies. Int J Cancer 2007;120(4):885–91.
59. Singh H, Demers AA, Nugent Z, et al. Risk of cervical abnormalities in women with inflammatory bowel disease: a population-based nested case-control study. Gastroenterology 2009;136(2):451–8.
60. Jess T, Horvath-Puho E, Fallingborg J, et al. Cancer risk in inflammatory bowel disease according to patient phenotype and treatment: a Danish population-based cohort study. Am J Gastroenterol 2013;108(12):1869–76.
61. Allegretti JR, Barnes EL, Cameron A. Are patients with inflammatory bowel disease on chronic immunosuppressive therapy at increased risk of cervical high-grade dysplasia/cancer? A meta-analysis. Inflamm Bowel Dis 2015;21(5): 1089–97.
62. Shwaartz C, Munger JA, Deliz JR, et al. Fistula-associated anorectal cancer in the setting of Crohn's disease. Dis Colon Rectum 2016;59(12):1168–73.
63. von Roon AC, Reese G, Teare J, et al. The risk of cancer in patients with Crohn's disease. Dis Colon Rectum 2007;50(6):839–55.
64. Lindstrom L, Lapidus A, Ost A, et al. Increased risk of colorectal cancer and dysplasia in patients with Crohn's colitis and primary sclerosing cholangitis. Dis Colon Rectum 2011;54(11):1392–7.
65. Askling J, Dickman PW, Karlen P, et al. Colorectal cancer rates among first-degree relatives of patients with inflammatory bowel disease: a population-based cohort study. Lancet 2001;357(9252):262–6.
66. Askling J, Brandt L, Lapidus A, et al. Risk of haematopoietic cancer in patients with inflammatory bowel disease. Gut 2005;54(5):617–22.

67. Lewis JD, Bilker WB, Brensinger C, et al. Inflammatory bowel disease is not associated with an increased risk of lymphoma. Gastroenterology 2001;121(5):1080–7.
68. Bernstein CN, Blanchard JF, Kliewer E, et al. Cancer risk in patients with inflammatory bowel disease: a population-based study. Cancer 2001;91(4):854–62.
69. Long MD, Herfarth HH, Pipkin CA, et al. Increased risk for non-melanoma skin cancer in patients with inflammatory bowel disease. Clin Gastroenterol Hepatol 2010;8(3):268–74.
70. Ariyaratnam J, Subramanian V. Association between thiopurine use and nonmelanoma skin cancers in patients with inflammatory bowel disease: a meta-analysis. Am J Gastroenterol 2014;109(2):163–9.

Sexuality, Fertility, and Pregnancy in Crohn's Disease

Jill K.J. Gaidos, MD[a], Sunanda V. Kane, MD, MSPH[b,*]

KEYWORDS

• Sexuality • Infertility • Pregnancy • Crohn's disease • Immunomodulators
• Biologics

KEY POINTS

- Fertility in men with inflammatory bowel disease (IBD) can be decreased by certain medications and by having active disease. In women with IBD, fertility is decreased in the setting of active disease and following surgery within the pelvis.
- Many factors influence sexuality in patients with Crohn's disease, including symptoms of active disease, extraintestinal manifestations of disease, medication side effects, and evidence of prior surgery.
- Having Crohn's disease has been associated with a higher risk for preterm delivery, small for gestational age infants, low birth weight babies, and stillbirth, but no increased risk for congenital anomalies. Being in a state of disease remission before conception is associated with the best pregnancy and neonatal outcomes.
- Other than methotrexate, most medications used to treat Crohn's disease are safe to continue throughout pregnancy.
- Infants with gestational exposure to anti–tumor necrosis factor medications should avoid live vaccines for the first 9 months of life or until the serum drug concentrations are undetectable.

INTRODUCTION

Crohn's disease (CD) is a chronic, transmural, inflammatory disease involving any area of the gastrointestinal tract, from mouth to anus. CD is commonly diagnosed in the late teens to early adulthood,[1] overlapping a time when people are discovering their sexuality, establishing relationships, and beginning family planning. The symptoms of CD

Disclosures: Dr J.K.J. Gaidos has no relevant commercial or financial conflicts of interest to disclose. Dr S.V. Kane serves as a consultant to AbbVie, Janssen, and Samsung Bioepis, and has research funding from UCB.
[a] GI/Hepatology Service, McGuire VA Medical Center, Virginia Commonwealth University, 111-N, 1201 Broad Rock Boulevard, Richmond, VA 23249, USA; [b] Mayo Clinic, 200 First Street Southwest, Rochester, MN 55905, USA
* Corresponding author.
E-mail address: Kane.Sunanda@mayo.edu

Gastroenterol Clin N Am 46 (2017) 531–546
http://dx.doi.org/10.1016/j.gtc.2017.05.007
gastro.theclinics.com

include abdominal pain, diarrhea, weight loss, and poor nutrition, and can include hair loss and other extraintestinal manifestations, including ulcerating skin lesions. Complications, including strictures, enterocutaneous fistulas, and perianal fistulas, often require surgical repair with up to 50% of patients with CD undergoing surgery by 10 years after their diagnosis,[2] which Sometimes results in a temporary or permanent ostomy or permanent scarring.

Many patients with inflammatory bowel disease (IBD), including CD and ulcerative colitis (UC), worry about the impact that IBD will have on their sexual functioning and body image.[3,4] In addition, several studies have shown that patients with IBD, both men and women, are afraid that having IBD will impair their sexual performance, decrease their libido, as well as negatively affect intimacy and relationship quality.[3–6] Further, many questions arise when patients are considering conception, particularly with regard to the safety of their medications during pregnancy. This article reviews the most current literature regarding the influence of CD on sexuality, fertility, and pregnancy so that providers are well prepared to address these concerns with their patients.

SEXUALITY

Sexuality is the ability to have sexual experiences and responses. Normal sexual function requires intact physiologic functions, including sex hormones, neurotransmitters, pelvic muscles, and genital blood flow; and psychological components, including personal and interpersonal factors. Physiologic impairments of sexual functioning lead to decreased sexual satisfaction, difficulty with arousal and orgasm, reduced lubrication and dyspareunia in women, and erectile dysfunction/impotence and retrograde ejaculation in men. Psychological difficulties can result in reduced sexual satisfaction and decreased interest in sexual intercourse.

There are many factors that affect sexuality and sexual function in patients with CD. Survey studies have shown that more than half of both men and women with IBD report difficulties with some aspect of sexual function,[7,8] although women seem to be more affected than men. In one study, more than half of the male and female subjects thought that having IBD had negatively affected their relationship status, but more women than men reported that having IBD had decreased their libido (67.1% of women vs 41.9% of men; $P = .0005$) and led to a decrease in sexual activity (66.3% of women vs 40.5% of men; $P<.0001$).[5] Another survey study of patients with IBD found that women overall had more concerns about their bodies, attractiveness, and having children, whereas women with CD were more likely than men with CD to have concerns about intimacy and sexual performance.[3] Several studies have reported higher rates of dyspareunia in women with IBD,[6,9] although other studies have suggested the rates are similar in controls.[10]

Disease activity, body image, and depression also play key roles in the sexuality of patients with CD. In women, active disease has been showed to result in low sexual desire,[7] whereas in men it has been found to affect libido, attractiveness, enjoyment, and frequency of sexual activity as well as causing difficulties with erection and ejaculation.[10,11] Symptoms associated with active CD can lead to impaired intimacy and sexual inactivity[9] as well as decreasing libido and feelings of attractiveness.[11] Having IBD led to a negative body image in more than two-thirds of respondents in one study, with higher rates in women (74.8% of women vs 51.4% of men; $P = .0007$) and in those with prior surgery (81.4% operated vs 51.3% no prior surgery; $P = .0003$).[5] Depression is a major contributor to sexual dysfunction in men and women with IBD.[7,10,12]

Medications are responsible for up to 25% of cases of impotence in the general population[13]; however, there are only a few cases of IBD medications as the cause, including sulfasalazine[14] and methotrexate.[15–17] Despite the limited evidence, approximately 40% of subjects in one study reported a negative impact of their IBD medications on their sexual activity or their libido, resulting in around 10% occasionally omitting doses.[5] One recent study found the use of corticosteroids in women and the use of biologic agents in men to be independent predictors of sexual dysfunction.[12] Erectile dysfunction is a common adverse side effect of antianxiety and antidepressant medications, which are frequent comorbidities seen in patients with IBD, as well as the use of opioid pain medications.

FERTILITY

Fertility is defined as the ability to conceive after a year of unprotected sexual intercourse, which requires proper function of the male and female sexual organs. Fertility differs from fecundability, which is the probability of conception with each menstrual cycle for a couple attempting conception.

In Men

Reduction in fertility is estimated to be as high at 50% in men with CD; however, no studies have shown any difference in reproductive capacity.[18] In particular, an early study found that almost half of the men with CD had oligospermia in the absence of sulfasalazine, as well as an increase in disordered sperm morphology and motility,[19] which the investigators attributed to disease activity, nutritional status, or other medications. Another study of semen analysis found a significant decrease in sperm quality in the cohort of men with CD taking sulfasalazine and methylprednisolone compared with a no-treatment cohort and a cohort taking sulfasalazine alone, which was attributed to active disease.[20] A survey study comparing family size in men with CD before and after diagnosis with age-matched, healthy controls found that the men with CD fathered fewer children after their CD diagnosis than the controls, regardless of medication use, including steroids or sulfasalazine.[21] The investigators concluded that there were lower fertility rates in the CD cohort, although it was not clear whether the subjects with CD were actively attempting conception. Another questionnaire study found that the mean number of pregnancies among the group of men with CD was significantly lower compared with the controls (2.14 ± 0.11; $P<.02$), but there was no difference in fecundability between the groups,[22] leading the investigators to conclude that there was no decrease in reproductive capacity.

The most common reversible cause for male infertility is medication use (**Table 1**). Sulfasalazine has been shown to cause qualitative and quantitative abnormalities of sperm, including oligospermia, abnormal sperm morphology, and decreased sperm motility.[23,24] Importantly, these abnormalities resolve within a few months after discontinuing the drug, with a median time to pregnancy of 2.5 months,[24] or after switching to another mesalamine medication.[25] There has been only 1 case report of infertility with mesalazine, which also resolved following cessation of that medication.[26] Other studies have not shown any impact on male fertility with mesalamine use.

Methotrexate is known to be contraindicated in pregnancy because of its teratogenicity; however, few studies have evaluated the impact of methotrexate on male reproductive capability. Animal studies have clearly shown an adverse impact on fertility with methotrexate use,[27] but the results of studies in humans have been contradictory. There are case reports of reversible oligospermia in men with psoriasis treated with

Table 1
Effect of inflammatory bowel disease medications on male sexual function, fertility, and pregnancy outcomes

Medication	Sexual Function	Fertility	Pregnancy Outcome	Recosmmendation
Sulfasalazine	Report of ED	Decreased, oligospermia, decreased motility, abnormal sperm morphology; reversible after cessation	Limited data, possible increase in congenital anomalies	Discontinue 2–3 mo before attempting conception
Other 5-ASAs	None reported	Cases of oligospermia	No adverse outcomes reported	Safe to continue
Steroids	None reported	None reported	None reported	Safe to continue
Azathioprine/6MP	None reported	None reported	Conflicting data, but no clear association	Safe to continue
Methotrexate	ED	Likely altered spermatogenesis	None reported, but limited data	Discontinue for at least 3 mo before attempting conception
Metronidazole	None reported	None reported	None reported	Safe to continue
Ciprofloxacin	None reported	Decreased fertility in rat models	None reported	Weigh risks vs benefits of use
Cyclosporine	None reported	Limited data, none reported	None reported	Safe to continue
Infliximab	None reported	Decreased sperm motility, unclear impact on fertility	None reported	Safe to continue
Adalimumab	None reported	None reported	None reported	Safe to continue
Certolizumab pegol	None reported	None reported	None reported	Safe to continue
Vedolizumab	None reported	None reported	None reported	Safe to continue
Ustekinumab	None reported	None reported	None reported	Safe to continue

Abbreviations: 5-ASAs, 5-aminosalycylates; 6MP, 6-mercaptopurine; ED, erectile dysfunction.

methotrexate,[28] although a study of 26 men with psoriasis on methotrexate found no seminal abnormalities.[29]

Other than medications, nutritional status, particularly zinc deficiency, has been proposed as a cause of infertility in men with IBD.[30] Other causes of male infertility in the general population also pertain to the IBD population, including tobacco and alcohol use.[31]

In Women

Fertility in women with medically managed, quiescent CD is not decreased compared with the general population.[32,33] However, active IBD and prior pelvic surgery, such as following an ileal pouch anal anastomosis, lead to significantly decreased fertility.[34,35] Methotrexate does not decrease fertility in women, but it is a teratogen and is recommended to be discontinued for at least 3 months, ideally 6 months, before attempting conception. No other IBD medications have been found to decrease fertility in women with IBD.

PREGNANCY

Effect of Pregnancy on Inflammatory Bowel Disease

Overall, pregnancy does not exacerbate IBD. Prior studies have shown that the rate of disease worsening is similar between pregnant and nonpregnant women with CD.[36] The risk of flare has been found to correlate closely with the degree of disease activity at conception. Less than one-third of women with inactive disease at conception experience worsening disease in pregnancy, compared with two-thirds of those with active disease at conception who continue to have active disease at the same severity or worse throughout pregnancy.[32,37,38] A recent meta-analysis including 1130 women with UC and 590 women with CD found that women with active disease at conception had twice the risk of having ongoing active or worsening disease throughout pregnancy compared with the risk of a flare in women with inactive disease at conception (for UC: RR, 2.0; 95% confidence interval [CI], 1.5–3; $P<.001$. For CD: RR, 2.0; 95% CI, 1.2–3.4; $P = .006$).[39] For optimal pregnancy and fetal outcomes (**Table 2**), the goal is to be in a steroid-free remission on a stable drug regimen that can be continued throughout pregnancy for at least 3 months before conception.

Table 2
Definitions of adverse pregnancy and neonatal outcomes

Term	Definition
Adverse pregnancy outcomes	• Induced/elective abortion • Spontaneous abortion/miscarriage • Ectopic pregnancy • Small for gestational age (defined as birth weight <10th percentile for gestational age) • Preterm birth (defined as delivery at <37 wk of gestation) • Stillbirth
Adverse fetal/neonatal outcomes	• Intrauterine growth restriction • Low birth weight (defined as weight of <2500 g) • Congenital anomalies • Newborn seizure • Neonatal intensive care unit admission • Infant mortality

Effect of inflammatory bowel disease on pregnancy

Having IBD, even quiescent disease, can result in higher rates of preterm delivery (ie, born at <37 weeks of gestation), small for gestational age (SGA) infants, low birth weight infants, or stillbirth (**Table 3**). A large community-based IBD study reported increased odds for preterm birth, SGA, or stillbirth (odds ratio [OR], 1.54; 95% CI, 1.00–2.38) and increased odds for spontaneous abortion (OR, 1.65; 95% CI, 1.09–2.48), not associated with medication use or with disease severity.[40] Importantly, several studies have found no increase in adverse fetal outcomes, specifically congenital anomalies, among infants born to women with IBD.[40,41] A population-based study of women with CD in Denmark and Sweden reported an increased risk of preterm birth, further increased among those with prior surgery; however, no increased risk of congenital anomalies or stillbirth.[42] Using a Swedish health registry to assess pregnancy outcomes among women with CD, a recent study also found an increased risk for low birth weight (adjusted OR [aOR], 1.86; 95% CI, 1.46–2.38), preterm birth (aOR, 1.65; 95% CI, 1.33–2.06), and, unlike in other studies, an increased risk for stillbirth (aOR, 2.93; 95% CI, 1.57–5.47).[43] A study that compared outcomes of pregnancies in a cohort of women before and after their diagnosis of IBD found a higher incidence of low birth weight (P = .048) and preterm birth (P = .008) after diagnosis.[44]

The risk of adverse outcomes increases with active CD. A recent study including 298 pregnancies in IBD found that active disease at conception results in almost 8-fold increased odds of relapse during pregnancy (aOR, 7.66; 95% CI, 3.77–15.54).[45] In the previously mentioned health registry study, the presence of active disease almost doubled the odds for preterm birth (aOR, 2.66; 95% CI, 1.89–3.74), doubled the odds for stillbirth (aOR, 4.48; 95% CI, 1.67–11.90), and almost tripled the odds for low birth weight (aOR, 3.30; 95% CI, 2.29–4.74).[43] These findings further stress the importance of disease remission during pregnancy.

Table 3
Pregnancy outcomes in Crohn's disease

Outcome	Odds	95% CI	Reference
Any adverse pregnancy outcome	OR, 1.54	1.00–2.38	Mahadevan et al,[40] 2007
	No increase		Bortoli et al,[100] 2011
SGA birth	OR, 1.46	1.14–1.88	Getahun et al,[101] 2014
Spontaneous preterm birth	OR, 1.32	1.0–1.76	Getahun et al,[101] 2014
	No increase		Bortoli et al,[100] 2011
	aOR, 1.65	1.33–2.06	Bröms et al,[43] 2014
	aOR, 2.66 (with active disease)	1.89–3.74	Bröms et al,[43] 2014
Preterm birth at 32–36 wk	POR, 1.76	1.51–2.05	Stephansson et al,[42] 2010
Preterm birth at <32 wk	POR, 1.86	1.38–2.52	Stephansson et al,[42] 2010
Low birth weight	aOR, 1.86	1.46–2.38	Bröms et al,[43] 2014
	aOR, 3.30 (with active disease)	2.29–4.74	Bröms et al,[43] 2014
Adverse conception outcome	OR, 1.63	1.09–2.48	Mahadevan. et al,[40] 2007
	No increase		Bortoli et al,[100] 2011
Neonatal death/stillbirth	aOR, 2.93	1.57–5.47	Bröms et al,[43] 2014
	aOR, 4.48 (with active disease)	1.67–11.90	Bröms et al,[43] 2014

Abbreviations: aOR, adjusted odds ratio; OR, odds ratio.

Medication use in pregnancy

Disease remission at the time of conception and throughout pregnancy is important for optimizing pregnancy and fetal outcomes, which, for most women with CD, requires that they continue their medications throughout pregnancy. One major concern for women with IBD is the impact their medications will have on fetal development, which can result in either medication nonadherence, discontinuation, or deciding not to conceive.[46,47] Preconception care has recently been shown to improve medication compliance and reduce disease relapses during pregnancy, leading to a decreased risk for low birth weight infants,[48] which shows the importance of discussing family planning and medication safety with women with IBD before conception. The rest of this article provides the most current evidence on the safety of the use of current medications for the treatment of CD during pregnancy (see **Table 3**). Recommendations regarding the safety of continuing these medications while breastfeeding are included in **Table 4**.

Aminosalicylates A few studies have reported adverse effects associated with the use of aminosalicylates, or 5-aminosalicylic acid (5-ASA) derivatives, during pregnancy; however, none were able to determine whether the adverse effects were medication induced or caused by ongoing disease activity.[49,50] A large meta-analysis including 642 pregnancies in women exposed to 5-ASA medications did not find any increased risk for adverse pregnancy or fetal outcomes.[51] However, 2 of the 5-ASA medications do warrant potential concern. Sulfasalazine crosses the placenta and has been shown to inhibit absorption and metabolism of folic acid, requiring an increase in folic acid supplementation to 2 mg daily preconception and during pregnancy to limit the impact on neural tube defects. In addition, Asacol HD has dibutyl phthalate in the coating of the medication, which is associated with urologic defects in animal studies when given in much higher doses. Given the potential for urogenital malformation, it is reasonable to recommend a switch to another 5-ASA medication in the preconception period.[52]

Corticosteroids Even women in disease remission before attempting conception are at risk of a flare during pregnancy, which may require the use of steroids for treatment. Prior studies have shown an association between oral clefts and intrauterine corticosteroid exposure in the first trimester[53,54]; however, these findings have not been replicated in more recent studies of patients with IBD.[36,38,41,44] Most of the evidence on the safety of corticosteroid use in pregnancy comes from the Pregnancy in Inflammatory Bowel Disease and Neonatal Outcomes (PIANO) study, which is a multicenter, prospective, observational registry following the outcomes of pregnant women with IBD and their infants for up to 4 years. As of 2014, this study included 969 women with IBD exposed to either intravenous (IV) or oral steroids during pregnancy and showed no increase in newborn infections or congenital anomalies; however, there was an associated increase in infants with low birth weight (aOR, 2.8; 95% CI, 1.3–6.1) and gestational diabetes (aOR, 2.8; 95% CI, 1.3–6.0).[55]

The use of IV steroids for the treatment of a disease flare during pregnancy has not been associated with an increase in adverse fetal outcomes.[56] If needed, prednisolone should be considered as a first choice for treatment if steroids are required for management during pregnancy because it does not cross the placenta as effectively as other steroid formulations. Budesonide is another option to consider given its high first-pass metabolism and fewer systemic effects. A small case series of patients with CD treated with budesonide throughout pregnancy found no increase in adverse fetal outcomes.[57] Avoiding steroids during pregnancy is best given the associated risk for low birth weight and gestational diabetes; however, controlling active inflammation is also important for improving pregnancy and fetal outcomes.

Table 4
Medication safety during pregnancy and breastfeeding

Medication	Safety in Pregnancy	Safety with Breastfeeding
5-ASA		
Mesalamine/mesalazine	Low risk	Low risk
Asacol HD	Likely low risk, contains DBP	Likely low risk
Sulfasalazine	Low risk, +2 g folic acid QD	Low risk
Corticosteroids	Low risk, risk of GD and LBW	Low risk
Antibiotics		
Ciprofloxacin	Low risk with short-term use	Avoid if possible, wait 48 h after dosing
Metronidazole	Low risk with short-term use	Avoid if possible, wait 12–24 h after dosing
Immunomodulators		
AZA/6MP	Low risk	Low risk
Cyclosporine	Low risk	Not compatible
Tacrolimus	Low risk	Limited evidence, seems low risk
Methotrexate	Contraindicated, stop 6 mo before conception	Contraindicated
Anti-TNF Agents		
Adalimumab	Low risk	Low risk
Certolizumab pegol	Low risk	Low risk
Infliximab	Low risk	Low risk
Anti-integrins		
Natalizumab	Discontinue 3 mo before conception	Limited evidence, likely compatible
Vedolizumab	Low risk	Limited evidence, likely compatible
Anti–IL-12/IL-23		
Ustekinumab	Limited evidence	Limited evidence, likely compatible
JAK Inhibitor		
Tofacitinib	Discontinue 2 mo before conception	Limited evidence, should be avoided

Abbreviations: 5-ASA, 5-aminosalycylate; 6MP, 6-mercaptopurine; anti-TNF, anti–tumor necrosis factor; AZA, azathioprine; DBP, dibutyl phthalate; GD, gestational diabetes; IL, interleukin; JAK, Janus kinase; LBW, low birth weight; QD, every day.

Antibiotics Ciprofloxacin and metronidazole are the most common antibiotics used in IBD. Use of quinolones, including ciprofloxacin, during pregnancy can result in newborn arthropathies caused by the drug's high affinity for cartilage and bone. However, a large meta-analysis, including 1433 women with exposure to fluoroquinolones during pregnancy, showed no increased odds of stillbirth, preterm birth, major malformations, or low birth weight.[58] Similarly, metronidazole use during pregnancy was previously associated with cleft lip and palate; however, a meta-analysis including almost 200,000 pregnant women with gestational exposure to metronidazole during the first trimester found no associated increase in birth defects.[59] Given the more recent evidence suggesting overall safety, short courses of ciprofloxacin or metronidazole can be safely given during pregnancy, although long-term treatment with either antibiotic is not recommended.[52]

Immunomodulators Two early studies reported an increased risk for congenital malformations following intrauterine exposure to thiopurines, including azathioprine and 6-mercaptopurine.[60,61] More recent studies have not found any increase in congenital malformations, or other adverse pregnancy or fetal outcomes, following exposure to thiopurines during pregnancy.[41,62–64] Importantly, a prospective study including 30 children with gestational exposure to thiopurines found no altered immune function or any developmental delays.[65] Based on the current evidence, the thiopurines seem safe to continue throughout pregnancy.

Other immunomodulators used less frequently to treat CD are the calcineurin inhibitors tacrolimus and cyclosporine. A review including 100 pregnancies with tacrolimus exposure found no associated increase in congenital malformations.[66] However, neonatal renal injury and hyperkalemia have been reported following gestational exposure to tacrolimus.[67] Use of cyclosporine during pregnancy has been associated with intrauterine growth restriction, preterm birth, as well as an increase in fetal infections.[68] Birth outcomes in 3 pregnant women following inpatient use of IV cyclosporine for acute IBD flares resulted in 2 preterm births and 1 spontaneous abortion at 15 weeks, most likely caused by active IBD than by cyclosporine use.[56] However, smaller studies of these medications have not shown any increase in pregnancy complications or congenital malformations with use during pregnancy.[69–72] As such, if these medications are needed to maintain disease remission in the mother, then it is likely safe to continue them during pregnancy.

Anti–tumor necrosis factor agents The anti–tumor necrosis factor (anti-TNF)–alpha medications that are approved for the treatment of CD include infliximab, adalimumab, and certolizumab pegol. In large series of patients exposed to anti-TNF medications, there have not been any associated adverse effects on outcomes of pregnancy.[73–75] In the ongoing PIANO registry, there are more than 500 women with exposure to anti-TNF agents during pregnancy, with no increase in congenital anomalies compared with the unexposed cohort of pregnant women.[64] Similarly, a systematic review including more than 1000 women with exposure to anti-TNF medication during pregnancy found no associated increase in adverse pregnancy outcomes or any increase in congenital anomalies.[76] Further, a meta-analysis with more than 1200 women with IBD treated with anti-TNF medications during pregnancy showed no increase in preterm delivery, low birth weight, or congenital anomalies compared with an unexposed cohort,[77] suggesting overall safety.

Reviewing safety reports of medication adverse events, treatment with a thiopurine combined with an anti-TNF medication was not associated with increased odds of adverse pregnancy or neonatal outcomes (OR, 0.97; 95% CI, 0.49–1.93).[78] However, data from the PIANO registry show increased odds for preterm delivery among women on combination therapy (OR, 2.4; 95% CI, 1.3–4.1) as well as an increase in infections at 1 year of age among infants with gestational exposure to combination therapy compared with infants in an unexposed cohort.[64] In contrast, several observational studies have not identified any increased infection rate among infants with gestational exposure to combination therapy compared with infants exposed to anti-TNF monotherapy.[76,79] The current recommendations regarding management of pregnant women on combination therapy are to consider switching to monotherapy on a case-by-case basis depending on the risk of disease relapse and patient preference.[52]

Anti–tumor necrosis factor agents infliximab and adalimumab are full monoclonal antibodies, which are actively transported across the placenta beginning at 20 weeks but predominantly in the third trimester, whereas certolizumab pegol is a pegylated FAB' fragment and is only passively transported across the placenta in the third trimester, resulting in much lower infant cord blood levels at birth.[80] Because of their active transfer, studies have shown that infant infliximab and adalimumab cord blood levels are 4 times higher than maternal levels at birth[81,82] and can be detected in some infants for up to 1 year[82]; however, this has not correlated with an increase in neonatal infections, neonatal intensive care unit admissions, or delay in achieving developmental milestones.[83] Given this active transfer, there is still some debate regarding the timing of the last dose of these medications to decrease the neonatal drug levels at the time of birth. Several European studies have suggested discontinuing biologic agents at 22 weeks' gestation in women with disease remission, although recent studies have suggested that patients in remission who discontinue treatment experience disease flares at similar rates to those who were not in remission.[84] Further, discontinuing treatment during pregnancy has also been shown to result in higher rates of disease relapse postpartum.[85] More importantly, recent studies have shown that exposure to anti-TNF medications during the third trimester does not negatively affect the infant growth rate, number of infections, immune development during the first year, or achievement of developmental milestones.[80,86] Given these more recent findings, some experts are now recommending continuing these medications throughout the third trimester.[87]

Because of the detectable drug concentrations in infants with intrauterine exposure to infliximab and adalimumab, these infants should not receive live vaccines for the first 9 months or until the drug concentrations are undetectable.[82] In the United States, these exposed infants should avoid the rotavirus vaccine, which is given in several doses starting at 2 months of age, but all other vaccinations can be administered on schedule. Outside the United States, this also means avoiding the live bacillus Calmette-Guérin vaccine for the first 9 months. In addition, pediatricians should be informed of the infant's anti-TNF exposure so that live vaccinations can be avoided and possible infections can be addressed early.[87]

Anti-integrins Two anti-integrin medications are approved for use in the treatment of CD. Natalizumab is an immunoglobulin (Ig) G4 monoclonal antibody to the $\alpha 4$ subunit present on both the $\alpha 4\beta 1$ and $\alpha 4\beta 7$ integrin molecules, which limits the adhesion and transmigration of leukocytes across blood vessels to areas of inflammation. Several small studies have been inconclusive regarding the risk of use in pregnancy. One case series reported anemia and thrombocytopenia in neonates following intrauterine exposure to natalizumab,[88] whereas other studies have not shown any increase in adverse pregnancy or fetal outcomes,[89–91] including after exposure in the third trimester.[80] The data to support the safety of natalizumab use in pregnancy remain limited. Subsequently, the current recommendations are for natalizumab to be discontinued for at least 3 months before conception.[90]

Vedolizumab, the second anti-integrin medication, is a monoclonal IgG1 antibody that targets only the $\alpha 4\beta 7$ integrin molecule, leading to directed treatment limited to the gastrointestinal mucosa. Because of its recent US Food and Drug Administration approval, the current data on safety in pregnancy are limited to exposure in 24 women involved in the vedolizumab clinical development program.[92] Recent evidence has shown that neonatal vedolizumab drug concentrations were lower than maternal drug levels in a small patient sample.[83] Further studies are clearly needed; however, given the mechanism of action, the risk of adverse outcomes is likely low and continuation of the medication during pregnancy is likely safe.

Anti–interleukin-12/interleukin-23 Ustekinumab is a humanized IgG1 monoclonal antibody that decreases cytokine activity by binding to the p40 subunit on both interleukin (IL)-12 and IL-23. It was recently approved for the treatment of CD but has been used to treat psoriasis and psoriatic arthritis for several years. The current evidence for the safety of use in pregnancy is limited to unpublished data from clinical trials[93] and a few case reports; all but one[94] of which showed no associated adverse effects.[95–97] Given the limited available data, the current recommendations are to avoid ustekinumab during pregnancy unless other medications that are compatible with pregnancy have not been effective.[98]

Tofacitinib Although the clinical trials are showing efficacy in treating UC but not CD, the next medication likely to be approved for the treatment of IBD is tofacitinib, which is a small molecule agent that reduces inflammation by inhibiting the Janus kinase (JAK) 3 receptor. It was recently approved for use in rheumatoid arthritis and experience with exposure in pregnancy is limited to 34 pregnancies that occurred during the clinical trials. Because of the limited data on safety, the current recommendations are to discontinue tofacitinib at least 2 months before conception.[99]

SUMMARY

Although most gastroenterologists rarely address these issues, patients with CD have concerns about the impact of their disease on their ability to have a normal sex life. Fertility is not negatively affected by CD. Medications, particularly sulfasalazine, commonly lead to infertility in men with IBD, whereas pelvic surgery significantly decreases fertility in women. Many factors influence the sexual health of men and women with CD but disease activity and depression are key causes of sexual dysfunction. CD is associated with an increased risk for some adverse pregnancy and neonatal outcomes; however, these outcomes are optimized by achieving disease remission before conception. Other than methotrexate, most of the commonly used medications to treat CD seem to be safe to continue throughout pregnancy. Infants with gestational exposure to anti-TNF medications should not be given live vaccines for the first 9 months of life or until drug concentrations are undetectable. Preconception care to discuss the importance of continuing IBD treatment throughout pregnancy has been shown to improve adherence to treatment and to decrease the rate of relapse in pregnant patients with IBD, resulting in improved fetal outcomes.[48]

REFERENCES

1. Keighley MR, Stockbrugger RW. Inflammatory bowel disease. Aliment Pharmacol Ther 2003;18(Suppl 3):66–70.
2. Bokemeyer B, Hardt J, Huppe D, et al. Clinical status, psychosocial impairments, medical treatment and health care costs for patients with inflammatory bowel disease [IBD] in Germany: an online IBD registry. J Crohns Colitis 2013;7:355–68.
3. Maunder R, Toner B, de Rooey E, et al. Influence of sex and disease on illness-related concerns in inflammatory bowel disease. Can J Gastroenterol 1999;13(9):728–32.
4. Carlsson E, Bosaeus I, Nordgren S. What concerns subjects with inflammatory bowel disease and an ileostomy? Scand J Gastroenterol 2003;38:978–84.
5. Muller KR, Prosser R, Bampton P, et al. Female gender and surgery impair relationships, body image, and sexuality in inflammatory bowel disease: patient perceptions. Inflamm Bowel Dis 2010;16(4):657–63.

6. Moody GA, Mayberry J. Perceived sexual dysfunction among patients with inflammatory bowel disease. Digestion 1993;54:256–60.
7. Timmer A, Kemptner D, Bauer A, et al. Determinants of female sexual function in inflammatory bowel disease: a survey based cross-sectional analysis. BMC Gastroenterol 2008;8:45–54.
8. O'Toole A, Winter D, Friedman S. Review article: the psychosexual impact of inflammatory bowel disease in male patients. Aliment Pharmacol Ther 2014;39: 1085–94.
9. Moody G, Probert C, Srivastava EM, et al. Sexual dysfunction amongst women with Crohn's disease: a hidden problem. Digestion 1992;52(3–4):179–83.
10. Timmer A, Bauer A, Dignass A, et al. Sexual function in persons with inflammatory bowel disease: a survey with matched controls. Clin Gastroenterol Hepatol 2007;5:87–94.
11. Timmer A, Bauer A, Kemptner D, et al. Determinants of male sexual function in inflammatory bowel disease: a survey-based cross-sectional analysis in 280 men. Inflamm Bowel Dis 2007;13:1236–43.
12. Marin L, Manosa M, Garcia-Planella E, et al. Sexual function and patients' perceptions in inflammatory bowel disease: a case-control survey. J Gastroenterol 2013;48:713–20.
13. Beeley L. Drug-induced sexual dysfunction and infertility. Adverse Drug React Acute Poisoning Rev 1984;3:23–42.
14. Ireland A, Jewell D. Sulfasalazine-induced impotence: a beneficial resolution with olsalazine? J Clin Gastroenterol 1989;11:711.
15. Thomas E, Koumouvi K, Blotman F. Impotence in a patient with rheumatoid arthritis treated with methotrexate. J Rheumatol 2000;27:1821–2.
16. Blackburn WD Jr, Alarcon G. Impotence in three rheumatoid arthritis patients treated with methotrexate. Arthritis Rheum 1989;32:1341–2.
17. Riba N, Morena F, Costa J, et al. Appearance of impotence in relation to the use of methotrexate. Med Clin (Barc) 1996;106:558.
18. Tavernier N, Fumery M, Peyrin-Biroulet L, et al. Systematic review: fertility in nonsurgically treated inflammatory bowel disease. Aliment Pharmacol Ther 2013; 38:847–53.
19. Farthing MJ, Dawson AM. Impaired semen quality in Crohn's disease-drugs, ill health, or undernutrition? Scand J Gastroenterol 1983;18:57–60.
20. Karbach U, Ewe K, Schramm P. Quality of semen in patients with Crohn's disease. Z Gastroenterol 1982;20(6):314–20.
21. Burnell D, Mayberry J, Calcraft BJ, et al. Male fertility in Crohn's disease. Postgrad Med J 1986;62:269–72.
22. Narendranathan M, Sandler R, Suchindran CM, et al. Male infertility in inflammatory bowel disease. J Clin Gastroenterol 1989;11(4):403–6.
23. Birnie GG, McLeod TIF, Watkinson G. Incidence of sulphasalazine-induced male infertility. Gut 1981;22:452–5.
24. O'Morain C, Smethurst P, Dore CJ, et al. Reversible male infertility due to sulphasalazine: studies in man and rat. Gut 1984;25:1078–84.
25. Riley SA, Lecarpentier J, Mani V, et al. Sulphasalazine induced seminal abnormalities in ulcerative colitis: results of mesalazine substitution. Gut 1987;28: 1008–12.
26. Chermesh I, Eliakim R. Mesalazine-induced reversible infertility in a young male. Dig Liver Dis 2004;36:551–2.

27. Saxena AK, Dhungel S, Bhattacharya S, et al. Effect of chronic low dose methotrexate on cellular proliferation during spermatogenesis in rats. Arch Androl 2004;50:33–5.
28. Sussman A, Leonard JM. Psoriasis, methotrexate, and oligospermia. Arch Dermatol 1980;116:215–7.
29. El-Beheiry A, El-Mansy E, Kamel N, et al. Methotrexate and fertility in men. Arch Androl 1979;3:177–9.
30. El-Tawil AM. Zinc deficiency in men with Crohn's disease may contribute to poor sperm function and male infertility. Andrologia 2003;35:337–41.
31. Feagins LA, Kane SV. Sexual and reproductive issues for men with inflammatory bowel disease. Am J Gastroenterol 2009;104:768–73.
32. Khosla R, Willoughby CD, Jewell DP. Crohn's disease and pregnancy. Gut 1984; 25:52–6.
33. Andres PG, Friedman LS. Epidemiology and natural course of inflammatory bowel disease. Gastroenterol Clin North Am 1999;28(2):255–81.
34. Ording Olsen K, Juul S, Berndtssen I, et al. Ulcerative colitis: female fecundity before diagnosis, during disease and after surgery compared to a population sample. Gastroenterology 2002;122(1):15–9.
35. Waljee A, Waljee J, Morris AM, et al. Threefold increased risk of infertility: a meta-analysis of infertility after ileal pouch anal anastomosis in ulcerative colitis. Gut 2006;55:1575–80.
36. Nielsen OH, Andreasson B, Bondesen S, et al. Pregnancy in Crohn's disease. Scand J Gastroenterol 1984;19(6):724–32.
37. Willoughby CP, Truelove SC. Ulcerative colitis and pregnancy. Gut 1980;21: 469–74.
38. Miller JP. Inflammatory bowel disease in pregnancy: a review. J R Soc Med 1986;79(4):221–5.
39. Abhyankar A, Ham M, Moss AC. Meta-analysis: the impact of disease activity at conception on disease activity during pregnancy in patients with inflammatory bowel disease. Aliment Pharmacol Ther 2013;38(5):460–6.
40. Mahadevan U, Sandborn W, Li D, et al. Pregnancy outcomes in women with inflammatory bowel disease: a large community-based study from Northern California. Gastroenterology 2007;133:1106–12.
41. Ban L, Tata L, Fiaschi L, et al. Limited risks of major congenital anomalies in children of mothers with IBD and effects of medications. Gastroenterology 2014; 146:76–84.
42. Stephansson O, Larsson H, Pedersen L, et al. Crohn's disease is a risk factor for preterm birth. Clin Gastroenterol Hepatol 2010;8(6):509–15.
43. Bröms G, Granath F, Linder M, et al. Birth outcomes in women with inflammatory bowel disease: effects of disease activity and drug exposure. Inflamm Bowel Dis 2014;20:1091–8.
44. Molnár T, Farkas K, Nagy F, et al. Pregnancy outcome in patients with inflammatory bowel disease according to the activity of the disease and the medical treatment: a case-control study. Scand J Gastroenterol 2010;45:1302–6.
45. de Lima-Karagiannis A, Zelinkova-Detkova Z, van der Woude CJ. The effects of active IBD during pregnancy in the era of novel IBD therapies. Am J Gastroenterol 2016;111:1305–12.
46. Mountifield R, Bampton P, Prosser R, et al. Fear and fertility in inflammatory bowel disease: a mismatch of perception and reality affects family planning decisions. Inflamm Bowel Dis 2009;15(5):720–5.

47. Zelikova Z, Mensink P, Dees J, et al. Reproductive wish represents an important factor in influencing therapeutic strategy in inflammatory bowel diseases. Scand J Gastroenterol 2010;45:46–50.
48. de Lima A, Zelinkova A, Mulders A, et al. Preconception care reduces relapse of inflammatory bowel disease during pregnancy. Clin Gastroenterol Hepatol 2016; 14:1285–91.
49. Diav-Citrin O, Park Y, Veerasuntharam G, et al. The safety of mesalamine in human pregnancy: a prospective controlled cohort study. Gastroenterology 1998; 144:23–8.
50. Nørgård B, Fonager K, Pedersen L, et al. Birth outcome in women exposed to 5-aminosalycylic acid during pregnancy: a Danish cohort study. Gut 2003;52: 243–7.
51. Rahimi R, Nikfar S, Rezale A, et al. Pregnancy outcome in women with inflammatory bowel disease following exposure to 5-aminosalicylic acid drugs: a meta-analysis. Reprod Toxicol 2008;25:271–5.
52. Nguyen GC, Seow C, Maxwell C, et al. The Toronto consensus statements for the management of inflammatory bowel disease in pregnancy. Gastroenterology 2016;150:734–57.
53. Park-Wylie L, Mazzotta P, Pastuszak A, et al. Birth defects after maternal exposure to corticosteroids: prospective cohort study and meta-analysis of epidemiological studies. Teratology 2000;62(6):385–92.
54. Pradat P, Robert-Gnansia E, Di Tanna GL, et al. First trimester exposure to corticosteroids and oral clefts. Birth Defects Res A Clin Mol Teratol 2003;67(12): 968–70.
55. Lin K, Martin CF, Dassopoules T, et al. Pregnancy outcomes amongst mothers with inflammatory bowel disease exposed to systemic corticosteroids: results of the PIANO registry. Gastroenterology 2015;146:S1.
56. Reddy D, Murphy SJ, Kane SV, et al. Relapses in inflammatory bowel disease during pregnancy: in-hospital management and birth outcomes. Am J Gastroenterol 2008;103:1203–9.
57. Beaulieu DB, Ananthakrishnan A, Issa M, et al. Budesonide induction and maintenance therapy for Crohn's disease during pregnancy. Inflamm Bowel Dis 2009;15(1):25–8.
58. Bar-Oz B, Moretti M, Boskovic R, et al. The safety of quinolones - A meta-analysis of pregnancy outcomes. Eur J Obstet Gynecol Reprod Biol 2009; 143:75–8.
59. Caro-Paton T, Carvajal A, Martin de Diego I, et al. Is metronidazole teratogenic? A meta-analysis. Br J Clin Pharmacol 1997;44:179–82.
60. Polifka JE, Friedman JM. Teratogen update: azathioprine and 6-mercaptopurine. Teratology 2002;65:240–61.
61. Nørgård B, Pedersen L, Fonager K, et al. Azathioprine, mercaptopurine and birth outcome: a population-based cohort study. Aliment Pharmacol Ther 2003;17:827–34.
62. Coelho J, Beaugerie L, Colombel JF, et al. Pregnancy outcome in patients with inflammatory bowel disease treated with thiopurines: cohort from the CESAME Study. Gut 2011;60:198–203.
63. Akbari M, Shah S, Velayos FS, et al. Systemic review and meta-analysis on the effects of thiopurines on birth outcomes from female and male patients with inflammatory bowel disease. Inflamm Bowel Dis 2013;19:15–22.

64. Mahadevan U, Martin C, Sandler RS, et al. PIANO: a 1000 patient prospective registry of pregnancy outcomes in women with IBD exposed to immunomodulators and biologic therapy. Gastroenterology 2012;142:S149.
65. De Meij TGJ, Jharap B, Kneepkens CMF, et al. Long-term follow-up of children exposed intrauterine to maternal thiopurine therapy during pregnancy in females with inflammatory bowel disease. Aliment Pharmacol Ther 2013;38:38–43.
66. Kainz A, Harabacz I, Cowlrisk IS, et al. Analysis of 100 pregnancy outcomes in women treated systemically with tacrolimus. Transpl Int 2000;13(Suppl 1): S299–300.
67. Jain A, Venkataramanan R, Fung JJ, et al. Pregnancy after liver transplantation under tacrolimus. Transplantation 1997;64:559–65.
68. Leroy C, Rigot J, Leroy M, et al. Immunosuppressive drugs and fertility. Orphanet J Rare Dis 2015;10:136–51.
69. Baumgart DC, Sturm A, Wiedenmann B, et al. Uneventful pregnancy and neonatal outcome with tacrolimus in refractory ulcerative colitis. Gut 2005;54:1822–3.
70. Nevers W, Pupco A, Koren G, et al. Safety of tacrolimus in pregnancy. Can Fam Physician 2014;60:905–6.
71. Westbrook RH, Yeoman A, Agarwal K, et al. Outcomes of pregnancy following liver transplantation: the King's College Hospital experience. Liver Transpl 2015;21(9):1153–9.
72. Bar-Oz B, Hackman R, Einarson T, et al. Pregnancy outcome after cyclosporine therapy during pregnancy: a meta-analysis. Transplantation 2001;71:1051–5.
73. Jürgens M, Brand S, Filik L, et al. Safety of adalimumab in Crohn's disease during pregnancy: case report and review of the literature. Inflamm Bowel Dis 2010; 16:1634–6.
74. Lichtenstein GR, Feagan B, Cohen RD, et al. Serious infection and mortality in patients with Crohn's disease: more than 5 years of follow-up in the TREAT registry. Am J Gastroenterol 2012;107:1409–22.
75. Mahadevan U, Vermeire S, Wolf DC, et al. Pregnancy outcomes after exposure to certolizumab pegol: updated results from safety surveillance. Gastroenterology 2015;148:S858–9.
76. Nielsen OH, Loftus EV Jr, Jess T. Safety of TNF-alpha inhibitors during IBD pregnancy: a systematic review. BMC Med 2013;11:174.
77. Narula N, Al-Dabbagh R, Dhillon A, et al. Anti-TNF alpha therapies are safe during pregnancy in women with inflammatory bowel disease: a systematic review and meta-analysis. Inflamm Bowel Dis 2014;20:1862–9.
78. Deepak P, Stobaugh DM. Maternal and foetal adverse events with tumour necrosis factor-alpha inhibitors in inflammatory bowel disease. Aliment Pharmacol Ther 2014;40:1035–43.
79. Bortlik M, Duricova D, Machkova N, et al. Impact of anti-tumor necrosis factor alpha antibodies administered to pregnant women with inflammatory bowel disease on long-term outcome of exposed children. Inflamm Bowel Dis 2014;20(3):495–501.
80. Mahadevan U, Martin CF, Dubinsky M, et al. Exposure to anti-TNFa therapy in the third trimester of pregnancy is not associated with increased adverse outcomes: results from the PIANO registry. Gastroenterology 2014;146:s170.
81. Mahadevan U, Wolf D, Dubinsky M, et al. Placental transfer of anti-tumor necrosis factor agents in pregnant patients with inflammatory bowel disease. Clin Gastroenterol Hepatol 2013;11:286–92.
82. Julsgaard M, Christensen LA, Gibson PR, et al. Concentrations of adalimumab and infliximab in mothers and newborns, and effects on infection. Gastroenterology 2016;151:110–9.

83. Mahadevan U, Martin C, Kane SV, et al. Do infant serum levels of biologic agents at birth correlate with risk of adverse outcomes? Results from the PIANO registry. Gastroenterology 2016;150:S91–2.
84. de Lima A, Zelinkova A, van der Ent C, et al. Tailored anti-TNF therapy during pregnancy in patients with IBD: maternal and fetal safety. Gut 2016;65:1261–8.
85. Seirafi M, de Vroey B, Amiot A, et al. Factors associated with pregnancy outcome in anti-TNF treated women with inflammatory bowel disease. Aliment Pharmacol Ther 2014;40:363–73.
86. Mahadevan U, Martin CF, Chambers C, et al. Achievement of developmental milestones among offspring of women with inflammatory bowel disease: the PIANO registry. Gastroenterology 2014;146:S1.
87. Mahadevan U, McConnell RA, Chambers CD. Drug safety and risk of adverse outcomes for pregnant patients with inflammatory bowel disease. Gastroenterology 2017;152:451–62.
88. Haghikia A, Langer-Gould A, Reliensmann G, et al. Natalizumab use during the third trimester of pregnancy. JAMA Neurol 2014;71(7):891–5.
89. Ebrahimi N, Herbstritt S, Gold R, et al. Pregnancy and fetal outcomes following natalizumab exposure in pregnancy. A prospective, controlled observational study. Mult Scler 2015;21(2):198–205.
90. Hellwig K, Haghikia A, Gold R. Pregnancy and natalizumab: results of an observational study in 35 accidental pregnancies during natalizumab treatment. Mult Scler 2011;17(8):958–63.
91. Mahadevan U, Nazareth M, Cristiano L, et al. Natalizumab use in pregnancy. Am J Gastroenterol 2008;103:s449.
92. Dubinsky M, Mahadevan U, Vermeire S, et al. Vedolizumab exposure in pregnancy: outcomes from clinical studies in inflammatory bowel disease. ECCO 2015. p. 563.
93. Data on file. Reports of pregnancy with ustekinumab: STE/inj/DoF/Sep2010/EMEA001.
94. Fotiadou C, Lazaridou E, Sotiriou E, et al. Spontaneous abortion during ustekinumab therapy. J Dermatol Case Rep 2012;6(4):105–7.
95. Alsenaid A, Prinz JC. Inadvertent pregnancy during ustekinumab therapy in a patient with plaque psoriasis and impetigo herpetiformis. J Eur Acad Dermatol Venereol 2016;30:488–90.
96. Rocha K, Piccinin MC, Kalache L, et al. Pregnancy during ustekinumab treatment for severe psoriasis. Dermatology 2015;231:103–4.
97. Sheeran C, Nicolopoulos J. Pregnancy outcomes of two patients exposed to ustekinumab in the first trimester. Australas J Dermatol 2014;55:235–6.
98. Gotestam Skorpen C, Hoeltzenbein M, Tincani A, et al. The EULAR points to consider for use of antirheumatic drugs before pregnancy, during pregnancy and lactation. Ann Rheum Dis 2016;75:795–810.
99. Levy RA, de Jesus GR, de Jesus NR, et al. Critical review of the current recommendations for the treatment of systemic inflammatory rheumatic diseases during pregnancy and lactation. Autoimmun Rev 2016;15:955–63.
100. Bortoli A, Pedersen N, Duricova D, et al. Pregnancy outcome in inflammatory bowel disease: prospective European case-control ECCO-EpiCom study, 2003-2006. Aliment Pharmacol Ther 2011;34:724–34.
101. Getahun D, Fassett M, Longstreth G, et al. Association between maternal inflammatory bowel disease and adverse perinatal outcomes. J Perinatol 2014;34:435–40.

Interdisciplinary Management of Perianal Crohn's Disease

Amy L. Lightner, MD[a,*], William A. Faubion, MD[b], Joel G. Fletcher, MD[c]

KEYWORDS

- Perianal fistulizing disease • Crohn's disease
- Combined medical and surgical management

KEY POINTS

- Perianal Crohn's disease (CD) is notoriously difficult to treat and often requires a multidisciplinary team of gastroenterologists, surgeons, and radiologist to best determine the management of the patient.
- Medical options for perianal CD most commonly include antibiotic therapy and biologic therapy.
- The primary surgical treatment is drainage of sepsis and placement of a seton for ongoing drainage.
- Many other surgical options, such as fistulotomy or advancement flaps, are not feasible if there is evidence of impaired wound healing or the presence of proctitis.
- Emerging stem cell–based therapies are promising, with safety and efficacy shown in several clinical trials.

INTRODUCTION

Perianal fistula is one of the most common manifestations of Crohn's disease (CD). At least 26% of patients with CD develop perianal fistulas in the first 2 decades following diagnosis,[1–4] particularly those with colonic and rectal involvement.[1] Achieving complete fistula healing is commonly an arduous process involving multiple medical and surgical treatments followed by multiple relapses. The resulting morbidity greatly affects patients' quality of life because of pain, discharge, and abscess formation, and often results in difficulty maintaining a job.

Disclosures: None.
[a] Division of Colon and Rectal Surgery, Mayo Clinic, 200 1st Street Southwest, Rochester, MN 55905, USA; [b] Division of Gastroenterology, Mayo Clinic, 200 1st Street Southwest, Rochester, MN 55905, USA; [c] Division of Radiology, Mayo Clinic, 200 1st Street Southwest, Rochester, MN 55905, USA
* Corresponding author.
E-mail address: Lightner.amy@mayo.edu

Gastroenterol Clin N Am 46 (2017) 547–562
http://dx.doi.org/10.1016/j.gtc.2017.05.008
0889-8553/17/

In approximately 10% of patients, a perianal fistula is the initial manifestation of CD.[1] The formation of a perianal fistula may precede the onset of intestinal CD by several years.[1,5] Of note, the presence of a fistula is an indicator of more aggressive disease that may require more frequent hospitalizations, higher incidence of surgery, and increased use of steroid treatment.[6] Perianal fistulas are notoriously difficult to treat. Given the significant morbidity associated with perianal fistulas, the diagnosis, assessment, and treatment of perianal fistulas mandates a multidisciplinary approach involving gastroenterologists, surgeons, and radiologists at a specialized referral center.

DIAGNOSIS

Diagnosis is most often initiated by the presence of drainage on physical examination, air or stool in the urine in the setting of fistulization to the bladder, or new onset of high-output liquid stool in the setting of an internal fistula. Following a careful history and physical examination, imaging is of paramount importance in diagnosis and classification of fistulas. Of the currently used methods for mapping fistula anatomy, examination under anesthesia (EUA), MRI of the pelvis, and endoanal ultrasonography (EUS) all show similar accuracies.[7–10] Although the gold standard for diagnosis remains undefined, when combining EUA and MRI, diagnostic accuracy approaches 100%.[10] In addition, an international consensus report has recommended the use of MRI (**Figs. 1** and **2**)[11,12] and clinical examination to assess fistula closure in clinical trials.[13]

Treatment Goals and Classification of Healing

The primary goal for the patient is to reduce or eliminate fistula secretion and abscess risk. In addition, avoidance of a stoma and fecal incontinence are critical to consider when treating a fistula.

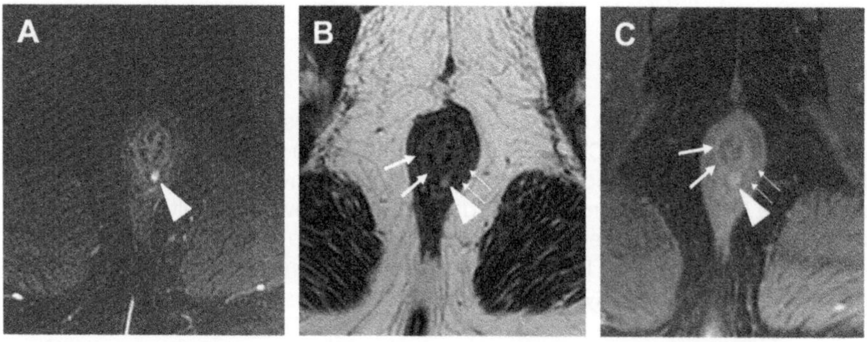

Fig. 1. Simple intersphincteric perianal fistula showing typical imaging characteristics. Axial T2-weighted fast spin-echo image with fat saturation (*A*) shows a hyperintense fistula (*A, arrowhead*). T2-weighted fast spin-echo image with fat saturation shows that the fistula (*B, arrowhead*) is located between the internal (*B, larger arrows*) and external anal sphincter (*B, small arrows*). After gadolinium enhancement, the internal anal sphincter (*C, large arrows*) enhances to a greater degree than the external anal sphincter (*C, small arrows*), which enhances similar to skeletal muscle. The intersphincteric fistula enhances avidly because of internal granulation tissue (*C, arrowhead*). Multiplanar T2-weighted fast spin-echo images without fat saturation permit classification of the fistula as an intersphincteric fistula that arises below the level of the puborectalis, and has an external opening along the left gluteal cleft.

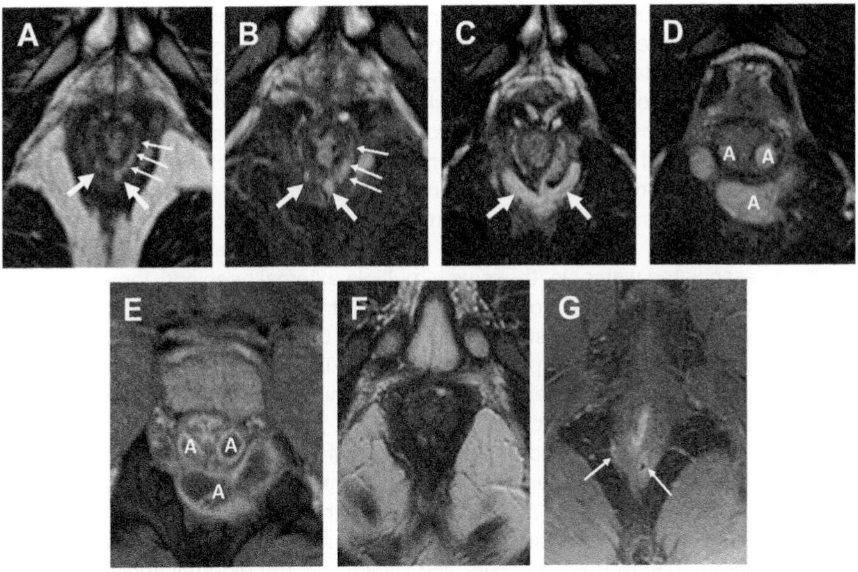

Fig. 2. Axial T2-weighted fast spin-echo images without and with fat saturation show 2 intersphincteric fistulas (*A, B, arrows*), 1 with a horseshoe ramification in the left intersphincteric space (*A, B, small arrows*). Axial T2-weighted fast spin-echo image more superiorly shows supralevator extensions involving the posterior anal space with horseshoe extensions bilaterally involving the external anal sphincter and levator (*C, arrows*). Axial fast spin-echo T2-weighted image (*D*) and T1-weighted images with fat saturation and gadolinium enhancement (*E*) show nonenhancing fluid, indicating that the horseshoe and intramural collections are abscesses (A). Follow-up MRI after incision and drainage of abscesses, placement of draining setons, and initiation of vedolizumab (*F, G*) show complete resolution of abscesses and diminution in size and abnormal signal associated with the fistulous tracts, with hypointense setons in place (*G, arrows*).

The results of treatment can be classified as closure, improvement, remission, or definitive fistula closure.[14] Closure of the individual fistula is considered the cessation of drainage when light manual compression is applied. Improvement refers to a reduction in the open or secreting fistula by greater than 50% compared with the baseline level on at least 2 consecutive examinations at least 1 month following fistula treatment. Remission refers to the closure of all fistulas in relation to the baseline level on at least 2 consecutive examinations, at least 1 month following the treatment intervention for the fistula. Definitive fistula closure refers to complete closure of the fistula, where probing to open the tract is not feasible and the fistula cannot be visualized on MRI.

Another simplified and commonly used classification of treatment success in perianal fistulas is clinical and radiographic healing. Clinical resolution refers to decreased drainage, or cessation of drainage in the case of complete clinical resolution. Radiographic healing refers to scarring or resolution of the fistula tract identified on initial imaging, which most commonly, and most accurately, is determined by MRI.

Classification of Perianal Fistula from Crohn's Disease (Expansion of the Parks Classification)

In approximately 10% of patients, a perianal fistula is the initial manifestation of CD.[1] The formation of perianal fistulas may precede the onset of intestinal CD by several years.[1] Patients with colonic CD, particularly those with active proctitis, have a significantly higher incidence of perianal fistulas than patients without colorectal disease. Perianal fistulas can be classified as low, high, simple, or complex. Low refers to perianal fistulas originating below the dentate line, whereas high fistulas originate above the dentate line. Simple fistulas are those that are low and painless with a single external opening and no evidence of rectovaginal involvement or anorectal stricture.[3] The definition of a complex fistula is not standardized but most clinicians agree that any fistula that is high transsphincteric, or when a fistulotomy would result in incontinence, the fistula should be considered to be complex. The definition also includes all those caused by CD, those associated with pain, those with multiple external openings, those involving a rectovaginal component, or those with anorectal stricture or active proctitis.

Parks and colleagues'[15] classification of perianal CD classifies anal fistulas based on their relationship to the anal sphincter complex.[15] The nomenclature reflects the fistula's relationship to the external sphincter: intersphincteric, transsphincteric, suprasphincteric, and extrasphincteric (**Fig. 3**).

An intersphincteric fistula occurs in 20% to 45% of cases[16] and does not penetrate the external sphincter. Parks and colleagues[15] described 7 subtypes of intersphincteric fistula, of which a high blind tract with an extension in the intersphincteric groove cephalad toward the rectum was the most common. A transsphincteric fistula occurs in 30% to 60% of cases and penetrates the external sphincter below the level of the puborectalis muscle, exiting into varying levels within the ischiorectal fossa. A suprasphincteric fistula occurs in 20% of cases, and describes a fistula tract that is over the top of the puborectalis, then turns down again through the levator plate to the ischiorectal fossa and finally out the skin. As this tract passes over the puborectalis, it is in the supralevator space, and abscess formation in this space can result in horseshoe extension around the rectum. Extrasphincteric fistula, which is the least

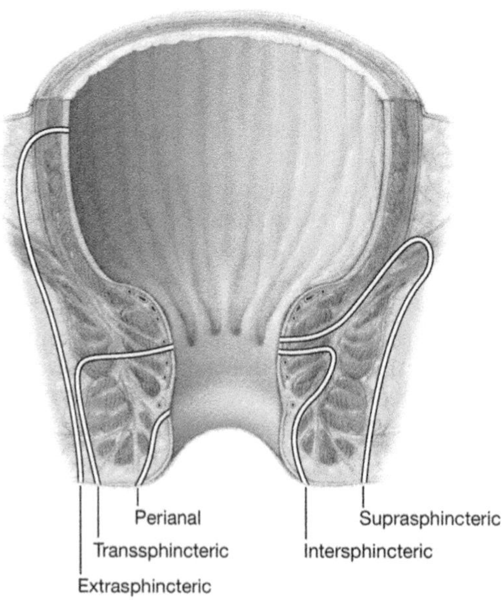

Fig. 3. Parks and colleagues'[15] classification of perianal CD classifies anal fistulas based on their relationship to the anal sphincter complex. The nomenclature reflects the fistula's relationship to the external sphincter: intersphincteric, transsphincteric, suprasphincteric, and extrasphincteric. (*Courtesy of* Mayo Foundation for Medical Education and Research; with permission.)

common, occurring in 2% to 5% of cases, passes from the perineal skin through the ischiorectal fat and levator muscles into the rectum.

Simple and complex fistula

Medical management The medical options for perianal fistulizing CD significantly changed after the introduction of anti–tumor necrosis factor (TNF) biologic therapy in refractory CD in the late 1990s. Before the landmark trial of infliximab in Crohn's-related fistulas,[14] the only real medical options for this complication were antibiotics. Despite a lack of controlled efficacy data, the use of oral antibiotic therapy for fistulas was well established. A small, double-blind, placebo controlled clinical trial showed more frequent response to ciprofloxacin 500 mg twice a day compared with metronidazole 500 mg twice a day; however, the differences were not significant in this very small pilot trial.[17] As referred to earlier, the emergence of the anti-TNF infliximab in patients with CD greatly improved medical response rates. Closure of fistulas occurred in 55% of patients over 3 months; however, the response was durable in only 36% of patients over 1 year.[14,18]Despite modest long-term remission rates, infliximab maintenance therapy leads to fewer hospitalizations and surgical procedures.[19]

The efficacy of the subsequent anti-TNF therapies, adalimumab and certolizumab, has been assessed to varying degrees of rigor in populations of patients either naive or refractory to infliximab. Blinded clinical trials and open-label experience of adalimumab in active CD showed similar efficacy to infliximab (approximately 40% rate of fistula healing) with sustained response over 2 years.[20,21] Subgroup analysis of fistulizing patients from PRECiSE 2 (PEGylated Antibody Fragment Evaluation in Crohn's Disease Safety and Efficacy), a randomized clinical trial of certolizumab in Crohn's disease, also reported a 36% remission rate at 26 weeks.[22] In general, the combination of an anti-TNF agent with ciprofloxacin has been reported to be more effective than either infliximab[23] or adalimumab[24] alone.

Emerging therapies for CD are now under study in this particularly refractory disease manifestation. Subgroup analysis for GEMINI II (Study of Vedolizumab [MLN0002] in Patients With Moderate to Severe Crohn's Disease), a registration trial for vedolizumab in CD, recently reported the probability of fistula closure at 52 weeks among the 57 patients with 1 or more draining fistulas to be 33%.[25] Notably, although the number of patients at risk was small, approximately half the patients had failed prior anti-TNF therapy, suggesting a highly refractory group of patients. Although the newest approved agent, ustekinumab, has yet to undergo formal prospective study in fistulas, recent publication of a multicenter open-label experience suggests effectiveness in fistulas as well.[26]

As discussed more fully later, the management of complex perianal CD is a synergistic exercise between the surgeon and gastrointestinal physician. Drainage of current sepsis and control of future abscess formation through seton placement is essential for optimized probability of healing. The published experience suggests that the presence of complex perianal fistulas warrants biologic therapy, and the bulk of the data reside in the anti-TNF experience. Furthermore, there seems to be an adjunctive role for combination therapy with antibiotics, and this is certainly true in the perioperative period around the control of perianal sepsis. The authors frequently provide 6 weeks to 3 months of antibiotic adjunctive therapy around the time of seton placement, and are vigilant for the long-term neurologic effects of metronidazole. Despite optimal drainage, long-term healing in response to the most effective medical regimens continues to be in the 40% range, indicating the continued need to innovate in this highly morbid condition.

Surgical options Whether the fistula is simple or complex, up to 90% of patients with perianal CD require operative treatment, and many require more than 1 operative intervention.[4] When operations for perianal CD are performed, it is often difficult to achieve complete healing, and surgical interventions put patients at risk for incontinence.[27] The high risk of incontinence is caused by the complex nature of CD, characterized by frequent diarrhea, and the need for multiple operative interventions that put the sphincter complex at risk. Patients with perianal CD are also at risk for prolonged fistula healing and frequent recurrences. In complex perianal fistulas, the durable remission rates, despite all available medical and surgical options, remain as low as 37%.[28] This number may even be higher because many studies are not able to provide long-term follow-up.[1,4,29–32]

Therefore, the risk of iatrogenic injury and poor wound healing combined with disappointing surgical treatment outcomes culminates in a conservative approach to the surgical management of perianal CD. Surgical treatment options are often based on the location and branching of the fistula and include seton placement, fistulotomy, fibrin glue or plug, advancement flaps, fecal diversion, and (as a last resort) proctectomy.

Incision and drainage of abscesses The most common operative intervention for perianal CD is incision and drainage of a perianal abscess or undrained fistula.[33] Although small (<1 cm) clinically silent abscesses found on imaging may be treated with medical therapy alone,[34] clinically symptomatic abscesses require incision and drainage to control sepsis.[35,36] Although many abscesses represent an underlying fistula tract, perianal abscesses can be a complication of infliximab treatment,[37] and the number of perianal abscesses has increased 3-fold since the approval of biologics for the treatment of CD.[38]

Seton placement A noncutting seton is the most effective treatment modality used for complex fistulas in CD to drain fistula tracts and prevent ongoing sepsis.[39–44] A noncutting seton is a nonabsorbable suture (or vessel loop) that is passed through a fistula tract and secured loosely in place, allowing the fistula tract to remain open and drain any ongoing source of sepsis (**Fig. 4**). The risk of sphincter damage is exceeding low, and setons can be left in place long term while medical treatments are used. In a randomized control trial, placement of a seton before infliximab induction produced improved perianal fistula healing compared with infliximab alone at 3 months.[14,18,45]

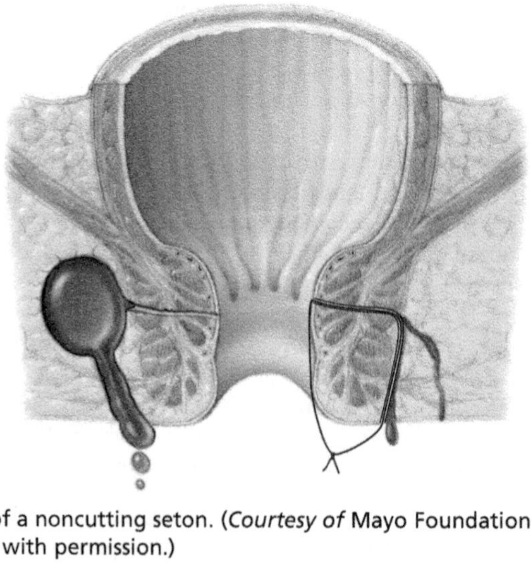

Fig. 4. Placement of a noncutting seton. (*Courtesy of* Mayo Foundation for Medical Education and Research; with permission.)

The difficulty with setons is the decision of when to remove them. However, when setons are removed, the recurrence rate of local sepsis is up to 70%[39,46] and rates of fistula recurrence may be as high as 80% at 10 years following seton placement.[9] Regardless, in general, setons can result in healing or can be seen as a bridge to a more definitive procedure in the setting of active perianal disease or proctitis.

Fistulotomy The use of a fistulotomy for perianal CD depends on the location of the amount of sphincter complex involved in the fistula (**Fig. 5**). For patients with a low fistula, not involving the sphincter complex, most studies report healing rates of 80% to 100%.[3] Without active proctitis, healing rates may be up to 95%, and recurrence rates only 15%.[47–49] However, with active proctocolitis, healing rates decreased from 83% to 27%,[50] showing the lack of efficacy in this clinical scenario. Therefore, for patients with active rectal disease, the authors recommend that the fistula should be treated with a non-cutting seton and concomitant medical therapy.[45] Caution should also be used in patients who have diarrhea, women with anterior fistulas, and patients with short anal canals.[36]

Similar results may be achieved in patients with simple intersphincteric and transphincteric fistulas,[44,46,48] despite the hesitation expressed by surgeons because of the risk of incontinence. However, once greater than one-third of a sphincter is involved, a fistulotomy is no longer appropriate, with more than 50% of patients expressing some degree of incontinence.[46]

Fibrin glue and fistula plug Fibrin glue and bioprosthetic anal fistula plugs have the advantage of avoiding sphincter injury, especially in high-risk patients with CD (**Figs. 6** and **7**). Fibrin glue is a mixture of fibrinogen and thrombin that is injected into the fistula tract with a catheter and results in a fibrin clot sealing the tract. This clot is thought to promote wound healing. Initial small series reported excellent healing rates.[11,12] However, the largest prospective randomized trial across 12 centers found clinical remission (absence of purulence with gentle compression) in 38% at 8 weeks compared with 16% in the observation group (P = .04).[51] This group did not assess healing with MRI or EUS, which suggests that this success rate may even be lower than the reported 38%. In addition, the lack of follow-up beyond 8 weeks leaves the durability of this treatment option in question. Although the use of fibrin glue is a low-risk option, the low overall healing rate and high risk of recurrence make this a less desirable treatment option.

Fistula plugs are a bioabsorbable matrix inserted into the fistula tract and sutured in place. They are designed for fistula healing while preserving continence.

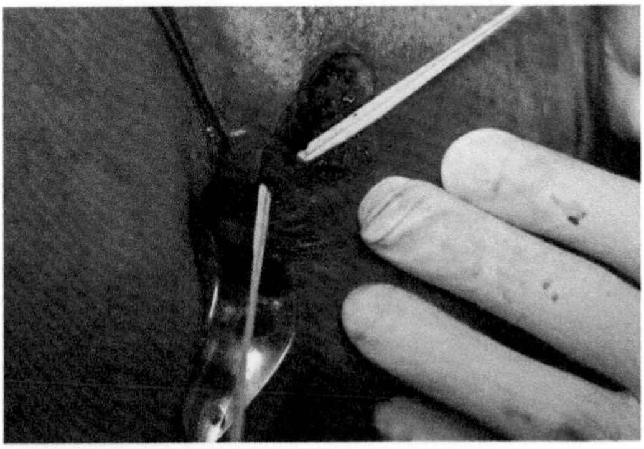

Fig. 5. Fistulotomy: opening of the fistula tract. (*Courtesy of* Mayo Foundation for Medical Education and Research; with permission.)

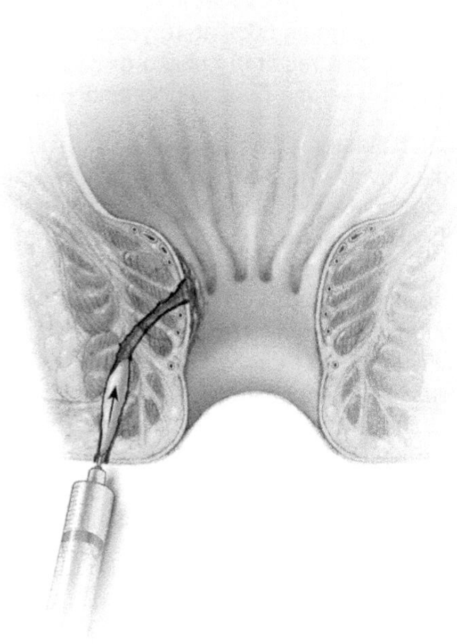

Fig. 6. Fibrin glue injection into a fistula tract. (*Courtesy of* Mayo Foundation for Medical Education and Research; with permission.)

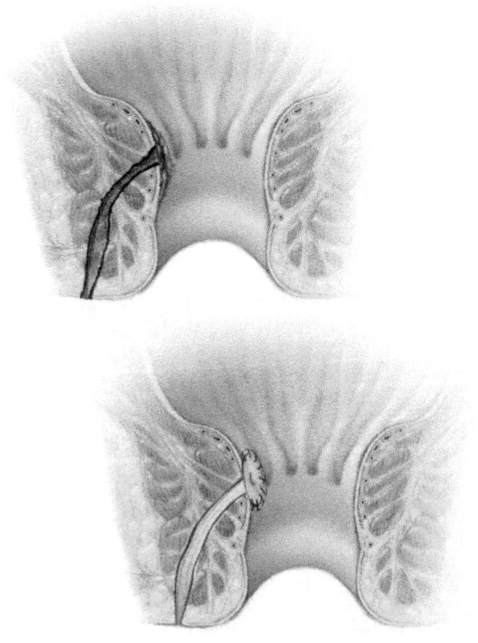

Fig. 7. Use of a fistula plug. (*Courtesy of* Mayo Foundation for Medical Education and Research; with permission.)

O'Connor and colleagues[52] reported an 80% closure rate of perianal fistulas after a median of 10 months' follow-up in a series of 20 patients with CD. The primary risk factor for failure was the presence of multiple fistulous tracts. Note that use of anti-TNF-α therapy did not correlate with outcomes.[52] Two subsequent systematic reviews regarding efficacy of the anal fistula plug for perianal CD showed a 55% success rate[53] and 58% success rate[54] of the procedure. The Surgisis and GORE BIO-A brand plugs were compared, and Surgisis had 60% healing (n = 48 of 80), whereas GORE had 25% healing (n = 1 of 4). Of the 5 studies that reported recurrence, 3 of 22 (13.6%) experienced recurrence after treatment of their fistulas. Despite moderate healing rates, incontinence has not been reported with the use of a plug.

Endorectal advancement flap An endorectal advancement flap involves creating a full-thickness or partial-thickness U-shaped flap of endogenous rectal tissue to cover the internal opening of a fistula (**Fig. 8**). Although the concept is to close off the high-pressure end of the fistula without division of any sphincter muscle, incontinence has been reported[30] at a rate of up to 10%,[55,56] and this risk increases with multiple flap repairs.[31,57,58] If the initial repair fails, there is an option to perform a second and third attempt. The efficacy of the repair is significantly decreased in patients with CD, and proctitis and anal stenoses are contraindications caused by poor healing.[31,59] Because of poor healing in this setting, some surgeons use a diverting stoma[60] before performing an endorectal advancement flap.

Rates of successful healing with this procedure are highly variable, reported anywhere from 25% to 64%.[30–32,39,60,61] In a systematic review of 35 studies including 1654 patients, the overall success rate of endorectal advancement flaps in CD was

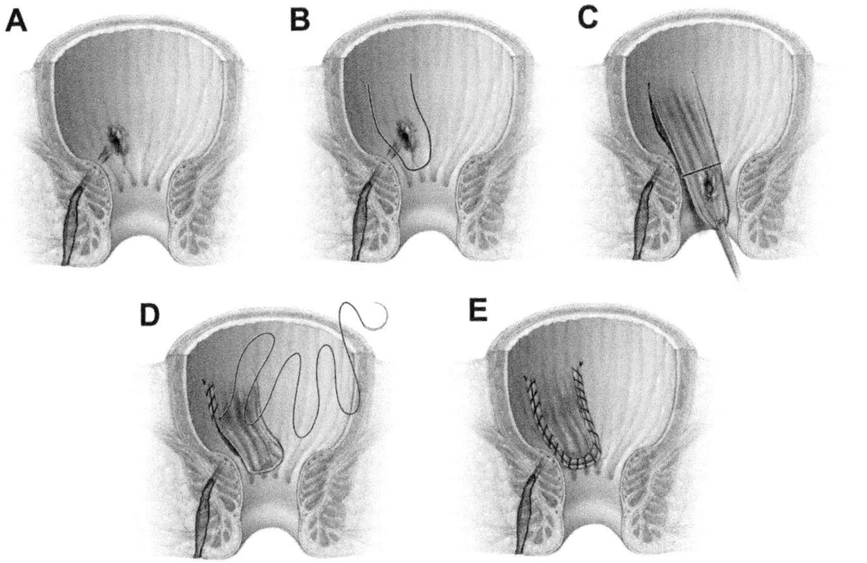

Fig. 8. An endorectal advancement flap involves creating a full-thickness or partial-thickness U-shaped flap of endogenous rectal tissue to cover the internal opening of a fistula. (*A*) Identification of the fistula tract, (*B*) currettting of the fistula tract, (*C*) creation of partial thickness rectal flap, (*D*) advancement of the flap over the internal opening of the fistula tract, and (*E*) mucosa now covering the internal opening of the fistula tract. (*Courtesy of* Mayo Foundation for Medical Education and Research; with permission.)

64% compared with 81% in patients without CD.[55] Only 3 of 16 studies reported on incontinence rates among patients with CD specifically; the reported rate at an average follow-up of 29 months was 9%. Although these reported success rates seem to offer a reasonable treatment approach, the authors recommend careful patient selection because of the poor healing associated with proctitis, and the risk of incontinence.

Ligation of intersphincteric tract procedure First described by Rojanasakul in 2007,[62] the ligation of intersphincteric fistula tract (LIFT) is a procedure designed to close complex fistulas with complete sphincter preservation. It is performed by making an incision at the intersphincteric groove, identifying the intersphincteric tract, ligating the ends at the internal and external sphincter sides, and removing the fistula tract between the 2 ligated openings[63] (**Fig. 9**). There are limited data on this technique in patients with CD because of the rare use in this patient population.

The largest series to date in patients with CD is a single-center series of 15 patients. Fistula healing was observed in 60% of patients at 2 months and 67% of patients at 1 year. There was no reported incontinence, suggesting that this may be a good surgical technique if no proctitis is present. In a series of 15 patients with CD, Gingold and

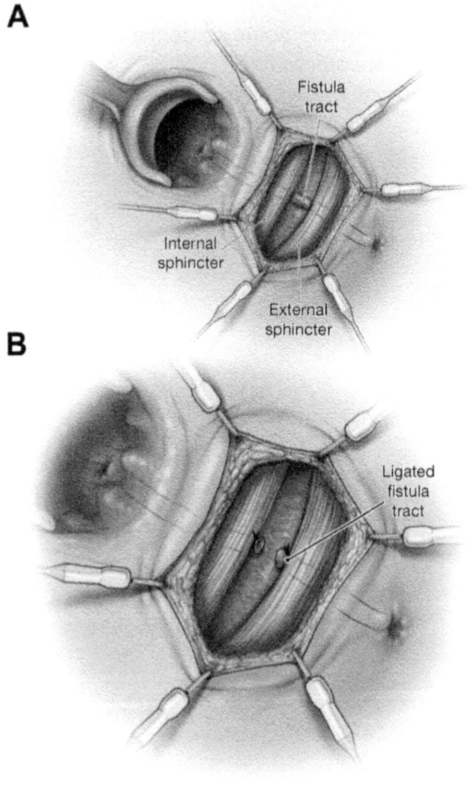

Fig. 9. LIFT procedure is a procedure designed to close complex fistulas with complete sphincter preservation. (*A*) Entering the space between the internal and external sphincter to identify the fistula tract, (*B*) The fistula tract is cut and trimmed. Suture ligation is performed on both ends, close to the internal and external sphincters. (*Courtesy of* Mayo Foundation for Medical Education and Research; with permission.)

colleagues[64] showed a 67% wound healing rate at 1-year follow-up without any fecal incontinence. Significant factors for long-term LIFT site healing were lateral versus midline location and longer mean fistula tract length.[64] Although additional data are needed regarding the LIFT procedure in the CD population, it seems to be a safe and effective surgical treatment option.

Fecal diversion The concept of fecal diversion is to divert the fecal stream from the fistula sites and allow healing. Although fecal diversion does improve long-term quality of life,[2] it has limited success for long-term perianal healing. In a large meta-analysis of 556 patients, 64% of patients experienced an early clinical response with perianal healing.[65] However, only 17% of patients had a successful restoration of bowel continuity, and, of these patients, 27% required rediversion or multiple subsequent interventions to treat their fistulas. Overall, 42% of patients ultimately required a proctectomy. The only factor found to be associated with restoration of continuity was absence of proctitis.

Proctectomy Proctectomy is seen as the last, and definitive, resort for healing perianal CD. Many patients undergo many attempts at intervention before succumbing to a proctectomy. In 1 series of 87 patients treated at St Mark's Hospital, the median number of treatment attempts before a proctectomy was 12, and the median time to proctectomy was 6.3 years.[29] The reported rates of proctectomy performed for perineal CD are 8% to 40%.[66] This rate is higher in patients with multiple operations for perianal disease,[33,58] the use of previous temporary fecal diversion (42%),[65] Crohn's colitis with rectal sparing (46%), and Crohn's colitis with proctitis (89%).[1] In our own long-term series of patients at Mayo Clinic with anorectal Crohn's, the rates of proctectomy at 10 and 20 years were 8.4% and 17.5%, respectively.[67]

If a proctectomy is needed, perineal wound management becomes a significant issue of concern. The authors have chosen as our standard an intersphincteric dissection to decrease postoperative surgical site morbidity.[67] In patients with severe perianal sepsis, a diverting laparoscopic ileostomy followed by proctocolectomy in 6 to 12 weeks results in fewer wound complications.[68] However, for those patients with large perineal defects or continued extensive sepsis, myocutaneous advancement flaps are likely the best option to obtain proper healing and closure.[69,70] In addition, rectus abdominis flaps seem to have better healing than gracilis flaps.[6,69]

Emerging therapies Mesenchymal stem cells (MSCs) are an emerging therapy that has shown great promise in phase I, II, and now III clinical trials. The initial phase I trial by Garcia-Olmo and colleagues[71] in Spain studied injection of autologous adipose-derived MSCs into 4 patients; 3 patients achieved healing (75%) at 9 weeks and there were no adverse events noted at 12-week and 22-week follow-up.[71] A later phase II study by the same group observed perianal fistula healing in 71% of the 7 patients treated with MSCs incorporated into fibrin glue versus 16% in those treated with fibrin group alone ($P<.001$).[72] Another phase II trial from a group in Korea found that autologous adipose-derived MSCs injected directly into perianal Crohn's fistula tracts with fibrin glue resulted in 82% healing at 2 months, with 88% of these patients having sustained healing at 1 year.[73] A recent phase III study of allogeneic adipose-derived MSCs found 50% (n = 53 of 107) healing in the MSC group compared with 34% in the placebo group (n = 36 of 105; $P = .024$) at 24 weeks.[74] In all clinical trials to date, there have been no adverse events related to the MSCs or the procedure for insertion, underscoring the safety of this treatment and the lack of risk for incontinence. Although these results are promising, the use of MSCs remains investigational and has not become a widespread treatment option.

PREDICTORS OF RECURRENCE

The strongest predictors of recurrence are active colitis, proctitis, and complex fistulas. Crohn's colitis is associated with a recurrence rate of 84% to 100%.[1,30,44,50] In a small series of 3 patients who attempted to treat perianal fistulas in the setting of severe colitis, none healed with a temporary stoma and biologic medications; all ended up requiring a permanent stoma.[75] One study of 513 patients with CD reported a 67% proctectomy rate in patients with proctitis versus 11% without macroscopic rectal involvement.[35] Complex fistulas also require an increased number of procedures and a high rate of fecal diversion.[30] In chronic, nonhealing fistulas, clinicians should always have a high index of suspicion for malignancy, and should consider biopsy of the tract[76]; half of malignancies are found to be adenocarcinoma and the other half are squamous cell carcinoma.[76]

SUMMARY

Fistulizing CD is a particularly morbid phenotype of CD, and affects nearly half of all patients with CD. If often portends an increased severity of disease with worse overall prognosis. Appropriate classification and anatomic mapping are critical for identifying effective treatment strategies. Much of the anatomic information comes from imaging, primarily MRI for perianal disease. Once the appropriate classification is given, treatment can ensue with a hope to alleviate symptoms or cure the fistula tract. Treatment may include a combination of medical management and surgical intervention. Emerging stem cell–based therapies present a promising option for the treatment of perianal disease. Given the challenge in effectively treating perianal CD, a multidisciplinary approach should be taken to maximize patient benefit.

REFERENCES

1. Hellers G, Bergstrand O, Ewerth S, et al. Occurrence and outcome after primary treatment of anal fistulae in Crohn's disease. Gut 1980;21(6):525–7.
2. Kasparek MS, Glatzle J, Temeltcheva T, et al. Long-term quality of life in patients with Crohn's disease and perianal fistulas: influence of fecal diversion. Dis Colon Rectum 2007;50(12):2067–74.
3. Sandborn WJ, Fazio VW, Feagan BG, et al, American Gastroenterological Association Clinical Practice Committee. AGA technical review on perianal Crohn's disease. Gastroenterology 2003;125(5):1508–30.
4. Schwartz DA, Loftus EV Jr, Tremaine WJ, et al. The natural history of fistulizing Crohn's disease in Olmsted County, Minnesota. Gastroenterology 2002;122(4):875–80.
5. Safar B, Sands D. Perianal Crohn's disease. Clin Colon Rectal Surg 2007;20(4):282–93.
6. Schaden D, Schauer G, Haas F, et al. Myocutaneous flaps and proctocolectomy in severe perianal Crohn's disease–a single stage procedure. Int J Colorectal Dis 2007;22(12):1453–7.
7. Beckingham IJ, Spencer JA, Ward J, et al. Prospective evaluation of dynamic contrast enhanced magnetic resonance imaging in the evaluation of fistula in ano. Br J Surg 1996;83(10):1396–8.
8. Beets-Tan RG, Beets GL, van der Hoop AG, et al. Preoperative MR imaging of anal fistulas: does it really help the surgeon? Radiology 2001;218(1):75–84.

9. Buchanan GN, Halligan S, Bartram CI, et al. Clinical examination, endosonography, and MR imaging in preoperative assessment of fistula in ano: comparison with outcome-based reference standard. Radiology 2004;233(3):674–81.
10. Schwartz DA, Wiersema MJ, Dudiak KM, et al. A comparison of endoscopic ultrasound, magnetic resonance imaging, and exam under anesthesia for evaluation of Crohn's perianal fistulas. Gastroenterology 2001;121(5):1064–72.
11. Abel ME, Chiu YS, Russell TR, et al. Autologous fibrin glue in the treatment of rectovaginal and complex fistulas. Dis Colon Rectum 1993;36(5):447–9.
12. Zmora O, Mizrahi N, Rotholtz N, et al. Fibrin glue sealing in the treatment of perineal fistulas. Dis Colon Rectum 2003;46(5):584–9.
13. Van Assche G, Dignass A, Reinisch W, et al. The second European evidence-based consensus on the diagnosis and management of Crohn's disease: special situations. J Crohns Colitis 2010;4(1):63–101.
14. Present DH, Rutgeerts P, Targan S, et al. Infliximab for the treatment of fistulas in patients with Crohn's disease. N Engl J Med 1999;340(18):1398–405.
15. Parks AG, Gordon PH, Hardcastle JD. A classification of fistula-in-ano. Br J Surg 1976;63(1):1–12.
16. Sileri P, Cadeddu F, D'Ugo S, et al. Surgery for fistula-in-ano in a specialist colorectal unit: a critical appraisal. BMC Gastroenterol 2011;11:120.
17. Thia KT, Mahadevan U, Feagan BG, et al. Ciprofloxacin or metronidazole for the treatment of perianal fistulas in patients with Crohn's disease: a randomized, double-blind, placebo-controlled pilot study. Inflamm Bowel Dis 2009;15(1):17–24.
18. Sands BE, Anderson FH, Bernstein CN, et al. Infliximab maintenance therapy for fistulizing Crohn's disease. N Engl J Med 2004;350(9):876–85.
19. Lichtenstein GR, Yan S, Bala M, et al. Infliximab maintenance treatment reduces hospitalizations, surgeries, and procedures in fistulizing Crohn's disease. Gastroenterology 2005;128(4):862–9.
20. Colombel JF, Schwartz DA, Sandborn WJ, et al. Adalimumab for the treatment of fistulas in patients with Crohn's disease. Gut 2009;58(7):940–8.
21. Lichtiger S, Binion DG, Wolf DC, et al. The CHOICE trial: adalimumab demonstrates safety, fistula healing, improved quality of life and increased work productivity in patients with Crohn's disease who failed prior infliximab therapy. Aliment Pharmacol Ther 2010;32(10):1228–39.
22. Schreiber S, Lawrance IC, Thomsen OO, et al. Randomised clinical trial: certolizumab pegol for fistulas in Crohn's disease - subgroup results from a placebo-controlled study. Aliment Pharmacol Ther 2011;33(2):185–93.
23. West RL, van der Woude CJ, Hansen BE, et al. Clinical and endosonographic effect of ciprofloxacin on the treatment of perianal fistulae in Crohn's disease with infliximab: a double-blind placebo-controlled study. Aliment Pharmacol Ther 2004;20(11–12):1329–36.
24. Dewint P, Hansen BE, Verhey E, et al. Adalimumab combined with ciprofloxacin is superior to adalimumab monotherapy in perianal fistula closure in Crohn's disease: a randomised, double-blind, placebo controlled trial (ADAFI). Gut 2014;63(2):292–9.
25. Feagan BG, Sandborn WJ, D'Haens G, et al. Randomised clinical trial: vercirnon, an oral CCR9 antagonist, vs. placebo as induction therapy in active Crohn's disease. Aliment Pharmacol Ther 2015;42(10):1170–81.
26. Khorrami S, Ginard D, Marin-Jimenez I, et al. Ustekinumab for the treatment of refractory Crohn's disease: the Spanish experience in a large multicentre open-label cohort. Inflamm Bowel Dis 2016;22(7):1662–9.

27. Keighley MR, Allan RN. Current status and influence of operation on perianal Crohn's disease. Int J Colorectal Dis 1986;1(2):104–7.
28. Molendijk I, Nuij VJ, van der Meulen-de Jong AE, et al. Disappointing durable remission rates in complex Crohn's disease fistula. Inflamm Bowel Dis 2014; 20(11):2022–8.
29. Bell SJ, Williams AB, Wiesel P, et al. The clinical course of fistulating Crohn's disease. Aliment Pharmacol Ther 2003;17(9):1145–51.
30. Makowiec F, Jehle EC, Starlinger M. Clinical course of perianal fistulas in Crohn's disease. Gut 1995;37(5):696–701.
31. Mizrahi N, Wexner SD, Zmora O, et al. Endorectal advancement flap: are there predictors of failure? Dis Colon Rectum 2002;45(12):1616–21.
32. Williamson PR, Hellinger MD, Larach SW, et al. Twenty-year review of the surgical management of perianal Crohn's disease. Dis Colon Rectum 1995;38(4):389–92.
33. Fichera A, Michelassi F. Surgical treatment of Crohn's disease. J Gastrointest Surg 2007;11(6):791–803.
34. Shenoy-Bhangle A, Nimkin K, Goldner D, et al. MRI predictors of treatment response for perianal fistulizing Crohn disease in children and young adults. Pediatr Radiol 2014;44(1):23–9.
35. Hurst RD, Molinari M, Chung TP, et al. Prospective study of the features, indications, and surgical treatment in 513 consecutive patients affected by Crohn's disease. Surgery 1997;122(4):661–7 [discussion: 667–8].
36. Judge TA, Lichtenstein GR. Treatment of fistulizing Crohn's disease. Gastroenterol Clin North Am 2004;33(2):421–54, xi-xii.
37. Poritz LS, Rowe WA, Koltun WA. Remicade does not abolish the need for surgery in fistulizing Crohn's disease. Dis Colon Rectum 2002;45(6):771–5.
38. Jones DW, Finlayson SR. Trends in surgery for Crohn's disease in the era of infliximab. Ann Surg 2010;252(2):307–12.
39. Faucheron JL, Saint-Marc O, Guibert L, et al. Long-term seton drainage for high anal fistulas in Crohn's disease–a sphincter-saving operation? Dis Colon Rectum 1996;39(2):208–11.
40. Halme L, Sainio AP. Factors related to frequency, type, and outcome of anal fistulas in Crohn's disease. Dis Colon Rectum 1995;38(1):55–9.
41. Pearl RK, Andrews JR, Orsay CP, et al. Role of the seton in the management of anorectal fistulas. Dis Colon Rectum 1993;36(6):573–7 [discussion: 577–9].
42. Sangwan YP, Schoetz DJ Jr, Murray JJ, et al. Perianal Crohn's disease. Results of local surgical treatment. Dis Colon Rectum 1996;39(5):529–35.
43. Thornton M, Solomon MJ. Long-term indwelling seton for complex anal fistulas in Crohn's disease. Dis Colon Rectum 2005;48(3):459–63.
44. Williams JG, Rothenberger DA, Nemer FD, et al. Fistula-in-ano in Crohn's disease. Results of aggressive surgical treatment. Dis Colon Rectum 1991;34(5):378–84.
45. Regueiro M, Mardini H. Treatment of perianal fistulizing Crohn's disease with infliximab alone or as an adjunct to exam under anesthesia with seton placement. Inflamm Bowel Dis 2003;9(2):98–103.
46. Williams JG, MacLeod CA, Rothenberger DA, et al. Seton treatment of high anal fistulae. Br J Surg 1991;78(10):1159–61.
47. Hobbiss JH, Schofield PF. Management of perianal Crohn's disease. J R Soc Med 1982;75(6):414–7.
48. Morrison JG, Gathright JB Jr, Ray JE, et al. Surgical management of anorectal fistulas in Crohn's disease. Dis Colon Rectum 1989;32(6):492–6.
49. Sohn N, Korelitz BI, Weinstein MA. Anorectal Crohn's disease: definitive surgery for fistulas and recurrent abscesses. Am J Surg 1980;139(3):394–7.

50. Nordgren S, Fasth S, Hulten L. Anal fistulas in Crohn's disease: incidence and outcome of surgical treatment. Int J Colorectal Dis 1992;7(4):214–8.
51. Grimaud JC, Munoz-Bongrand N, Siproudhis L, et al. Fibrin glue is effective healing perianal fistulas in patients with Crohn's disease. Gastroenterology 2010; 138(7):2275–81, 2281.e1.
52. O'Connor L, Champagne BJ, Ferguson MA, et al. Efficacy of anal fistula plug in closure of Crohn's anorectal fistulas. Dis Colon Rectum 2006;49(10):1569–73.
53. O'Riordan JM, Datta I, Johnston C, et al. A systematic review of the anal fistula plug for patients with Crohn's and non-Crohn's related fistula-in-ano. Dis Colon Rectum 2012;55(3):351–8.
54. Nasseri Y, Cassella L, Berns M, et al. The anal fistula plug in Crohn's disease patients with fistula-in-ano: a systematic review. Colorectal Dis 2016;18(4):351–6.
55. Soltani A, Kaiser AM. Endorectal advancement flap for cryptoglandular or Crohn's fistula-in-ano. Dis Colon Rectum 2010;53(4):486–95.
56. van der Hagen SJ, Baeten CG, Soeters PB, et al. Anti-TNF-alpha (infliximab) used as induction treatment in case of active proctitis in a multistep strategy followed by definitive surgery of complex anal fistulas in Crohn's disease: a preliminary report. Dis Colon Rectum 2005;48(4):758–67.
57. Joo JS, Weiss EG, Nogueras JJ, et al. Endorectal advancement flap in perianal Crohn's disease. Am Surg 1998;64(2):147–50.
58. Michelassi F, Melis M, Rubin M, et al. Surgical treatment of anorectal complications in Crohn's disease. Surgery 2000;128(4):597–603.
59. Sonoda T, Hull T, Piedmonte MR, et al. Outcomes of primary repair of anorectal and rectovaginal fistulas using the endorectal advancement flap. Dis Colon Rectum 2002;45(12):1622–8.
60. Fazio VW, Aufses AH Jr. Evolution of surgery for Crohn's disease: a century of progress. Dis Colon Rectum 1999;42(8):979–88.
61. Makowiec F, Jehle EC, Becker HD, et al. Clinical course after transanal advancement flap repair of perianal fistula in patients with Crohn's disease. Br J Surg 1995;82(5):603–6.
62. Rojanasakul A. LIFT procedure: a simplified technique for fistula-in-ano. Tech Coloproctol 2009;13(3):237–40.
63. Rojanasakul A, Pattanaarun J, Sahakitrungruang C, et al. Total anal sphincter saving technique for fistula-in-ano; the ligation of intersphincteric fistula tract. J Med Assoc Thai 2007;90(3):581–6.
64. Gingold DS, Murrell ZA, Fleshner PR. A prospective evaluation of the ligation of the intersphincteric tract procedure for complex anal fistula in patients with Crohn's disease. Ann Surg 2014;260(6):1057–61.
65. Singh S, Ding NS, Mathis KL, et al. Systematic review with meta-analysis: faecal diversion for management of perianal Crohn's disease. Aliment Pharmacol Ther 2015;42(7):783–92.
66. Steele SR, Kumar R, Feingold DL, et al. Practice parameters for the management of perianal abscess and fistula-in-ano. Dis Colon Rectum 2011;54(12):1465–74.
67. Wolff BG, Culp CE, Beart RW Jr, et al. Anorectal Crohn's disease. A long-term perspective. Dis Colon Rectum 1985;28(10):709–11.
68. Mennigen R, Heptner B, Senninger N, et al. Temporary fecal diversion in the management of colorectal and perianal Crohn's disease. Gastroenterol Res Pract 2015;2015:286315.
69. Collie MH, Potter MA, Bartolo DC. Myocutaneous flaps promote perineal healing in inflammatory bowel disease. Br J Surg 2005;92(6):740–1.

70. Windhofer C, Michlits W, Heuberger A, et al. Perineal reconstruction after rectal and anal disease using the local fascio-cutaneous-infragluteal flap: a new and reliable technique. Surgery 2011;149(2):284–90.
71. Garcia-Olmo D, Garcia-Arranz M, Herreros D, et al. A phase I clinical trial of the treatment of Crohn's fistula by adipose mesenchymal stem cell transplantation. Dis Colon Rectum 2005;48(7):1416–23.
72. Garcia-Olmo D, Herreros D, Pascual I, et al. Expanded adipose-derived stem cells for the treatment of complex perianal fistula: a phase II clinical trial. Dis Colon Rectum 2009;52(1):79–86.
73. Lee WY, Park KJ, Cho YB, et al. Autologous adipose tissue-derived stem cells treatment demonstrated favorable and sustainable therapeutic effect for Crohn's fistula. Stem Cells 2013;31(11):2575–81.
74. Panes J, Garcia-Olmo D, Van Assche G, et al. Expanded allogeneic adipose-derived mesenchymal stem cells (Cx601) for complex perianal fistulas in Crohn's disease: a phase 3 randomised, double-blind controlled trial. Lancet 2016; 388(10051):1281–90.
75. Uzzan M, Stefanescu C, Maggiori L, et al. Case series: does a combination of anti-TNF antibodies and transient ileal fecal stream diversion in severe Crohn's colitis with perianal fistula prevent definitive stoma? Am J Gastroenterol 2013; 108(10):1666–8.
76. Ky A, Sohn N, Weinstein MA, et al. Carcinoma arising in anorectal fistulas of Crohn's disease. Dis Colon Rectum 1998;41(8):992–6.

Management of Crohn's Disease After Surgical Resection

Siddharth Singh, MD, MS[a,b,*], Geoffrey C. Nguyen, MD, PhD[c,d,*]

KEYWORDS

• Crohn's disease • Surgery • Prevention • Recurrence

KEY POINTS

- Approximately 25% to 35% of patients require repeat surgery after initial resection for Crohn's disease.
- Smoking, multiple prior surgeries, and penetrating or perianal disease are risk factors associated with disease recurrence.
- Early initiation of anti–tumor necrosis factor agents and immunomodulators within 4 to 8 weeks of surgery is consistently effective in decreasing risk of recurrence of Crohn's disease, whereas the benefit of mesalamine is uncertain.
- Regardless of initial approach to prevention of recurrence of Crohn's disease, active colonoscopic surveillance for early detection of endoscopic recurrence within 6 to 12 months of surgery is recommended.
- In the absence of endoscopic recurrence, noninflammatory causes should be sought for gastrointestinal symptoms such as bile acid malabsorption and small intestinal bacterial overgrowth.

INTRODUCTION

Crohn's disease (CD) is a chronically relapsing inflammatory condition of the gut that leads to complications requiring intestinal resection. Even though surgery often leads to resolution of symptoms, a meta-analysis of population-based cohorts of patients with CD who had undergone initial surgery showed that nearly a quarter of patients

---

Disclosure: Dr S. Singh has received a research grant from Pfizer.
[a] Division of Gastroenterology, University of California San Diego, 9452 Medical Center Drive, ACTRI 1W501, La Jolla, CA 92093, USA; [b] Division of Biomedical Informatics, University of California San Diego, 9452 Medical Center Drive, ACTRI 1W501, La Jolla, CA 92093, USA; [c] Joseph and Wolf Lebovic Health Complex, Mount Sinai Hospital Centre for Inflammatory Bowel Disease, Mount Sinai Hospital, University of Toronto, Suite 437, 600 University Avenue, Toronto, Ontario M5G 1x5, Canada; [d] Institute for Clinical Evaluative Sciences, 155 College Street, Suite 424, Toronto, Ontario M5T 3M6, Canada
* Corresponding authors. Division of Gastroenterology, University of California San Diego, 9452 Medical Center Drive, ACTRI 1W501, La Jolla, CA 92093.
E-mail addresses: sis040@ucsd.edu (S.S.); Geoff.Nguyen@Utoronto.Ca (G.C.N.)

Gastroenterol Clin N Am 46 (2017) 563–575
http://dx.doi.org/10.1016/j.gtc.2017.05.011 gastro.theclinics.com

required a subsequent surgery within 5 years of their first surgery and 35% within a decade.[1] Surgical recurrence is often preceded by clinical recurrence, defined as the presence of inflammatory bowel disease (IBD)–related symptoms, and is observed in 28% to 50% of patients within 5 years.[2] Even before the onset of symptoms, there is endoscopic recurrence just proximal to anastomosis, which serves as a harbinger of need for subsequent surgery, and is observed in 50% to 90% of patients within 5 years of surgery. Significant advances in medical therapy have led to a steady decline in rates of first surgery for CD over the last several decades.[3,4] Although cumulative rates of second intestinal surgery initially decreased between 1970 and the late 1980s, they have not continued to decrease since then.[1,4,5] Thus, there is an opportunity to optimize postoperative management of CD through risk stratification, postoperative surveillance of endoscopic recurrence, and prophylactic medical therapy.

RISK STRATIFICATION OF POSTOPERATIVE RECURRENCE

Risk stratification for disease recurrence following resective surgery is the first critical step in optimizing postoperative outcomes. The identification of high-risk individuals could prompt early medical prophylaxis, whereas low-risk individuals may adopt a more conservative wait-and-monitor approach. Several phenotypic characteristics are associated with increased risk of recurrence. Individuals who underwent initial bowel surgery for fistulizing disease have been shown across multiple observational studies and meta-analyses to have increased risk of endoscopic and surgical recurrence.[6,7] Similarly, the presence of perianal fistula has been linked with increased recurrent surgery.[8] A prior history of 2 or more resective surgeries has also been consistently shown to be associated with higher rates of postoperative endoscopic and surgical recurrence.[9] Numerous studies have also shown that active tobacco smokers have a greater than 2-fold risk of clinical and surgical recurrence compared with nonsmokers and ex-smokers.[10] Other clinical factors that may predispose to disease recurrence include shorter disease duration (<10 years), isolated small bowel or continuous ileocolonic involvement, and young age at diagnosis (<30 years).[2,8]

Although clinicians have an understanding of the clinical factors that are associated with postoperative disease recurrence, there are currently no risk models that quantify such risk based on the number and relative weighting of predisposing factors.[11] In general, postoperative patients with CD should be considered at higher risk for recurrence if they have had 2 or more prior resective surgeries, have fistulizing or perianal disease, or are active smokers.[12]

ASSESSING FOR ENDOSCOPIC RECURRENCE

Endoscopic recurrence frequently precedes clinical recurrence and occurs in as many as 80% to 90% of postoperative patients within 5 years.[2,13–15] Ileocolonoscopy is usually used to assess for recurrent endoscopic lesions in the neoterminal ileum and is classified using the Rutgeerts score (**Fig. 1**). Endoscopic recurrence is defined as a Rutgeerts score of i2 or greater (at least 5 aphthous lesions with normal intervening mucosa), which predicts clinical recurrence.[16] Only 5% of postoperative patients with a Rutgeerts score of i0 or i1 go on to develop recurrent IBD-related symptoms at 3 years. In contrast, the 3-year rate of clinical recurrence is 15%, 40%, and 90% for those with i2, i3, and i4 recurrence, respectively. Note that, although the Rutgeerts score has been used to guide medical treatment, it has never been formally validated in postoperative treatment trials. Moreover, the interrater reliability of the Rutgeerts

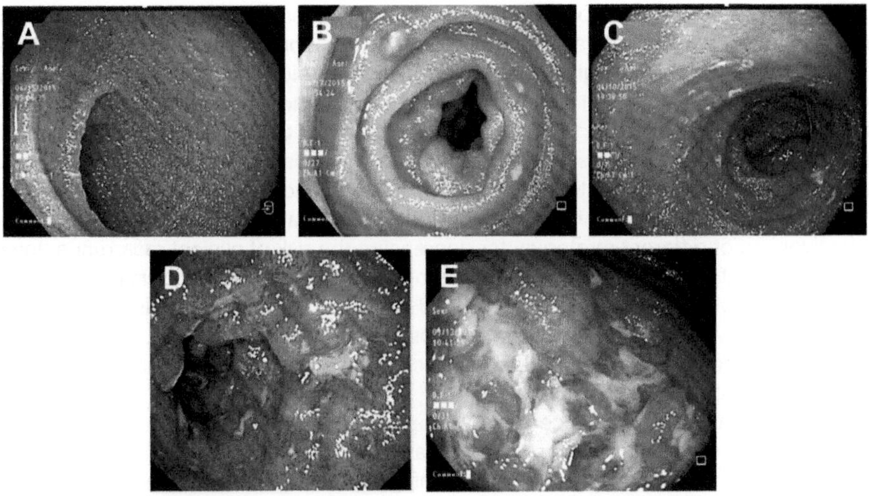

Fig. 1. Rutgeerts score for grading endoscopic recurrence of CD. (*A*) i0, no aphthous lesions; (*B*) i1, fewer than or equal to 5 aphthous lesions; (*C*) i2, more than 5 aphthous lesions with normal intervening mucosa, and skip areas of larger lesions; (*D*) i3, diffuse aphthous ileitis; (*E*) i4, diffuse inflammation with large ulcers, nodules, and/or strictures. (*Courtesy of* Dr Miguel Reguerio, University of Pittsburgh, Pittsburgh, PA.)

score for detecting recurrence (≥i2 vs i2) is only moderate and may result in inappropriate therapeutic decisions.[17]

TIMING OF INITIATION OF PROPHYLACTIC THERAPY

Given differences in the risk of recurrence based on presence or absence of risk factors, different strategies have been proposed regarding timing of initiation of these medications. Although early use of these medications, within 4 to 8 weeks after surgical resection, is very effective in decreasing the risk of endoscopic and clinical recurrence of CD over the next 1 to 2 years, there is potential for overtreatment with associated risks, costs, and inconvenience of therapy, with this approach, because a subset of patients, particularly those at low risk, may not develop recurrence, regardless of therapy.[12] In these patients, a strategy of endoscopy-guided therapy, wherein treatment is initiated only after established endoscopic recurrence within 6 to 12 months of surgical resection, may be optimal. These strategies were compared in a single small randomized controlled trial (RCT) of 63 patients with surgically induced remission, in which patients were randomized to either routine early pharmacologic prophylaxis within 2 weeks of surgery (n = 32) or endoscopy-guided initiation of therapy (treat only patients with endoscopic recurrence of CD in colonoscopy performed within 6–12 months of surgery) (n = 31).[18] Patients in both arms received weight-based azathioprine therapy. There was no significant difference in the rates of clinical remission (62% vs 55%; *P* = .54) or endoscopic remission (50% vs 42%; *P* = .52) at 2 years between the two groups. There were no surgical recurrences in either arm. In contrast with patients in the routine early postoperative prophylaxis group, who all received medications, only 14 out of 31 patients in the endoscopy-guided therapy group required pharmacologic intervention; 17 patients (54.8%) were able to avoid medications for at least 2 years. However, this trial was at high risk of bias because there were baseline differences in prognostic factors (higher rates of smokers in the early-prophylaxis group vs the endoscopy-guided group [53% vs 29%]; higher proportion of patients with presurgical thiopurine exposure in the routine postoperative prophylaxis group), and had a high attrition rate (33%). The trial was terminated early because of low recruitment (only 63 of the proposed 200 patients randomized), and hence was significantly underpowered to detect true differences in the strategies. Also, because the risk of disease recurrence is closely linked to the choice of pharmacologic prophylactic agent, these results cannot be directly extrapolated to pharmacologic agents other than azathioprine. Decision analyses comparing the cost-effectiveness of different strategies for decreasing the risk of clinical recurrence have suggested that, although routine early postoperative prophylaxis with infliximab may be more effective than endoscopy-guided infliximab therapy, it was significantly more expensive, with an incremental cost-effectiveness ratio of $629,500 per quality-adjusted life year (QALY) gained, which is substantially more than the standard thresholds for cost-effectiveness.[19]

Hence, the available evidence does not optimally inform on the ideal approach to the strategy of routine early postoperative prophylaxis for all patients, or endoscopy-guided therapy for a subset of patients with established endoscopic recurrence, and the approach to postoperative prophylaxis should tailored based on risk factors for disease recurrence and patients' values and preferences. In a qualitative cross-sectional interview-based study of 127 patients with CD evaluating patients' preferences, Kennedy and colleagues[20] observed that about 55% patients thought that type and severity of medication-related side effects were the most important aspects in determining choice of postoperative maintenance therapy, whereas 36% thought that effectiveness of therapy was most important. In addition, even when presented with a hypothetical scenario in which a postoperative prophylactic therapy (eg, 5-aminosalicylate [5-ASA]) was equivalent to no therapy (ie, 5-ASA did not decrease the risk of disease recurrence), 10% of participants still preferred 5-ASA to no therapy, because the patients thought that they were actively doing something about their disease or had more control over it. Keeping these factors in mind, the American Gastroenterological Association (AGA) in their recent guidelines on management of CD after surgical resection suggested early pharmacologic prophylaxis rather than endoscopy-guided pharmacologic treatment, based on very low-quality evidence, because most patients who undergo surgical resection have 1 or more risk factors for recurrence.[11] The guidelines also suggested that, "patients, particularly those at lower risk of recurrence, who place a higher value on avoiding the small risks of pharmacological prophylaxis and a lower value on the potential risk of early disease recurrence, may reasonably select endoscopy-guided pharmacological treatment over routine prophylaxis."[11] However, for those patients who choose to forego early postoperative prophylaxis, the guidelines strongly recommended endoscopy be performed 6 to 12 months after surgical resection to assess for endoscopic recurrence.

PHARMACOLOGIC AGENTS FOR PREVENTION OF RECURRENCE OF CROHN'S DISEASE

Several different medications, conventionally used in the management of active CD, have been shown to decrease the risk of recurrence of CD after surgical resection with variable efficacy. In a comprehensive synthesis of 21 RCTs including 2006 patients with CD, through network meta-analysis, Singh and colleagues[21] estimated the relative efficacy of all pharmacologic interventions. They observed that (1) antibiotics and immunomodulators alone or in combination, and anti–tumor necrosis factor (TNF) monotherapy, but not budesonide, decreased the risk of short-term ($\sim$1 year) clinical and endoscopic recurrence; (2) 5-ASA decreased the risk of clinical but not endoscopic recurrence; (3) anti-TNF monotherapy seemed to be the most efficacious pharmacologic intervention for postoperative prophylaxis, with large effect sizes relative to all other strategies (clinical recurrence relative risk [RR], 0.02–0.20; endoscopic recurrence RR, 0.005–0.04); (4) antibiotic monotherapy and immunomodulator monotherapy seemed to have similar efficacy, with comparable rates of serious adverse events warranting medication discontinuation. **Fig. 2** shows the relative efficacy of different medications compared with placebo for decreasing the risk of clinical and endoscopic recurrence 1 year after surgical resection.

Since the publication of this network meta-analysis, 2 key trials on efficacy of anti-TNF and 6-mercaptopurine for pharmacologic prophylaxis have been published, and have suggested that the observed magnitude of benefit with prophylactic therapy is probably smaller than previously reported in smaller trials. In the PREVENT study, Reguiero and colleagues[22] randomized 297 patients who had undergone ileocolonic resection to infliximab (5 mg/kg) or placebo every 8 weeks for 104 weeks, within 45 days of surgery. All patients had at least 1 of the following risk factors for recurrence: prior intestinal resection within 10 years, more than 2 prior resections, resection for a penetrating CD complication, history of perianal fistulizing CD or smoking. The primary end point of the trial was clinical recurrence, defined as a composite outcome consisting of a CD Activity Index (CDAI) score greater than 200 and a greater than or

A

Intervention	Risk ratio	Lower limit	Upper limit
Anti-TNF monotherapy	0.04	0.01	0.15
IMM + Antibiotics	0.11	0.03	0.41
Immunomodulators	0.36	0.20	0.64
Antibiotics	0.26	0.11	0.61
Mesalamine	0.60	0.40	0.89
Budesonide	0.93	0.45	1.90

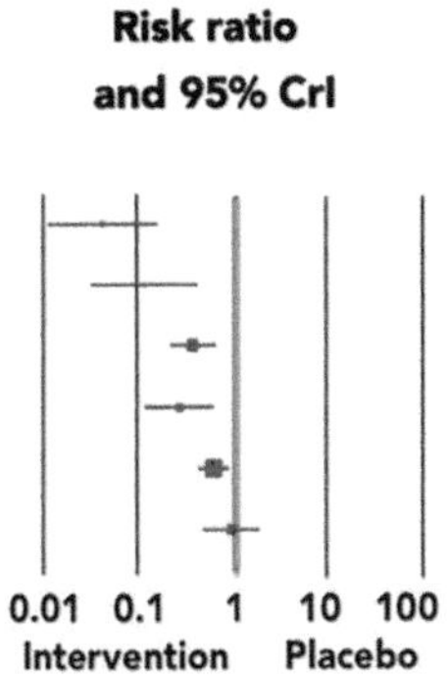

B

Intervention	Risk ratio	Lower limit	Upper limit
Anti-TNF monotherapy	0.01	0.00	0.09
IMM + Antibiotics	0.16	0.05	0.50
Immunomodulators	0.33	0.16	0.68
Antibiotics	0.41	0.18	0.93
Mesalamine	0.67	0.42	1.07
Budesonide	0.79	0.35	1.80

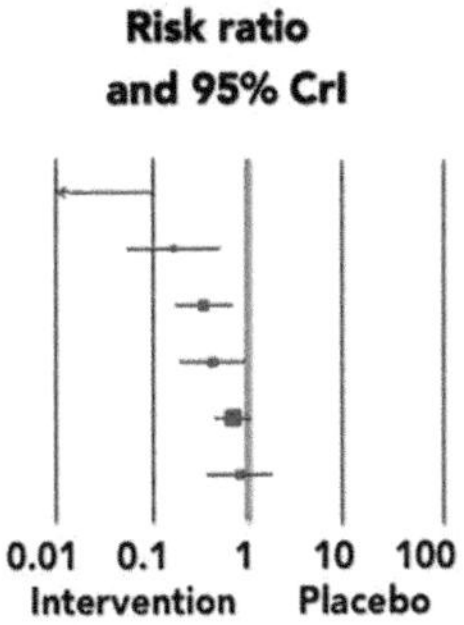

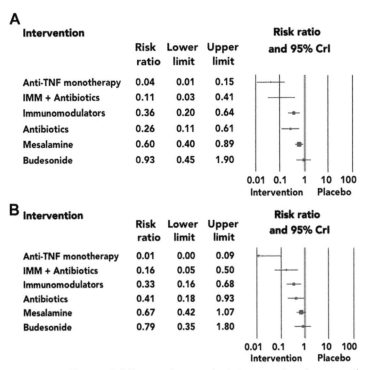

Fig. 2. Comparative efficacy of different pharmacologic interventions in prevention of (*A*) clinical and (*B*) endoscopic recurrence of CD. CrI, credible intervals; IMM, immunomodulators. (*Adapted from* Singh S, Garg SK, Pardi DS, Wang Z, Murad MH, Loftus EV Jr. Comparative efficacy of pharmacologic interventions in preventing relapse of Crohn's disease after surgery: a systematic review and meta-analysis. Gastroenterology 2015;148;64–76.)

equal to 70-point increase from baseline, and endoscopic recurrence (Rutgeerts score ≥ i2, determined by a central reader) or development of a new or redraining fistula or abscess, before or at week 76. Overall, the risk of clinical recurrence was numerically, but not statistically, lower, in infliximab-treated patients compared with placebo-treated patients (20% vs 13%; *P* = .10). The risk of endoscopic recurrence (defined based on Rutgeerts score ≥ i2, development of a new or redraining fistula or abscess, or treatment failure) was significantly lower in infliximab-treated patients (60% vs 31%; *P*<.01); similarly, the risk of severe endoscopic recurrence (i3/i4) was also significantly lower in infliximab-treated patients (7% vs 32%; *P*<.01). In the TOPPIC (Trial Of Prevention of Post-operative Crohn's disease) trial, 240 patients with CD at 29 centers in the United Kingdom were randomized to either weight-based 6-mercaptopurine (n = 128) or placebo (n = 112) after surgical resection for prevention of recurrence and followed for 3 years.[23] The investigators observed that risk of clinical recurrence (defined as CDAI score >150 and a 100-point increase from baseline, and the need for antiinflammatory rescue treatment or primary surgical intervention) was numerically, but not statistically, lower in 6-MP–treated patients (13% vs 23%; *P* = .07). Similar to the PREVENT study, more 6-MP–treated patients maintained complete endoscopic remission (Rutgeerts score, i0) compared with placebo-treated patients (36% vs 18%; *P* = .01) within 1 year. Note that smoking was a significant effect modifier; in a stratum of smokers, 6-MP significantly reduced risk of clinical recurrence compared with placebo (10% vs 36%; *P*<.01), but not in nonsmoking patients (who are at a lower risk of recurrence) (13% vs 16%; *P* = not significant).

The role of 5-ASAs in the prevention of disease recurrence in postoperative setting merits consideration. Although meta-analyses suggest that 5-ASAs reduce clinical recurrence, there is low confidence in these effect estimates, because of the low number of events and suspected publication bias; moreover, there is very low-quality evidence to support that 5-ASAs reduce the risk of endoscopic recurrence.[12,24] Hence, taken together with the lack of benefit of 5-ASAs for inducing or maintaining remission in patients with luminal CD, based on several large RCTs and meta-analyses, the AGA guidelines suggest against the use of 5-ASAs for postoperative prophylaxis.[11]

Most RCT-level data are limited in duration of follow-up and are unable to inform comment on the risk of surgical recurrence with different therapies. Observational studies, which carry inherent limitations of confounding by indication, have shown that anti-TNF and azathioprine therapy may decrease the risk of surgical recurrence. In a long-term, open-label follow-up of the first trial of infliximab for postoperative prophylaxis in CD, the observed rate of surgical recurrence was significantly lower in patients who received infliximab for most of the follow-up period compared with patients who received infliximab for a shorter duration of follow-up (20% vs 64%; *P* = .047).[25] In a matched case-control single-center Korean study, over a median 3-year follow-up, patients receiving postoperative anti-TNF prophylaxis within 2 months of surgery had a significantly lower risk of surgical recurrence compared with patients who did not receive an anti-TNF.[26] In a retrospective cohort study of 567 postsurgical patients with CD treated with different medications postoperatively, 42% developed surgical recurrence over a median 70 months; thiopurine use was independently associated with lower risk of surgical recurrence.[27] Similarly, in a separate retrospective cohort study, Papay and colleagues[28] observed that long-term use of azathioprine (>36 months) following surgical resection might be protective against surgical recurrence of CD. Of note, the timing of initiation of azathioprine after surgical resection is not known in the last 2 studies, making it unclear whether the protective effect truly represents the impact of routine early postoperative azathioprine prophylaxis.

In a cost-effectiveness analysis, Ananthakrishnan and colleagues[19] evaluated the comparative cost-effectiveness of 5 strategies for decreasing risk of clinical recurrence 1 year after surgically induced remission of CD (no treatment, early azathioprine monotherapy, early antibiotic monotherapy, routine early infliximab, and tailored endoscopy-guided therapy with infliximab) in which there was no early postoperative prophylaxis but infliximab was initiated only in patients with endoscopic recurrence at 6 months following surgical resection.[19] Early infliximab therapy was the most effective strategy, but antibiotic monotherapy was the most cost-effective strategy. Routine early infliximab monotherapy was not deemed cost-effective across the entire spectrum of hypothetical disease recurrence rates ($6,667,000/QALY in low risk, $1,266,801/QALY in high risk, $722,348/QALY in the highest risk group, compared with antibiotics). However, in sensitivity analysis, extending the time horizon to 3 years in the very-high-risk scenario (risk of clinical recurrence at 1 year, 78%), the cost per QALY gained with routine early infliximab decreased to $459,158/QALY compared with antibiotic monotherapy.

With these multiple options, the AGA guidelines suggest using anti-TNF therapy and/or thiopurines rather than other agents for postoperative prophylaxis, based on moderate quality of evidence, and suggest against using 5-ASA, probiotics, or budesonide for postoperative prophylaxis.[11] The guidelines acknowledge that patients' acceptance of risk of disease recurrence and risks associated with a medication varies widely, with some patients placing higher value on preventing disease recurrence than on medication risks, and others placing a higher value on avoiding medication risks than on risk of disease recurrence; physicians are unlikely to be able to select the most appropriate treatment option for their patients based on clinical and demographic data alone, and, hence, shared decision making on risks and benefits in the context of patients' values and preferences is inherently important in the management of CD after surgical resection. In lieu of this, the guidelines suggest that, "patients at lower risk of disease recurrence or who place a high value on avoiding the small risk of adverse events of thiopurines and/or anti-TNF treatment and a low value on a modestly increased risk of disease recurrence may reasonably choose nitroimidazole antibiotics (for 3–12 months)." However, the benefit of short-term antibiotics may not be sustained.

Although there are limited data on the role of combination therapy with anti-TNF agents and a thiopurine or methotrexate in the postoperative setting, indirect evidence derived from the effect of combination therapy on maintenance of remission in patients with luminal CD with medically induced remission suggests that this combination is likely to be effective in patients with CD with surgically induced remission. Likewise, there is no study on the anti-integrin agent vedolizumab in the postoperative setting, but it is likely to be effective.

COLONOSCOPIC SURVEILLANCE AFTER SURGICAL RESECTION

Regardless of what strategy is chosen in the early postoperative period, colonoscopic surveillance is warranted in 6 to 12 months to assess for presence and severity of endoscopic recurrence in the neoterminal ileum, to guide further management. In the pivotal POCER (Post-operative Crohn's Endoscopic Recurrence Study) trial, 184 patients with surgically induced remission (83.3% at high risk of disease recurrence) were randomized to either an active management strategy involving colonoscopy at 6 months with algorithmic treatment step-up if asymptomatic endoscopic recurrence was identified (n = 122) versus no routine endoscopic monitoring and continuation of the early postoperative management strategy (n = 62).[29] Early postoperative management included 3 months of metronidazole therapy for all patients, and high-risk patients additionally received thiopurine or adalimumab (if they were intolerant to thiopurines). In the arm randomized to active management, patients with endoscopic recurrence at 6 months, treatment step-up involved starting a thiopurine (for low-risk patients who preintervention received only 3 months of metronidazole), adding standard-dose adalimumab to a thiopurine (for patients who were on thiopurine monotherapy), or escalating to weekly adalimumab (for patients who were on standard-dose adalimumab before intervention). During the study, 47 patients in the active management arm had evidence of endoscopic recurrence at 6 months and required treatment step-up. Using this active management strategy, rates of endoscopic (RR, 0.73; 95% confidence interval [CI], 0.56–0.95, respectively) but not clinical recurrence (RR, 0.82; 95% CI, 0.56–1.18) at 18 months were significantly lower, compared with patients who did not receive colonoscopic surveillance within 6 months. No surgical recurrences were noted over 18 months. Despite treatment step-up in the active management arm (in 47 out of 122 patients with evidence of endoscopic recurrence at 6 months), endoscopic remission could be recaptured in only 18 (38.5%) of these patients. This finding suggests that a significant proportion of patients may develop permanent intestinal damage early after surgical resection, despite postoperative prophylaxis, which may not be adequately recaptured with treatment step-up.

Based on these findings, the AGA guidelines suggest routine postoperative endoscopic monitoring at 6 to 12 months rather than no monitoring, in patients who are on postoperative pharmacologic prophylaxis (weak recommendation), acknowledging that patients who are already on long-term prophylactic therapy may be at lower risk of asymptomatic endoscopic recurrence at 6 months, and have a low likelihood of requiring treatment escalation; these patients may reasonably choose to forego the inconvenience and small risks of colonoscopic surveillance.[11] In contrast, in patients with surgically induced remission of CD, not on pharmacologic prophylaxis, the AGA strongly recommends routine postoperative endoscopic monitoring at 6 to 12 months rather than no monitoring. These patients are most likely to benefit from early identification of asymptomatic endoscopic recurrence and treatment initiation to minimize the long-term risk of clinical and surgical recurrence. There are limited data on frequency of continued endoscopic monitoring after the first colonoscopy in patients without evidence of endoscopic recurrence.

Noninvasive biomarkers to detect endoscopic recurrence, such as fecal calprotectin, are being studied. In a post-hoc analysis of the POCER study, fecal calprotectin level greater than or equal to 100 μg/g indicated endoscopic recurrence with 89% sensitivity and 58% specificity, with a negative predictive value of 91%; based on this, colonoscopy could have been avoided in 47% of patients.[30] In a meta-analysis of 10 studies, the pooled sensitivity and specificity of fecal calprotectin for assessing suspected endoscopic recurrence was 0.82 and 0.61, respectively.[31] At present, these biomarkers have suboptimal performance characteristics, and hence are not recommended for use in clinical practice. Future studies comparing different active management surveillance strategies with endoscopic versus biochemical monitoring are warranted.

TREATMENT OF ESTABLISHED ENDOSCOPIC RECURRENCE

As described earlier, clinically silent endoscopic recurrence of CD is common in patients with surgically induced remission, being observed in 30% to 90% of patients within 12 months of surgery and almost universally by 5 years. Patients with endoscopic recurrence are at high risk of progression to clinical and surgical recurrence, and endoscopic remission is considered to be an appropriate surrogate marker for preventing future surgical recurrence. However, there is a dearth of direct evidence informing on the best management approach for these patients. In an RCT of 78 asymptomatic patients with CD with endoscopic recurrence after surgical recurrence, comparing azathioprine and mesalamine, risks of clinical (RR, 0.10; 95% CI, 0.01–1.81) and endoscopic recurrence (RR, 0.83; 95% CI, 0.58–1.20) were numerically but not statistically lower in azathioprine-treated patients.[32] In a 3-arm prospective cohort study, 26 patients were treated with either mesalamine 3 g/d, azathioprine 50 mg/d, or infliximab and were followed for 6 months.[33] The observed rate of clinical (RR, 0.11; 95% CI, 0.02–0.85) and endoscopic recurrence (RR, 0.56; 95% CI, 0.38–0.83) was lower in infliximab-treated patients compared with mesalamine-treated patients. Although recurrence was lower with infliximab even compared with azathioprine, these results were not statistically significantly different. In the absence of direct evidence, indirect evidence from trials of maintenance therapy in patients with medically induced remission of luminal CD may be used to inform approach to management. These data support the use of immunomodulators and/or anti-TNF therapy for treatment of asymptomatic endoscopic recurrence.

PROPOSED MANAGEMENT ALGORITHM

In summarizing this evidence for the management of CD after surgical resection, the authors propose the following algorithm (**Fig. 3**). In high-risk patients, early postoperative prophylaxis with the most effective agent (anti-TNF monotherapy or in combination with immunomodulators) is prudent, with active colonoscopic surveillance in 6 months, with intention to step up therapy if there is endoscopic recurrence. In contrast, in low-risk patients, particularly those who are concerned about medication side effects, endoscopy-guided therapy may be appropriate, wherein patients routinely undergo colonoscopy within 6 months of surgical resection, and then start therapy if there is endoscopic recurrence.

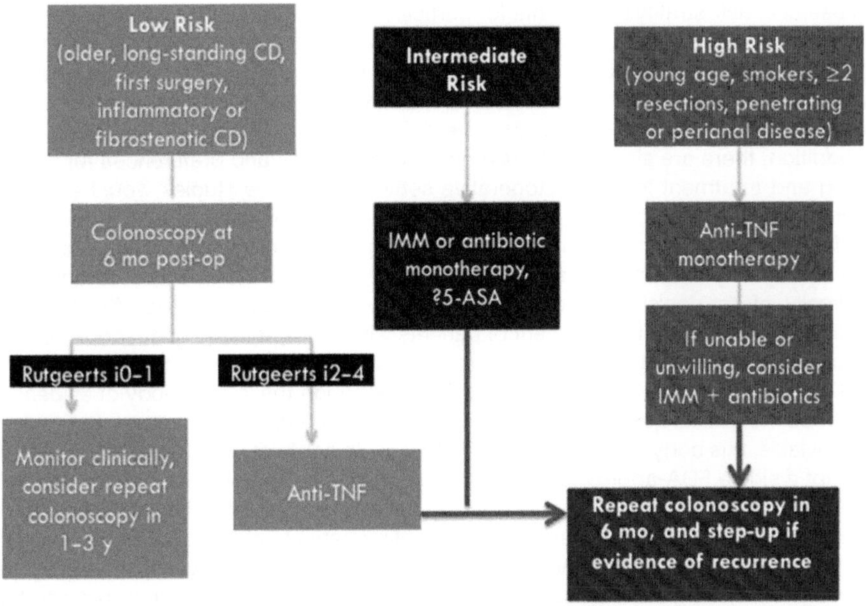

Fig. 3. Proposed algorithm for management of Crohn's disease after surgical resection. Post-op, postoperative.

GASTROINTESTINAL SYMPTOMS IN ABSENCE OF ENDOSCOPIC RECURRENCE

With altered anatomy following surgical resection, patients may experience gastrointestinal symptoms even in the absence of CD-related inflammation. Diarrhea following surgical resection should not be assumed to be caused by recurrence of CD. Potential noninflammatory causes for diarrhea include:

- Gastrointestinal infections like *Clostridium difficile*
- Noninfectious diarrhea caused by bile acid malabsorption, particularly if less than 100 cm of terminal ileum has been resected
- Small intestinal bacterial overgrowth, especially following resection of the ileocecal valve
- Irritable bowel syndrome

Likewise, abdominal pain should not automatically be attributed to recurrence of CD. Nonspecific postsurgical pain, irritable bowel syndrome, anastomotic stricture, or adhesions may also contribute to abdominal pain. Hence, in any symptomatic patient following surgical resection, due diligence in confirming the presence of CD-related inflammation should be followed before starting antiinflammatory therapy.

KNOWLEDGE GAPS AND FUTURE DIRECTIONS

There are several key questions in the management of CD after surgical resection that merit further study. First, although there is universal agreement that the risk of disease recurrence is highly variable among patients, based on presence or absence of certain risk factors, there is no validated risk prediction score that can inform patients and providers on the absolute risk of disease recurrence. A validated risk score could facilitate informed decision making and help patients and providers choose between endoscopy-guided therapy versus routine early postoperative pharmacologic prophylaxis, and, if the latter is chosen, the best choice of pharmacologic agent; it may also be useful in risk-stratifying patients for participation in clinical trials. Second, there is limited availability of data on the safety and cost-effectiveness of different postoperative management strategies. Although there is no reason to think that medication safety, for example, should be different in the postoperative setting, trade-offs between benefits and harms are likely to be different in this setting than in luminal CD. In addition, there are also limited data on patients' values and preferences for monitoring and treatment in the postoperative setting and future studies would also aid shared decision making. Third, the question regarding routine early postoperative prophylaxis versus endoscopy-guided treatment was informed by 1 small RCT yielding a very low quality of evidence, and additional well-designed studies are warranted to optimally inform decisions. Likewise, the question on the comparative effectiveness of different agents for management of patients with asymptomatic endoscopic recurrence in the postoperative setting was informed by indirect evidence from luminal CD, and also merits dedicated studies. In addition, although the largest body of evidence informed the clinical question regarding the choice of therapy for routine postoperative prophylaxis, this body of evidence has limitations. In contrast with luminal CD, there is still not a single FDA-approved medication to prevent recurrence of CD after surgical resection. Several factors are likely to be drivers of this, including underpowered studies, the lack of reliable markers for predicting patients at high risk of recurrence, limitations in measuring clinical recurrence, and the absence of a validated surrogate marker for key long-term outcomes such as surgery and hospitalization that can be measured within the typical duration of a trial. The result is that evidence encompasses heterogeneous trials enriched with patients who may not benefit from interventions; imprecise clinical outcome measurements (eg, CDAI) that often assess factors other than CD activity; and reliance on objective outcomes (Rutgeerts score) that are likely, but not yet established, surrogates of key long-term outcomes such as repeat surgery and hospitalization. In addition, with high rates of disease recurrence following surgical resection in patients with CD, placebo-controlled trials may not be ethical in this setting.

REFERENCES

1. Frolkis AD, Lipton DS, Fiest KM, et al. Cumulative incidence of second intestinal resection in Crohn's disease: a systematic review and meta-analysis of population-based studies. Am J Gastroenterol 2014;109(11):1739–48.
2. Buisson A, Chevaux JB, Allen PB, et al. Review article: the natural history of post-operative Crohn's disease recurrence. Aliment Pharmacol Ther 2012;35(6): 625–33.
3. Nguyen GC, Nugent Z, Shaw S, et al. Outcomes of patients with Crohn's disease improved from 1988 to 2008 and were associated with increased specialist care. Gastroenterology 2011;141(1):90–7.
4. Frolkis AD, Dykeman J, Negron ME, et al. Risk of surgery for inflammatory bowel diseases has decreased over time: a systematic review and meta-analysis of population-based studies. Gastroenterology 2013;145(5):996–1006.
5. Nguyen GC, Saibil F, Steinhart AH, et al. Postoperative health-care utilization in Crohn's disease: the impact of specialist care. Am J Gastroenterol 2012; 107(10):1522–9.
6. Simillis C, Yamamoto T, Reese GE, et al. A meta-analysis comparing incidence of recurrence and indication for reoperation after surgery for perforating versus non-perforating Crohn's disease. Am J Gastroenterol 2008;103(1):196–205.
7. Lautenbach E, Berlin JA, Lichtenstein GR. Risk factors for early postoperative recurrence of Crohn's disease. Gastroenterology 1998;115(2):259–67.
8. Bernell O, Lapidus A, Hellers G. Risk factors for surgery and postoperative recurrence in Crohn's disease. Ann Surg 2000;231(1):38–45.
9. Pascua M, Su C, Lewis JD, et al. Meta-analysis: factors predicting post-operative recurrence with placebo therapy in patients with Crohn's disease. Aliment Pharmacol Ther 2008;28(5):545–56.
10. Reese GE, Nanidis T, Borysiewicz C, et al. The effect of smoking after surgery for Crohn's disease: a meta-analysis of observational studies. Int J Colorectal Dis 2008;23(12):1213–21.
11. Nguyen GC, Loftus EV Jr, Hirano I, et al. American Gastroenterological Association Institute guideline on the management of Crohn's disease after surgical resection. Gastroenterology 2017;152(1):271–5.
12. Regueiro M, Velayos F, Greer JB, et al. American Gastroenterological Association Institute technical review on the management of Crohn's disease after surgical resection. Gastroenterology 2017;152(1):277–95.e273.
13. Tytgat GN, Mulder CJ, Brummelkamp WH. Endoscopic lesions in Crohn's disease early after ileocecal resection. Endoscopy 1988;20(5):260–2.
14. Olaison G, Smedh K, Sjodahl R. Natural course of Crohn's disease after ileocolic resection: endoscopically visualised ileal ulcers preceding symptoms. Gut 1992; 33(3):331–5.
15. Rutgeerts P, Geboes K, Vantrappen G, et al. Natural history of recurrent Crohn's disease at the ileocolonic anastomosis after curative surgery. Gut 1984;25(6): 665–72.

16. Rutgeerts P, Geboes K, Vantrappen G, et al. Predictability of the postoperative course of Crohn's disease. Gastroenterology 1990;99(4):956–63.
17. Marteau P, Laharie D, Colombel JF, et al. Inter-observer variation study of the Rutgeerts score to assess endoscopic recurrence after surgery for Crohn's disease. J Crohns Colitis 2016;10(9):1001–5.
18. Ferrante M, Papamichael K, Duricova D, et al. Systematic versus endoscopy-driven treatment with azathioprine to prevent postoperative ileal Crohn's disease recurrence. J Crohns Colitis 2015;9(8):617–24.
19. Ananthakrishnan AN, Hur C, Juillerat P, et al. Strategies for the prevention of postoperative recurrence in Crohn's disease: results of a decision analysis. Am J Gastroenterol 2011;106(11):2009–17.
20. Kennedy ED, To T, Steinhart AH, et al. Do patients consider postoperative maintenance therapy for Crohn's disease worthwhile? Inflamm Bowel Dis 2008;14(2):224–35.
21. Singh S, Garg SK, Pardi DS, et al. Comparative efficacy of pharmacologic interventions in preventing relapse of Crohn's disease after surgery: a systematic review and network meta-analysis. Gastroenterology 2015;148(1):64–76.e62 [quiz: e14].
22. Regueiro M, Feagan BG, Zou B, et al. Infliximab reduces endoscopic, but not clinical, recurrence of Crohn's disease after ileocolonic resection. Gastroenterology 2016;150(7):1568–78.
23. Mowat CA I, Cahill A, Smith M, et al. Mercaptopurine versus placebo to prevent recurrence of Crohn's disease after surgical resection (TOPPIC): a multicentre, double-blind, randomised controlled trial. Lancet Gastroenterol Hepatol 2016;1(4):273–82.
24. Ford AC, Achkar JP, Khan KJ, et al. Efficacy of 5-aminosalicylates in ulcerative colitis: systematic review and meta-analysis. Am J Gastroenterol 2011;106(4):601–16.
25. Regueiro M, Kip KE, Baidoo L, et al. Postoperative therapy with infliximab prevents long-term Crohn's disease recurrence. Clin Gastroenterol Hepatol 2014;12(9):1494–502.e1491.
26. Araki T, Uchida K, Okita Y, et al. Impact of postoperative infliximab maintenance therapy on preventing the surgical recurrence of Crohn's disease: a single-center paired case-control study. Surg Today 2014;44(2):291–6.
27. van Loo ES, Vosseberg NW, van der Heide F, et al. Thiopurines are associated with a reduction in surgical re-resections in patients with Crohn's disease: a long-term follow-up study in a regional and academic cohort. Inflamm Bowel Dis 2013;19(13):2801–8.
28. Papay P, Reinisch W, Ho E, et al. The impact of thiopurines on the risk of surgical recurrence in patients with Crohn's disease after first intestinal surgery. Am J Gastroenterol 2010;105(5):1158–64.
29. De Cruz P, Kamm MA, Hamilton AL, et al. Crohn's disease management after intestinal resection: a randomised trial. Lancet 2015;385(9976):1406–17.
30. Wright EK, Kamm MA, De Cruz P, et al. Measurement of fecal calprotectin improves monitoring and detection of recurrence of Crohn's disease after surgery. Gastroenterology 2015;148(5):938–47.e931.
31. Qiu Y, Mao R, Chen BL, et al. Fecal calprotectin for evaluating postoperative recurrence of Crohn's disease: a meta-analysis of prospective studies. Inflamm Bowel Dis 2015;21(2):315–22.
32. Reinisch W, Angelberger S, Petritsch W, et al. Azathioprine versus mesalazine for prevention of postoperative clinical recurrence in patients with Crohn's disease

with endoscopic recurrence: efficacy and safety results of a randomised, double-blind, double-dummy, multicentre trial. Gut 2010;59(6):752–9.
33. Yamamoto T, Umegae S, Matsumoto K. Impact of infliximab therapy after early endoscopic recurrence following ileocolonic resection of Crohn's disease: a prospective pilot study. Inflamm Bowel Dis 2009;15(10):1460–6.

Targeting Specific Immunologic Pathways in Crohn's Disease

Guilherme Piovezani Ramos, MD[a], William A. Faubion, MD[b], Konstantinos A. Papadakis, MD[b,*]

KEYWORDS

- Crohn's disease • Inflammatory bowel diseases • Immunology • Target therapy

KEY POINTS

- New therapeutic agents are intended to control disease activity by inhibiting different extracellular, intracellular, and even intranuclear targets involved in the abnormal inflammatory pathways.
- Leukocyte migration in inflammatory bowel disease can be prevented by blocking of leukocyte integrins and cellular adhesion molecules expressed in the intestinal vascular endothelium.
- Interleukin (IL)-12 and IL-23 are dimeric cytokines that share the p40 subunit. Anti-p40 agents are effective in controlling the Th1/Th17 predominant response of Crohn's disease (CD).
- The Janus kinase–signal transducer and activator of transcription factors pathways are responsible for intracellular and intranuclear signaling for inflammatory cytokines and have been exploited as potential targets for immune regulation in CD.
- Novel perspectives for the management of CD besides the administration of antiinflammatory cytokines and cell-based therapies may include the modulation of epigenetic targets.

INTRODUCTION

Inflammatory bowel diseases, Crohn's disease (CD), and ulcerative colitis (UC) are characterized by chronic and relapsing inflammation of different segments of the gastrointestinal tract. The exact cause remains unknown, but the working hypothesis is that inflammatory bowel disease (IBD) results from a combination of genetic and

---

Disclosures: None.
Grant Support: None.
[a] Department of Internal Medicine, College of Medicine, Mayo Clinic, 200 First Street Southwest, Rochester, MN 55905, USA; [b] Division of Gastroenterology and Hepatology, College of Medicine, Mayo Clinic, 200 First Street Southwest, Rochester, MN 55905, USA
* Corresponding author. Division of Gastroenterology and Hepatology, Mayo Clinic College of Medicine, Mayo Clinic, 200 First Street Southwest, Rochester, MN 55905.
E-mail address: Papadakis.konstantinos@mayo.edu

Gastroenterol Clin N Am 46 (2017) 577–588
http://dx.doi.org/10.1016/j.gtc.2017.05.009
gastro.theclinics.com

environmental factors, immune deregulation, barrier dysfunction, and changes in the intestinal microbiome.[1–3] The efficacy of current therapies that target cytokines, most notably tumor necrosis factor alpha (TNF-α), has validated the essential role of cytokine pathways in the development of UC and CD inflammation.[4–6] Nevertheless, not all patients treated with TNF-α inhibitors achieve remission and many may even lose response over-time, showing that development of new therapies is warranted.[5,7,8] Understanding of the different immunologic pathways that are involved in intestinal damage is crucial for the development of new therapies that can maximize patient response (**Fig. 1**). New therapeutic agents, currently in development, are intended to control disease activity by approaching different extracellular, intracellular, and even intranuclear targets involved in the abnormal inflammatory response (**Table 1**).

EXTRACELLULAR TARGETS: LEUKOCYTE MIGRATION

After being activated in induction sites, such as mucosal lymphoid follicles and Peyer patches, leukocytes traffic to effector sites, such as the lamina propria, where inflammation takes place. This process is mediated by binding of integrin molecules located on leukocyte surfaces to cellular adhesion molecules (CAMs) expressed on the

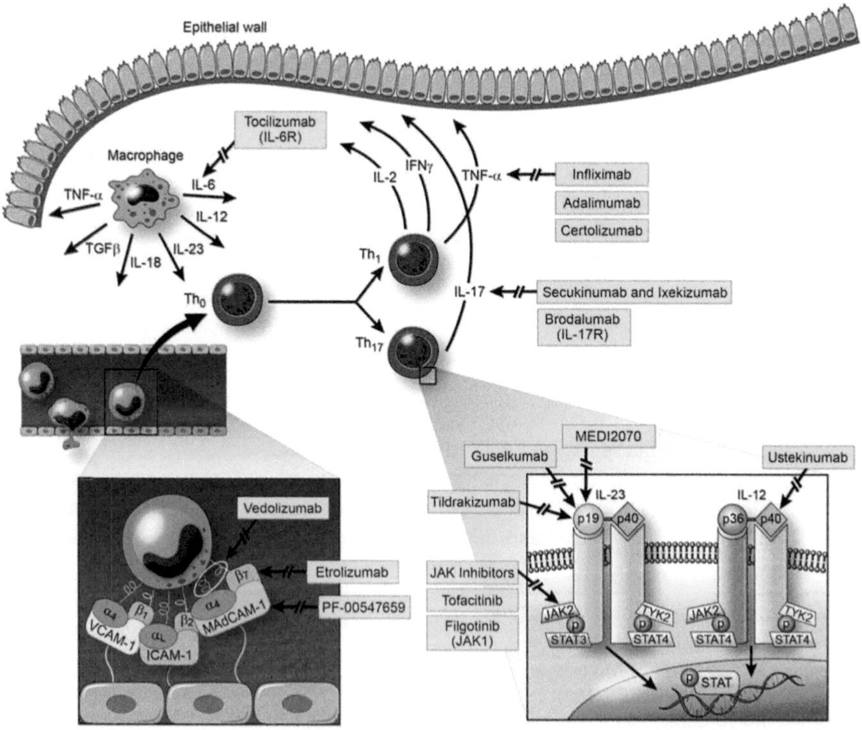

Fig. 1. Immunologic pathways involved in CD inflammation with its respective therapeutic agents. ICAM, intracellular adhesion molecule; IFN-γ, interferon gamma; IL, interleukin; IL-17R, IL-17 receptor; IL-6R, IL-6 receptor; JAK, Janus kinase; MAdCAM, mucosal addressin cellular adhesion molecule; STAT, signal transducer and activator of transcription factor; TGF-β, transforming growth factor beta; Th, T-helper cell; TYK, tyrosine kinase; VCAM, vascular cell adhesion molecule.

Table 1
New therapies for Crohn disease and their respective immunologic targets

Target		Therapeutic Agent
Extracellular		
(1) Leukocyte migration	$\alpha_4\beta_7$ Integrin	Vedolizumab, Abrilumab (AMG 181)
	β_7 Integrin	Etrolizumab
	MAdCAM-1	PF-00547659
	CCR9	Vercirnon
	S1P receptor	Ozanimod
(2) Cytokine inhibitors	TNF-α	Infliximab
		Adalimumab
		Certolizumab pegol
	IL-12/IL–IL23 (p40 subunit)	Ustekinumab
		Briakinumab
	IL-23 (p19 subunit)	Tildrakizumab (MK-3222) Guselkumab, Brazikumab (MEDI2070), Risankizumab (BI 655066)
	IL-17A	Secukinumab
		Ixekizumab
	IL-17R	Brodalumab (AMG 827)
	IL-6R	Tocilizumab
(3) Antiinflammatory agents	F8–IL-10	Dekavil
	SMAD7	Mongersen
Intracellular and Intranuclear		
(1) JAK inhibitors	JAK1, JAK2, JAK3	Tofacitinib
	JAK1	Filgotinib, Upadacitinib (ABT-494)
	JAK1, JAK2	Baricitinib

Abbreviations: CCR9, chemokine receptor 9; IL, interleukin; IL-17R, IL-17 receptor; IL-6R, IL-6-receptor; JAK, Janus kinase; MAdCAM, mucosal addressin cellular adhesion molecule; S1P, sphingosine 1-phosphate.

surface of endothelial cells. Furthermore, chemokines produced by endothelial, stromal, or epithelial cells during inflammation can also act as chemoattractants through integrin activation on the rolling leukocytes to promote their activation and migration across the endothelium.[9,10]

Integrins are heterodimeric receptors expressed on the surface of circulating leukocytes that are composed of an α and β subunit.[9] Several forms of α and β subunits exist and may combine to generate different combinations of integrin molecules expressed on human leukocytes. These combinations can be specific to a particular type of leukocyte or determine the target tissue for leukocyte trafficking. The integrins $\alpha_L\beta_2$, $\alpha_4\beta_1$, $\alpha_4\beta_7$, and $\alpha_E\beta_7$ are markers that interact with different adhesions molecules for specific leukocyte trafficking to the intestine, a property that is particularly important for IBD therapies that target leukocyte trafficking to the inflamed gut.[9] Natalizumab, a humanized anti-α_4 monoclonal antibody (mAb) originally developed for treatment of multiple sclerosis, was the first anti-integrin approved for use in CD.[11,12] By targeting the α_4 subunit, it not only inhibits the $\alpha_4\beta_7$ integrin T-cell trafficking in the inflamed intestine but also the $\alpha_4\beta_1$ integrin, which promotes trafficking of lymphocytes to the central nervous system.[10] This property may be associated with the risk of significant adverse effect of this medication; safety data have revealed the risk of developing JC virus–associated progressive multifocal leukoencephalopathy.[13] Vedolizumab is an antibody approved for the treatment of IBD that targets the $\alpha_4\beta_7$

integrin, which in theory should eliminate any associated risk of progressive multifocal leukoencephalopathy because $\alpha_4\beta_7$ is specifically expressed on T cells that home to the intestine.[14] Another therapy currently in development, etrolizumab, is a humanized anti-β_7 mAb, which, in addition to blocking lymphocyte recruitment via $\alpha_4\beta_7$ integrin, such as vedolizumab, also interferes with a different integrin, $\alpha_E\beta_7$ and its ligand E-cadherin, responsible for recruitment of intraepithelial lymphocytes and a subset of lamina propria lymphocytes.[15]

The integrin ligands expressed on the surface of vascular endothelial cells are CAMs. In particular, 3 CAMs are known to play a role in leukocyte trafficking to the inflamed intestine during active phases of IBD: intracellular adhesion molecule (ICAM)-1, mucosal addressin CAM (MAdCAM), and vascular cell adhesion molecule (VCAM)-1. ICAM-1 is induced on exposure to proinflammatory cytokines and causes firm adhesion, activation, and migration of leukocytes by interacting with the $\alpha L\beta 2$ integrin. VCAM-1 is also only expressed by cytokine stimulation and acts via 2 integrin ligands, $\alpha_4\beta_1$ or $\alpha_4\beta_7$.[10,15] PF-00547659 is an anti–MAdCAM-1 mAb currently under clinical development. Phase II studies have indicated that PF-00547659 is effective, safe, and well tolerated in patients with moderate to severe UC.[16] In patients with moderate to severe CD, PF-00547659 treatment showed an increased response, although not statistically significant, compared with placebo.[17] Phase III studies will address the issue of whether this strategy will be effective in CD.

An alternative approach to inhibiting lymphocyte recruitment is blockade of intestinal-specific chemokine-receptor complexes that act as chemoattractants for receptors in circulating lymphocytes. Vercirnon, a selective inhibitor of the chemokine receptor CCR9, expressed on the cell surface of gut-homing T cells, interacts with the small intestinal lymphocyte chemoattractant CCL25; however, this agent was found not to be effective in a placebo-controlled induction trial in active CD.[18] Eldelumab (BMS-936557 or MDX-1100) is another example that targets interferon-gamma–inducible protein (IP)-10 (CXCL10), an intestinal chemokine secreted by intestinal mucosal macrophages, lymphocytes, and endothelial cells that binds to the CXCR3 chemokine receptor on activated T lymphocytes.[19] However, eldelumab was ineffective in a placebo-controlled phase 2 study of patients with active UC.[20] In addition, a novel approach has been the effort to prevent leukocyte trafficking by targeting receptors that control lymphocyte egression from lymph nodes, such as the sphingosine 1-phosphate (S1P) receptor. Ozanimod is an S1P receptor modulator, which has been tested in patients with UC and is currently undergoing phase-2 clinical trials for induction of remission of patients with moderately to severely active CD.[21,22]

EXTRACELLULAR TARGETS: BEYOND TUMOR NECROSIS FACTOR ALPHA INHIBITORS

Even though UC and CD share many inflammatory pathway characteristics, they differ clinically, endoscopically, and histopathologically as a result of distinct immunologic processes associated with each disease entity. The intercalated transmural inflammation characteristic of CD is the result of an excessive T-helper (Th) type 1 and 17 response, whereas an excessive Th2 response drives the uniform mucosal inflammation seen in patients with UC.[1] Most new biomolecules for IBD therapy are designed to reduce pathogenic T-cell activation and its effects by inhibiting the actions of proinflammatory cytokines, such as TNF-α. New therapies are intended to address additional components involved upstream in these pathways, in order to reduce the final pathways of intestinal inflammation.

The differentiation of Th1 and Th17 in CD disease occurs in response to the production of IL-12, IL-18, IL-23, and transforming growth factor beta (TGF-β) by antigen presenting cells (APC) and macrophages. In turn, Th1 and Th17 cells secrete the proinflammatory cytokines IL-2, IL-17, INF-γ, and TNF-α. These cytokines feed into a self-sustaining amplification cycle whereby they stimulate APC, macrophages, fibroblasts, and endothelial cells to produce TNF-α, IL-1, IL-6, IL-8, IL-12, and IL-18.[1,3,8,23]

In addition to this pathway regulation, IL-12 and IL-23 have been extensively studied in IBD. The IL-12 molecule is composed of 2 subunits, IL-12p40 and IL-12p35, which signal through the IL-12 receptor (IL-12R), also composed of 2 subunits, IL-12R1 and IL-12R2. IL-23 is also a heterodimeric cytokine that shares the IL-12p40 subunit in addition to a second unique subunit, IL-23p19, making it capable of signaling through the IL-23R but also the IL-12R1.[24,25] Initial experimental observation suggested that mice deficient in IL-12p40 would be resistant to experimentally induced autoimmune conditions, including colitis, whereas mice deficient in the IL-12p35 subunit showed no protection, or even showed exacerbated disease, in some models.[26] It was later determined that mice deficient in IL-23 but not IL-12 are resistant to experimental immune-mediated diseases and that these two cytokines share the p19 subunit.[27] Several therapeutic agents targeting these cytokines are under development or have been already approved for the treatment of CD. Ustekinumab (Stelara) is an IL-12p40 inhibitor that was recently approved by the US Food and Drug Administration for the treatment of moderate to severe CD.[28] Briakinumab is a different Ab therapy that also targets the p40 subunit common to both IL-12 and IL-23 ; however, this was found to be ineffective for Crohn's disease in a randomized, placebo-controlled phase 2 trial.[29] Tildrakizumab (MK-3222 formerly SCH-900222), guselkumab, brazikumab (MEDI2070), and risankizumab (BI 655066), by targeting the p19 subunit (which is not part of IL-12), are designed to block IL-23, but not IL-12. These agents are in different phases of development for the treatment of several immune-mediated diseases, such as psoriasis and CD.[30–32] MEDI2070 was found in a phase II trial to be significantly better than placebo to induce clinical response in CD.[31] Risankizumab was recently found to be significantly better than placebo at inducing clinical remission in patients with moderate to severe CD in a phase 2a trial.[33] IL-12/IL-23p40 deficiencies have been associated with increased risk of mycobacterial infections, invasive salmonellosis, and mucocutaneous candida infections, which result from impaired IL-12–mediated interferon gamma (IFN-γ) responses.[24,25] Therefore, potential risks of these novel therapies should include infectious complications caused by intracellular pathogens that depend on robust Th1 immune responses for clearance.

Recent studies have shown that p40 inhibitors, such as ustekinumab (Stelara), control intestinal inflammation not by IL-12 blockage but by their effect on IL-23 and its downstream cytokines, such as IL-17A.[34] IL-17A is increased in the intestinal mucosa and fecal samples of patients with active CD.[35] In contrast, animal models of colitis have also suggested that IL-17A may play a protective role in IBD.[36] Secukinumab is an anti–IL-17A that has been recently tested in patients with CD.[37] Even though it had been shown to have good response in patients with psoriasis and rheumatoid arthritis, it was associated with a worsening response compared with placebo in patients with CD.[38] The reason for this response is still unclear, but it has been hypothesized that IL-17A may also play a role in protecting barrier integrity and regulatory T-cell function, which are crucial for mucosal homeostasis. Other therapies that interfere with IL-17 function or secretion are currently in different stages of development but their efficacy in CD is questionable.

In addition to targeting IL-12/IL-23/IL-17 pathways, other recent approaches have attempted to inhibit proinflammatory cytokines that are at increased levels in inflamed mucosa in CD, most notably IL-6. IL-6 is a pleiotropic cytokine with central roles in immune regulation and inflammation. It can also transduce its signal into cells lacking

IL-6 receptors, by forming a complex with its soluble IL-6R (sIL-6R) to activate cells via the receptor subunit gp130, which can be detected on the cell surface, in a process called trans-signaling.[39] IL-6 is known to contribute to Th17 differentiation and increased levels of IL-6 and soluble IL-6R have been reported in the serum and intestinal samples of patients with active IBD.[40,41] In animal models of colitis, administration of monoclonal IL-6R antibodies suppressed the expression of ICAM-1 and VCAM-1 in the intestinal vascular endothelium in addition to reducing colonic expression of TNF-α and other proinflammatory cytokines.[42] Therefore, blocking the IL-6 signaling pathway has been considered a potential new therapeutic strategy for managing CD. In parallel with these proinflammatory effects, IL-6 also affects the homeostasis of the epithelial barrier, and its inhibition could be detrimental, which may explain the mixed data obtained in patients with moderate to severe active UC treated with tocilizumab, a humanized monoclonal antibody against IL-6R.[43]

INTRACELLULAR AND INTRANUCLEAR TARGETS: JANUS KINASE/SIGNAL TRANSDUCER AND ACTIVATOR OF TRANSCRIPTION FACTORS PATHWAYS

An alternative approach to reduce the inflammatory response in CD is to block the downstream signaling pathways mediated by the aforementioned cytokines.

Janus kinases (JAK) play a key role in the intracellular signaling of several cytokines and therefore constitute attractive potential therapeutic targets. JAKs are a family of tyrosine kinases that consists of 4 proteins: JAK1, JAK2, JAK3, and TYK2.[44] Working as pairs, they mediate the intracellular communication between the receptor for cytokines and the intranuclear molecules, namely signal transducer and activator of transcription factors (STATs). Following direct activation by the JAKs and also working in pairs, STATs migrate to the nucleus to stimulate gene transcription. Seven proteins comprise the STAT family: STAT1, STAT2, STAT3, STAT4, STAT5a, STAT5b, and STAT6.[44,45] The combination of pairs of the 4 different JAKs with pairs of the 7 different STATs allows specific patterns of response linked to different cytokine pathways.

For example, IL-12 and IL-23 bind to their respective membrane receptors and directly activate JAK2 and TYK2, which recruit STAT3 and STAT4 to stimulate the transcription of genes responsible for mediating functions of the Th1/Th17 response.[25,44] In a different example, IL-6 signals through JAK1, JAK2, and TYK2, followed by STAT3-mediated activation of transcription of proinflammatory genes.[44] Multiple other cytokines involved in the Th responses in CD have been linked to specific JAK-STAT. Via JAK1 and JAK2 targeting, these agents can inhibit all cytokine receptors containing the γc chain, the β common chain (βc, used by IL-3, IL-5, and granulocyte-macrophage colony-stimulating factor), and gp130 (used by IL-6 family cytokines), as well as interferons, interleukins (IL-12, IL-23, IL-27), and the hormonelike cytokines.[45] These examples show the pleiotropy of functions that different combinations of JAK/STAT pathways can have based on the cytokines they mediate the signaling from, which opens a wide spectrum of possibilities for potential immune regulation therapies in IBD.

Tofacitinib was the first JAK inhibitor tested and later approved in humans with inflammatory disorders.[46] It was initially thought to be selective to JAK3, but has also been shown to interfere with JAK1-mediated and JAK2-mediated intracellular functions.[45] Tofacitinib was first tested in patients with moderate to severe UC, showing a higher likelihood of achieving clinical response and remission compared with placebo.[47] In contrast, in a cohort of patients with moderate to severe CD, no difference in the percentage of patients who achieved clinical responses or remission was noted when comparing tofacitinib and placebo.[48] The short duration of the former study as well as the significant side effect profile in the setting of multiple JAK inhibition (eg, anemia with JAK2 inhibition), which limited the doses used, may explain this difference. At present, several more selective JAK inhibitors are being tested for CD and other inflammatory or malignant conditions, including asthma and myeloproliferative diseases. Filgotinib is an example of a JAK-1 selective inhibitor, which was shown to effectively induce CD remission in a recent phase 2 study.[49]

Because many growth factors and hormones also use JAK-STAT to regulate their function, inhibition of a specific protein may have concomitant, undesired side effects on different organ systems. For example, granulocyte growth factor and erythropoietin act via JAK2, and anemia with mild neutropenia has been a common side effect associated with these therapies.[45] Cardiovascular events in patients on tofacitinib have been reported, but its association with hypercholesterolemia has previously been reported in patients with RA treated with tofacitinib and still needs further clarification.[50] Even within the intestinal epithelium, JAKs are crucial for the maintenance of the epithelial barrier and compromise of this would pose risks of infections and also exposure to intraluminal agents that could aggravate and promote inflammation. Infection rates with tofacitinib have been higher than those with placebo. These infections included mainly upper respiratory infections and viral gastroenteritis, but cases of opportunistic infections such as tuberculosis, cytomegalovirus, and *Pneumocystis jiroveci* pneumonia have also been reported.[45] Hence, the goal of more selectively targeting a single JAK remains a more attractive strategy with selective immune system inhibition while minimizing adverse events. JAK3 is a particularly attractive therapeutic target, because its deficiency did not affect nonimmunologic organs or tissues, indicating that the adverse-effect profile of a selective JAK3 inhibitor could be more favorable.

In alignment with JAK inhibitors, considerable effort is currently being expended for the development of STAT inhibitors in order to control transcription of proinflammatory genes and hence control inflammation. Conceptually, targeting of STAT may be achieved by blocking phosphorylation, disrupting the SH2 domains that mediate binding to phosphorylated receptors and dimerization, or interfering with DNA binding. Current STAT inhibitors that have been applied for clinical use are designed to interfere with DNA binding of these molecules and are currently available to use in various malignancies, mostly targeting STAT1 and STAT3.[45] Animal studies have shown that STAT inhibitors are effective in the treatment of autoimmune disease.[51] For example, STAT1 mediates interferon signaling and is critical for apoptosis, cell death, and defense against pathogens, whereas STAT3 also has important diverse roles in barrier function and host defense, as well as inhibiting tumorigenesis. The similarity of STAT1 and STAT3 molecules, as well as issues of bioavailability, in vivo efficacy, and selectivity, have been the main challenges in the development of these therapies. Empiric targeting of STAT is another strategy that has been used. Drugs, such as fludarabine and pyrimethamine, have been repurposed as STAT inhibitors; however, the mechanism of action through which they interfere with STAT-mediated function remains incompletely understood.[45]

NEW PERSPECTIVES

Most new therapies for CD are designed to reduce the pathogenic T-cell activation and its effects by inhibiting the actions of proinflammatory cytokines and cell migration. There are ongoing studies that attempt to achieve disease remission by targeting novel cytokine pathways (p40 and p19 subunits) of the IL-12/IL-23 and IL-23 cytokines, respectively, using antisense oligonucleotides targeting SMAD7 (Mongersen), or even modulation of intranuclear transcription (JAK/STAT inhibitors) and epigenetic targets.

Some of these approaches may work by restoring the balance between proinflammatory and antiinflammatory cytokines. Antiinflammatory cytokines that have been developed as potential IBD therapies include IL-10, IL-11, and IFN-β; however, results so far have not been promising. IL-10 exert its antiinflammatory action by activating different signaling pathways, and it has been suggested that IL-10 could still represent an important potential therapeutic agent in IBD.[52] Dekavil is an immunocytokine consisting of a targeting antibody fused to the antiinflammatory cytokine IL-10, which is currently on phase II clinical trials in combination with methotrexate for therapy for rheumatoid arthritis, and investigations in IBD indications are being considered.[53] Furthermore, it is known that CD-related inflammation is characterized by reduced activity of the immunosuppressive cytokine TGF-β1 caused by high levels of SMAD7, an inhibitor of TGF-β1 signaling. Mongersen, an oral SMAD7 antisense oligonucleotide, has been shown in preliminary studies to be effective at inducing remission compared with placebo; however, further studies are still required to show efficacy of this therapeutic strategy in CD.[54]

As mentioned previously, T cells play a central role in intestinal inflammation, therefore controlling T-cell activation and the balance between proliferation and apoptosis has been directed as a potential target in IBD and other autoimmune diseases. The use of cell-based therapies to stimulate, control, or replace aberrant immune responses has also been studied in the context of IBD. To this end, therapies involving stem cells or autologous immune cells are currently under development for IBD and other autoimmune diseases.[55] For example, the use of autologous nonmyeloablative hematopoietic stem cell transplant in patients with severe CD resulted in disease remission.[56] Stem cells have also been used specifically to address the problem of fistulas, with studies showing complete closure in up to 70% of patients.[57] Furthermore, the use of regulatory T cells (Tregs) has also been proposed as an alternative to control excessive inflammation in CD. In animal models, Tregs have not only been shown to prevent colitis but, when dysfunctional, they have been associated with increased risks of developing multiple autoimmune diseases.[58] Epigenetic markers have been shown to mediate important Treg and T-effector cell–mediated inflammatory function. For example, EZH2 has recently been reported to be involved in Treg FOXP3-mediated suppressive functions and its absence has been associated with the development of colitis in murine models.[59] Even though epigenetic targets are currently under study in the setting of various malignancies, these therapies have yet to be investigated in IBD.

Multiple therapies are currently being tested or are under development in order to optimize disease control and reduce the inflammatory burden in patients with CD. Future studies should consider the development of new therapies, but also exploring the efficacy of combination agents targeting different pathways may improve disease outcomes. In addition, inflammatory responses vary from patient to patient as well as over time in a single patient; hence, future therapeutic strategies should be designed to explore a more individualized treatment approach based on specific features of each individual's inflammatory response.

REFERENCES

1. Bouma G, Strober W. The immunological and genetic basis of inflammatory bowel disease. Nat Rev Immunol 2003;3(7):521–33.

2. Khor B, Gardet A, Xavier RJ. Genetics and pathogenesis of inflammatory bowel disease. Nature 2011;474(7351):307–17.
3. Xavier RJ, Podolsky DK. Unravelling the pathogenesis of inflammatory bowel disease. Nature 2007;448(7152):427–34.
4. St-Pierre J, Chadee K. How the discovery of TNF-alpha has advanced gastrointestinal diseases and treatment regimes. Dig Dis Sci 2014;59(4):712–5.
5. Peyrin-Biroulet L, Lemann M. Review article: remission rates achievable by current therapies for inflammatory bowel disease. Aliment Pharmacol Ther 2011;33(8):870–9.
6. Cader MZ, Kaser A. Recent advances in inflammatory bowel disease: mucosal immune cells in intestinal inflammation. Gut 2013;62(11):1653–64.
7. Atreya R, Neurath MF. New therapeutic strategies for treatment of inflammatory bowel disease. Mucosal Immunol 2008;1(3):175–82.
8. Danese S. New therapies for inflammatory bowel disease: from the bench to the bedside. Gut 2012;61(6):918–32.
9. Arseneau KO, Cominelli F. Targeting leukocyte trafficking for the treatment of inflammatory bowel disease. Clin Pharmacol Ther 2015;97(1):22–8.
10. Danese S, Panes J. Development of drugs to target interactions between leukocytes and endothelial cells and treatment algorithms for inflammatory bowel diseases. Gastroenterology 2014;147(5):981–9.
11. Sandborn WJ, Colombel JF, Enns R, et al. Natalizumab induction and maintenance therapy for Crohn's disease. N Engl J Med 2005;353(18):1912–25.
12. Targan SR, Feagan BG, Fedorak RN, et al. Natalizumab for the treatment of active Crohn's disease: results of the ENCORE trial. Gastroenterology 2007;132(5):1672–83.
13. Yednock TA, Cannon C, Fritz LC, et al. Prevention of experimental autoimmune encephalomyelitis by antibodies against alpha 4 beta 1 integrin. Nature 1992;356(6364):63–6.
14. Jovani M, Danese S. Vedolizumab for the treatment of IBD: a selective therapeutic approach targeting pathogenic a4b7 cells. Curr Drug Targets 2013;14(12):1433–43.
15. Vermeire S, O'Byrne S, Keir M, et al. Etrolizumab as induction therapy for ulcerative colitis: a randomised, controlled, phase 2 trial. Lancet 2014;384(9940):309–18.
16. Vermeire S, Ghosh S, Panes J, et al. The mucosal addressin cell adhesion molecule antibody PF-00547,659 in ulcerative colitis: a randomised study. Gut 2011;60(8):1068–75.
17. Sandborn W, Lee SD, Tarabar D, et al. 825 Anti-MAdCAM-1 antibody (PF-00547659) for active refractory Crohn's disease: results of the OPERA study. Gastroenterology 2015;148(4):S–162.
18. Feagan BG, Sandborn WJ, D'Haens G, et al. Randomised clinical trial: vercirnon, an oral CCR9 antagonist, vs. placebo as induction therapy in active Crohn's disease. Aliment Pharmacol Ther 2015;42(10):1170–81.
19. Ostvik AE, Granlund A, Gustafsson BI, et al. Mucosal toll-like receptor 3-dependent synthesis of complement factor B and systemic complement activation in inflammatory bowel disease. Inflamm Bowel Dis 2014;20(6):995–1003.
20. Sandborn WJ, Colombel JF, Ghosh S, et al. Eldelumab (anti-IP-10) induction therapy for ulcerative colitis: a randomised, placebo-controlled, phase 2b study. J Crohns Colitis 2016;10:418–28.
21. Sandborn WJ, Feagan BG, Wolf DC, et al. Ozanimod induction and maintenance treatment for ulcerative colitis. N Engl J Med 2016;374(18):1754–62.

22. Scott FL, Clemons B, Brooks J, et al. Ozanimod (RPC1063) is a potent sphingosine-1-phosphate receptor-1 (S1P1) and receptor-5 (S1P5) agonist with autoimmune disease-modifying activity. Br J Pharmacol 2016;173(11): 1778–92.
23. Nanau RM, Neuman MG. Metabolome and inflammasome in inflammatory bowel disease. Transl Res 2012;160(1):1–28.
24. McGovern D, Powrie F. The IL23 axis plays a key role in the pathogenesis of IBD. Gut 2007;56(10):1333–6.
25. Teng MW, Bowman EP, McElwee JJ, et al. IL-12 and IL-23 cytokines: from discovery to targeted therapies for immune-mediated inflammatory diseases. Nat Med 2015;21(7):719–29.
26. Murphy CA, Langrish CL, Chen Y, et al. Divergent pro- and antiinflammatory roles for IL-23 and IL-12 in joint autoimmune inflammation. J Exp Med 2003;198(12): 1951–7.
27. Oppmann B, Lesley R, Blom B, et al. Novel p19 protein engages IL-12p40 to form a cytokine, IL-23, with biological activities similar as well as distinct from IL-12. Immunity 2000;13(5):715–25.
28. Feagan BG, Sandborn WJ, Gasink C, et al. Ustekinumab as induction and maintenance therapy for Crohn's disease. N Engl J Med 2016;375(20):1946–60.
29. Panaccione R, Sandborn WJ, Gordon GL, et al. Briakinumab for treatment of Crohn's disease: results of a randomized trial. Inflamm Bowel Dis 2015;21(6): 1329–40.
30. Blauvelt A, Papp KA, Griffiths CEM, et al. Efficacy and safety of guselkumab, an anti-interleukin-23 monoclonal antibody, compared with adalimumab for the continuous treatment of patients with moderate to severe psoriasis: results from the phase III, double-blinded, placebo- and active comparator–controlled VOYAGE 1 trial. J Am Acad Dermatol 2017;76(3):405–17.
31. Sands BE, Chen J, Feagan BG, et al. Efficacy and safety of MEDI2070, an antibody against interleukin 23, in patients with moderate to severe Crohn's disease: a phase 2a study. Gastroenterology 2017. [Epub ahead of print].
32. Tausend W, Downing C, Tyring S. Systematic review of interleukin-12, interleukin-17, and interleukin-23 pathway inhibitors for the treatment of moderate-to-severe chronic plaque psoriasis: ustekinumab, briakinumab, tildrakizumab, guselkumab, secukinumab, ixekizumab, and brodalumab. J Cutan Med Surg 2014; 18(3):156–69.
33. Feagan BG, Sandborn WJ, D'Haens G, et al. Induction therapy with the selective interleukin-23 inhibitor risankizumab in patients with moderate-to-severe Crohn's disease: a randomized, double-blind, placebo-controlled phase 2 study. Lancet 2017;389:1699–709.
34. Yen D, Cheung J, Scheerens H, et al. IL-23 is essential for T cell–mediated colitis and promotes inflammation via IL-17 and IL-6. J Clin Invest 2006;116(5):1310–6.
35. Fujino S, Andoh A, Bamba S, et al. Increased expression of interleukin 17 in inflammatory bowel disease. Gut 2003;52(1):65–70.
36. O'Connor W Jr, Kamanaka M, Booth CJ, et al. A protective function for interleukin 17A in T cell-mediated intestinal inflammation. Nat Immunol 2009;10(6):603–9.
37. Hueber W, Sands BE, Lewitzky S, et al. Secukinumab, a human anti-IL-17A monoclonal antibody, for moderate to severe Crohn's disease: unexpected results of a randomised, double-blind placebo-controlled trial. Gut 2012;61(12):1693–700.
38. Hueber W, Patel DD, Dryja T, et al. Effects of AIN457, a fully human antibody to interleukin-17A, on psoriasis, rheumatoid arthritis, and uveitis. Sci Transl Med 2010;2(52):52ra72.

39. Jones SA, Horiuchi S, Topley N, et al. The soluble interleukin 6 receptor: mechanisms of production and implications in disease. FASEB J 2001;15(1):43–58.
40. Hosokawa T, Kusugami K, Ina K, et al. Interleukin-6 and soluble interleukin-6 receptor in the colonic mucosa of inflammatory bowel disease. J Gastroenterol Hepatol 1999;14(10):987–96.
41. Mitsuyama K, Toyonaga A, Sasaki E, et al. Soluble interleukin-6 receptors in inflammatory bowel disease: relation to circulating interleukin-6. Gut 1995;36(1): 45–9.
42. Yamamoto M, Yoshizaki K, Kishimoto T, et al. IL-6 is required for the development of Th1 cell-mediated murine colitis. J Immunol 2000;164(9):4878–82.
43. Ito H, Takazoe M, Fukuda Y, et al. A pilot randomized trial of a human anti-interleukin-6 receptor monoclonal antibody in active Crohn's disease. Gastroenterology 2004;126(4):989–96.
44. Galien R. Janus kinases in inflammatory bowel disease: four kinases for multiple purposes. Pharmacol Rep 2016;68(4):789–96.
45. O'Shea JJ, Schwartz DM, Villarino AV, et al. The JAK-STAT pathway: impact on human disease and therapeutic intervention. Annu Rev Med 2015;66:311–28.
46. Kremer JM, Bloom BJ, Breedveld FC, et al. The safety and efficacy of a JAK inhibitor in patients with active rheumatoid arthritis: results of a double-blind, placebo-controlled phase IIa trial of three dosage levels of CP-690,550 versus placebo. Arthritis Rheum 2009;60(7):1895–905.
47. Sandborn WJ, Ghosh S, Panes J, et al. Tofacitinib, an oral Janus kinase inhibitor, in active ulcerative colitis. N Engl J Med 2012;367(7):616–24.
48. Sandborn WJ, Ghosh S, Panes J, et al. A phase 2 study of tofacitinib, an oral Janus kinase inhibitor, in patients with Crohn's disease. Clin Gastroenterol Hepatol 2014;12(9):1485–93.e2.
49. Vermeire S, Schreiber S, Petryka R, et al. Clinical remission in patients with moderate-to-severe Crohn's disease treated with filgotinib (the FITZROY study): results from a phase 2, double-blind, randomised, placebo-controlled trial. Lancet 2017;389(10066):266–75.
50. Gabay C, McInnes IB, Kavanaugh A, et al. Comparison of lipid and lipid-associated cardiovascular risk marker changes after treatment with tocilizumab or adalimumab in patients with rheumatoid arthritis. Ann Rheum Dis 2016; 75(10):1806–12.
51. Park J-S, Kwok S-K, Lim M-A, et al. STA-21, a promising STAT-3 inhibitor that reciprocally regulates Th17 and Treg cells, inhibits osteoclastogenesis in mice and humans and alleviates autoimmune inflammation in an experimental model of rheumatoid arthritis. Arthritis Rheumatol 2014;66(4):918–29.
52. Kelsall B. Interleukin-10 in inflammatory bowel disease. N Engl J Med 2009; 361(21):2091–3.
53. Schwager K, Kaspar M, Bootz F, et al. Preclinical characterization of DEKAVIL (F8-IL10), a novel clinical-stage immunocytokine which inhibits the progression of collagen-induced arthritis. Arthritis Res Ther 2009;11(5):R142.
54. Monteleone G, Neurath MF, Ardizzone S, et al. Mongersen, an oral SMAD7 antisense oligonucleotide, and Crohn's disease. N Engl J Med 2015;372(12): 1104–13.
55. Dave M, Mehta K, Luther J, et al. Mesenchymal stem cell therapy for inflammatory bowel disease: a systematic review and meta-analysis. Inflamm Bowel Dis 2015; 21(11):2696–707.

56. Burt RK, Craig RM, Milanetti F, et al. Autologous nonmyeloablative hematopoietic stem cell transplantation in patients with severe anti-TNF refractory Crohn's disease: long-term follow-up. Blood 2010;116(26):6123–32.
57. Ciccocioppo R, Bernardo ME, Sgarella A, et al. Autologous bone marrow-derived mesenchymal stromal cells in the treatment of fistulising Crohn's disease. Gut 2011;60(6):788–98.
58. Himmel ME, Yao Y, Orban PC, et al. Regulatory T-cell therapy for inflammatory bowel disease: more questions than answers. Immunology 2012;136(2):115–22.
59. Sarmento OF, Svingen PA, Xiong Y, et al. The role of the histone methyltransferase enhancer of zeste homolog 2 (EZH2) in the pathobiological mechanisms underlying inflammatory bowel disease (IBD). J Biol Chem 2016;292(2):706–22.

Use of Anti–Tumor Necrosis Factors and Anti-Integrins in the Treatment of Crohn's Disease

Raina Shivashankar, MD[a], Darrell S. Pardi, MD[b,*]

KEYWORDS

• Crohn's disease • Treatment • Biologics • Anti-TNFs • Anti-integrins

KEY POINTS

- Anti–tumor necrosis factors (TNFs) are effective in induction and maintenance of remission in patients with moderate to severe Crohn's disease (CD).
- Anti-TNFs are effective in improving long-term outcomes (ie, rates of hospitalization, surgery, and health-related quality of life [HRQoL]) in patients with CD.
- Anti-integrins are effective in induction and maintenance of remission in patients with CD.
- There are limited data on long-term outcomes with the use of anti-integrins; however, some data suggest benefits in HRQoL.
- Anti-TNFs are effective for fistula closure; currently there are limited data on the use of anti-integrins for this indication.

INTRODUCTION

Crohn's disease (CD) is a chronic inflammatory disease that can affect the entire length of the gastrointestinal tract. The incidence of CD is increasing, and currently it is estimated there are approximately 780,000 Americans with CD. Patients with CD may experience complications such as strictures and fistulae, and therefore they often require aggressive therapy with the major aim of preventing long-term complications and surgery. This article separately discusses the clinical efficacy, long-term outcomes, safety, and comparative effectiveness of both anti–tumor necrosis factor (anti-TNF) alpha and anti-integrin biologics. In addition, it discusses indirect comparisons of anti-TNFs and anti-integrins.

Disclosures: Dr D.S. Pardi has received research grants from Janssen (CO168UCO4002) and Takeda (Z01-58001).

[a] Division of Gastroenterology, University of Pennsylvania, 3400 Civic Center Boulevard, 4th Floor, South Pavilion, Philadelphia, PA 19104, USA; [b] Division of Gastroenterology and Hepatology, Mayo Clinic, 200 First Street Southwest, Rochester, MN 55905, USA

* Corresponding author.

E-mail address: pardi.darrell@mayo.edu

Gastroenterol Clin N Am 46 (2017) 589–601
http://dx.doi.org/10.1016/j.gtc.2017.05.012
gastro.theclinics.com

ANTI–TUMOR NECROSIS FACTORS

The cause of CD is uncertain, and likely involves a complex interplay of genetics and the environment. Active CD is characterized by an inflammatory infiltrate of the gut lamina propria, which in turn increases levels of proinflammatory cytokines, including TNF-α.[1] Studies have shown that monoclonal antibodies targeting TNF-α are effective at induction and maintenance of remission in CD.[2]

The overall goal of CD therapy is to achieve corticosteroid-free clinical remission and mucosal healing, and to decrease long-term complications requiring hospitalization and surgery. Compared with mesalamine, corticosteroids, and immunomodulators, anti-TNFs are more effective at achieving these goals. For example, infliximab has been shown to decrease hospitalization and surgery rates,[3,4] whereas mesalamine, corticosteroids, and immunomodulators have not.

Three anti-TNFs have been approved for the treatment of CD: infliximab (IFX), adalimumab (ADA), and certolizumab pegol (CZP).[5] IFX is a chimeric monoclonal immunoglobulin G (IgG) 1 antibody targeted against TNF; it is infused intravenously with a weight-based dose of 5 mg/kg at weeks 0, 2, and 6 for induction, followed by 5 mg/kg every 8 weeks for maintenance therapy. ADA is a fully humanized, monoclonal IgG1 antibody against TNF administered subcutaneously with a loading dose of 160 mg and 80 mg at weeks 0 and 2 for induction, followed by 40 mg every 2 weeks for maintenance of remission. CZP contains the Fab fragment of a humanized anti-TNF monoclonal antibody; it is administered subcutaneously with a loading dosing of 400 mg at weeks 0, 2, and 4 followed by 400 mg every 4 weeks for maintenance.

Clinical Remission

Randomized controlled trials (RCTs) for IFX, ADA, and CZP induction therapy in patients with moderate to severe CD have defined clinical remission as a Crohn's Disease Activity Index (CDAI) less than 150. Remission rates at weeks 4 to 12 were 33% to 72% for IFX[6–8]; 21% to 43% for ADA (36%–43% in anti-TNF–naive patients, 21%–26% in anti-TNF–exposed patients)[9–11]; and 22% to 29.2% for CZP (22%–26.4% in anti-TNF–naive patients, 29.2% in anti-TNF–exposed patients).[12–14] The relative risk (RR) of failure to achieve remission with anti-TNF compared with placebo in active CD was 0.87 (95% confidence interval [CI], 0.80–0.94; *P* = .001). The number needed to treat (NNT) with anti-TNF to achieve remission in active CD was 8 (95% CI, 6–17).[15] As opposed to IFX and ADA studies, there was no significant difference between CZP and placebo at week 12 in induction of remission in patients with active CD.[14]

In patients who respond to induction with anti-TNFs, continued anti-TNF therapy is more effective than placebo for maintenance of remission.[2] Meta-analysis of the RCTs of anti-TNFs for maintenance of remission (through weeks 26–60) has shown a 29% decreased risk of relapse compared with placebo with an NNT of 4 (95% CI, 3–5).[15]

Treatment of Fistulae

Anti-TNFs are effective in treating CD-related fistulae. When studies that involved short durations (4 weeks) of fistula treatment were excluded, meta-analysis showed that anti-TNFs have a significantly higher rate of fistula healing compared with placebo (RR of fistulae remaining unhealed = 0.80; 95% CI, 0.65–0.98).[15] IFX is the only anti-TNF that has been studied with fistula healing as the primary end point in an RCT of patients with penetrating CD.[16,17] Rates of fistula closure were significantly higher in patients receiving IFX compared with placebo (55% vs 13%; *P* = .001).[16] IFX also was superior to placebo for maintaining fistula closure (36% vs 19% at week 54; *P* = .009).[17] Rates of partial fistula closure, which was defined as at least 50% reduction in the number of draining fistulae, are high[5]; 62% of IFX-treated patients (compared with 26% of placebo-treated patients) achieved partial response ($P = .002$).[5,16]

Post hoc analyses of RCTs of ADA and CZP have assessed fistula closure as secondary end points. At weeks 18 to 56, complete fistula closure rates were 33% for ADA (vs 13% for placebo-treated patients) and 30% to 54% for CZP (vs 31%–43% for placebo-treated patients).[13,18,19] In the GAIN (Gauging Adalimumab Efficacy in Infliximab Nonresponders) study of ADA efficacy in patients with prior intolerance to IFX or loss of response, partial fistula closure (reduction of number of draining fistulae by ≥50% at 2 weeks) was seen in 20% of ADA-treated patients versus 15% of placebo patients.[5,10]

Mucosal Healing

Mucosal healing has been associated with corticosteroid-free clinical remission, decreased rates of surgery, and fewer hospitalizations.[3,20–22] In a population-based cohort from Sweden (the Inflammatory Bowel South-Eastern Norway [IBSEN] study), patients with CD who achieved mucosal healing one year after diagnosis had decreased rates of steroid requirement, less inflammation, and a trend toward lower risk of surgical resection over the next 7 years compared with those with continued endoscopic disease activity.[23] A recent meta-analysis showed significantly higher odds for achieving long-term clinical remission (odds ratio [OR] = 2.8; 95% CI, 1.91–4.1) and avoiding CD-related surgeries (OR = 2.22; 95% CI, 0.86–5.69) in patients who achieved mucosal healing compared with those who did not.[22]

In the SONIC (Study of Biologic and Immunomodulator Naive Patients in Crohn's Disease) trial, mucosal healing was achieved in 44% of patients treated with combination therapy compared with 30% of patients treated with IFX monotherapy and 16% in those treated with azathioprine monotherapy.[6] In the EXTEND (Extend the Safety and Efficacy of Adalimumab through Endoscopic Healing) trial, mucosal healing was achieved in 27% of ADA-treated patients (vs 13% of placebo-treated patients) at week 12; at week 52, the rates were 24% and 0%, respectively.[24] In the MUSIC (Endoscopic MUcoSal Improvement in Patients with Active Crohn's Disease Treated with certolizumab pegol) trial, mucosal healing was achieved in 10% of CZP-treated patients (vs 4% with placebo) at week 10; at week 54 the rates were 14% and 8%, respectively.[25] The variations in healing may in part be caused by the different definitions of mucosal healing used in these trials.[5]

Long-Term Outcomes

The efficacy of anti-TNF agents in patients with CD has influenced long-term outcomes of disease, specifically the need for hospitalization and surgery. Previous tertiary referral data before the anti-TNF era estimated the need for surgery to be 75% to 80% within 20 years of CD diagnosis.[3,26] Population-based estimates from Norway suggested a cumulative probability of 38% within 10 years of CD diagnosis before the use of biologics[27]; in a population-based cohort from Olmsted County, Minnesota, the rate was slightly higher at 48% at 10 years.[28] In a subset of patients who were started on anti-TNF agents from an updated incidence cohort from Olmsted County (1970–2010), the rate of CD-related surgery was 19% after 5 years from initial CD diagnosis, supporting a beneficial effect of anti-TNFs on the risk of surgery.[29] A recent population-based study from Denmark showed the overall use of anti-TNFs to be 23.5%. The 7-year cumulative risk of intestinal resection was 28.5%, whereas surgical rate before the use of anti-TNFs was estimated to be 49% at 5 years.[30] Overall, from population-based estimates, it seems that there may be a decreased risk of surgery with use of anti-TNFs.

Similarly, RCTs have also found a decrease in surgery and hospitalization in patients with CD treated with anti-TNFs. The ACCENT I (A Crohn's Disease Clinical Trial

Evaluating Infliximab in a New Long-term Treatment Regimen) trial found that patients with moderate to severe CD with scheduled IFX (vs episodic IFX) were significantly less likely to require hospitalization or surgery.[5,31] In ACCENT II (A Crohn's disease Clinical trial Evaluating infliximab in a New Long-term Treatment regimen in patients with fistulising Crohn's disease) maintenance therapy with IFX led to significantly fewer hospitalization days, number of hospitalizations, and surgeries compared with treatment with placebo.[5,32]

Studies on ADA have shown similar results. In the CHARM (Crohn's trial of the fully Human antibody Adalimumab for Remission Maintenance) trial, patients who received ADA maintenance therapy had 48% fewer CD-related hospitalizations than those who received placebo.[33] There also was a decrease in CD-related surgeries compared with placebo.

Improvement in rates of hospitalization and surgery in patients with CD treated with IFX and ADA was also shown in a systematic review and meta-analysis.[34] In addition, when data from individual studies were pooled to make an indirect comparison, azathioprine alone was inferior to IFX and ADA at preventing CD-related hospitalization. However, only 1 trial was included for azathioprine in this study.

There are limited data on the impact of CZP on hospitalization and surgery. A comparative effectiveness study including anti-TNF–naive patients with CD suggested that IFX was superior to CZP in reducing both all-cause hospitalizations and CD-related hospitalizations.[35] When CZP-treated patients were compared with ADA-treated patients, there was a statistically significantly higher risk of all-cause hospitalization in those treated with CZP compared with ADA; the risks of CD-related hospitalization were numerically higher in CZP-treated patients compared with ADA-treated patients, although this was not statistically significant.[35] IFX-treated and ADA-treated patients had fewer abdominal surgeries than the CZP-treated group, although the differences were not statistically significant.

Safety

In RCTs of maintenance therapy, the reported rate of serious adverse events (AEs) was 22% to 28% for IFX (vs 29% for placebo),[36] 8% to 9.2% for ADA (vs 15.3%–24% for placebo),[11,18] and 6% to 10% for CZP (vs 7% for placebo).[13,19] The reported rate of serious infections was 4% to 5% for IFX (vs 4% for placebo),[6,36] 2.7% to 4% for ADA (vs 3.4%–8% for placebo),[11,18] and 2% to 3% for CZP (vs <1% for placebo).[13,19] There were no statistically significant differences in AEs between IFX, ADA, or CZP, and placebo in the respective studies.[13,18,36]

There have been no direct safety comparisons between IFX, ADA, and CZP. In 1 indirect analysis, there was no significant difference in the risk of serious infections requiring hospitalization between patients I treated with FX, ADA, and CZP.[35]

Quality of Life

Many studies have shown the benefit of anti-TNF therapy in improving health-related quality of life (HRQoL) in CD. In the ACCENT I study, patients who received IFX maintenance therapy achieved improvement in Inflammatory Bowel Disease Questionnaire (IBDQ) and Short Form 36 (SF-36) scores compared with those who received a single dose of IFX.[37]

In the CHARM trial, patients on ADA had statistically significant improvements in all HRQoL measures.[38] Those who continued ADA maintenance therapy had less fatigue, less depression, greater improvement in the IBDQ, greater SF-36 physical component scores, and less abdominal pain compared with placebo.[38] In the CARE (Crohn's treatment with Adalimumab, Patient Response to a Safety and Efficacy Study) trial,

ADA improved HRQoL and work productivity in both IFX-naive and IFX-exposed patients.

In addition, similar improvements on HRQoL were seen in CZP-treated patients with CD who previously lost response to IFX.[39] HRQoL, work productivity, and daily activity improved in those who received CZP maintenance therapy through week 26 of treatment, with improvements seen as early as week 6.

Comparative effectiveness

There have been no direct head-to-head comparisons of individual anti-TNFs against one another. However, a few retrospective cohort studies have sought to determine the comparative effectiveness of these agents. A study of Medicare beneficiaries found no significant difference between IFX and ADA in the number of patients who remained on the drug after week 26 (a surrogate marker of effectiveness), rates of hospitalizations, or the need for surgery.[40] In the minority of patients who were younger than 65 years old, IFX was superior to ADA in terms of lowering the risk of surgery.[40]

In a retrospective cohort study of a nationwide administrative claims database, Singh and colleagues[35] found that IFX-treated patients had a lower risk of CD-related hospitalizations, abdominal surgery, and corticosteroid use compared with ADA-treated patients. Compared with CZP-treated patients, IFX-treated patients had a lower risk of all-cause and CD-related hospitalization. The risk of all-cause hospitalization was significantly higher in CZP-treated patients compared with ADA-treated patients. CZP-treated patients also had higher risk of CD-related hospitalization and abdominal surgery than ADA-treated patients, but these differences were not statistically significant.[35] Overall, IFX-treated patients had better patient-related outcomes (lower CD-related hospitalizations, surgery, and corticosteroid use) compared with patients treated with both ADA or CZP as the first anti-TNF.[35]

A network meta-analysis found that IFX and ADA may be superior to CZP in biologic-naive patients with CD.[41] IFX (RR, 6.11; 95% credible interval [CrI], 2.49–18.29) and ADA (RR, 2.98; 95% CrI, 1.12–8.18) were more likely to induce remission than placebo, but CZP (RR, 1.48; 95% CrI, 0.76–2.93) was not. Similar results were found for maintenance of remission.

In addition, 2 other network meta-analyses provide indirect evidence of the benefits of anti-TNFs in patients with CD.[42,43] In one, all 3 anti-TNFs were superior to placebo for induction and maintenance of remission. For induction, there was a nonsignificant trend for IFX rather than ADA and CZP; among the subcutaneous anti-TNFs, ADA was superior to CZP (RR, 2.93; 95% CrI, 1.21–7.75).[42] In the third network meta-analysis, IFX plus azathioprine (OR, 3.1; 95% CrI, 1.4–7.7) and ADA (OR, 2.1; 95% CRI, 1.0–4.6) were superior to CZP for induction of remission.[43] For maintenance, ADA and IFX plus azathioprine were superior to CZP.[43] However, given the different conclusions of these 3 network meta-analyses and the lack of head-to-head comparisons, the confidence in these estimates is low.

ANTI-INTEGRINS

The migration of proinflammatory T cells into the gut mediates the inflammation that characterizes CD.[44,45] Activated effector T cells target the gut by interaction between surface-expressed α4β1 and α4β7 integrins on lymphocytes and adhesion molecules, which are present on endothelial cells. The interaction of these molecules allows movement of T cells out of the blood stream and into the gastrointestinal tract, and therefore blockade of α4β7 integrin has been targeted to prevent the downstream inflammatory cascade. Natalizumab (NAT) and vedolizumab (VDZ) are anti-integrin agents that have been approved for the treatment of CD.

NAT is a humanized IgG4 monoclonal antibody that targets the a4-integrin subunit of both α4β1 and α4β7 on the surface of lymphocytes and prevents binding to VCAM-1 (vascular cell adhesion molecule – 1) and MadCAM-1 receptors on the endothelium.[46] The interaction between α4β1 and VCAM-1 prevents trafficking of lymphocytes to the central nervous system, and the interaction of α4β7 and MadCAM-1 (Mucosal vascular addressin cell adhesion molecule 1) is gut specific.[46] NAT is an intravenous infusion that is administered at a dose of 300 mg at weeks 0, 4, and 8 for induction, followed by 300 mg intravenously every 4 weeks thereafter.

In contrast, VDZ is a gut-specific humanized IgG1 monoclonal antibody to α4β7 integrin that selectively regulates lymphocyte trafficking to the gut.[47] VDZ is infused intravenously at 300 mg at weeks 0, 2, 6 for induction, followed by 300 mg every 8 weeks thereafter.

Clinical Remission

The ENACT-1 (Efficacy of Natalizumab as Active Crohn's Therapy) study assessed the efficacy of NAT for induction of remission in patients with moderate to severe CD. Patients treated with NAT and placebo had similar rates of response (56% vs 49%; P = .05) and remission (37% vs 30%; P = .12) at week 10.[48]

Subsequently, the ENCORE (Efficacy of Natalizumab in Crohn's Disease Response and Remission) trial assessed patients with moderate to severe CD and active inflammation as defined by increased C-reactive protein (CRP) levels (>2.87 mg/L).[45] Compared with those who received placebo, NAT-treated patients had a significantly higher response rate at week 8 sustained through week 12 (48% compared with 32%; P<.001). Sustained remission was noted in 26% of NAT-treated patients compared with 16% of placebo-treated patients (P = .002). Week 4 response and remission rates also were significantly higher for NAT-treated patients compared with placebo. Therefore, patients treated with NAT had an early and sustained response through week 12.[45,46] Differences in outcomes between the ENACT-1 and ENCORE studies may be attributed to the subgroup analysis and differences in study design.

The ENACT-1 study delivered a fixed dose of NAT. In contrast, Ghosh and colleagues[49] studied weight-based dosing of NAT in patients with moderate to severe CD. Patients who received NAT had significantly higher rates of response and remission at several time points without a clear dose response.[49] In addition, a meta-analysis including these and other studies showed that NAT was significantly better than placebo for induction of remission in active CD (34.6% compared with 22.7%; NNT = 11).[15]

In the GEMINI-2 study, patients with moderate to severe CD treated with VDZ were significantly more likely to be in clinical remission than patients treated with placebo. However, there was no significant difference in CDAI-100 response at week 6.[47] Also, compared with placebo, there was no significant change in CRP concentration between week 0 and week 6 in patients treated with VDZ. A meta-analysis found fewer failures of induction of remission with VDZ and NAT compared with placebo (RR, 0.87; 95% CI, 0.84–0.91); the effect size for VDZ (RR, 0.87; 95% CI, 0.79–0.95) and NAT (RR, 0.86; 95% CI, 0.8–0.93) were similar.[50] The NNT with VDZ to achieve induction of remission was 10.[50]

Sands and colleagues[51] conducted a pooled analysis of patients with moderate to severe CD from the GEMINI-3 trial to assess the efficacy and safety of VDZ in patients who were previously exposed to anti-TNFs compared with those who were anti-TNF naive. In anti-TNF–naive patients, the effects of VDZ on induction of clinical remission were seen earlier (week 6) than in those who were previously exposed to anti-TNF agents (week 10). In both groups, clinical response with VDZ was higher than in the placebo-treated groups at weeks 6 and 10.[51] Also, there was no difference in VDZ efficacy when the number of previous anti-TNF agents used is taken into account.[51] Therefore, in CD the effects of VDZ may not be evident quickly, especially in patients previously on anti-TNFs, and therefore it is recommended that patients should be continued on VDZ at least through the first maintenance dose (week 14) to assess whether any benefit has occurred.

Chandar and colleagues[50] recently conducted a systematic review and meta-analysis including 8 trials (5 comparing NAT with placebo and 3 comparing VDZ with placebo) to assess the efficacy and safety of anti-integrins in the treatment of patients with CD. NAT was superior to placebo for induction of remission (RR of treatment failure, 0.86; 95% CI, 0.80–0.93). NAT was also effective in inducing remission in anti-TNF–naive (RR, 0.87; 95% CI, 0.75–1.00) and anti-TNF–exposed patients (RR, 0.86; 95% CI, 0.76–0.99).[50]

The ENACT-2 (Evaluation of Natalizumab as Continuous Therapy) trial showed that NAT was effective as maintenance therapy for CD from week 20 through week 60.[45,48] For maintenance of remission, a meta-analysis showed that NAT was superior to placebo in preventing a disease flare in CD at week 60 (39.2% vs 15%).[15] In the maintenance phase of the GEMINI 2 study, VDZ (300 mg every 8 weeks) maintained statistically significantly higher rates of clinical remission, CDAI-100 response, and glucocorticoid-free remission than placebo.[47]

A few open- label studies have reported the efficacy of VDZ in CD.[52,53] In a retrospective cohort study from 7 medical centers, the US VICTORY (Vedolizumab for Health OuTComes in InflammatORY Bowel Diseases) Consortium studied the efficacy of VDZ treatment of moderate to severe CD in usual clinical practice.[52] Most patients (90%) were previously treated with anti-TNFs. Cumulative rates of clinical remission at 6, 12, and 18 months of therapy were 18%, 35%, and 54%, respectively.[52] Patients with severe disease, active perianal disease, previous or active smoking, and previous anti-TNF use were less likely to achieve clinical remission. Most clinical response occurred after 6 months of treatment.

In patients who lose response to VDZ every 8 weeks, dose escalation to every 4 weeks may be beneficial. In one study, at 28 weeks after dose escalation 54% of patients were in clinical response and 23% were in clinical remission.[53] After 100 weeks of therapy, clinical response and remission rates were 35% and 19%, respectively. This trend was seen regardless of exposure to prior anti-TNF.

Treatment of Fistulae

In the GEMINI-2 trial, there was a significantly greater benefit for VDZ than for placebo for fistula closure (41.2% vs 11.1%) at week 52.[47] There was no significant difference in VDZ every 4 weeks (22.7%) compared with placebo.[47] These data suggest a treatment benefit for fistula closure; however, these data are limited and further studies are required to assess this end point. There is a paucity of data for NAT in fistula healing because the ENACT-1/ENACT-2[48] and ENCORE[45] studies did not enroll patients with draining fistulae.

At present, because there are stronger long-term data for fistula healing with anti-TNFs, it is reasonable to use anti-TNFs as first-line therapy for patients with fistulizing CD. Future prospective studies would be helpful in elucidating the effect of anti-integrins on CD fistula closure.

Mucosal Healing

There are limited data on mucosal healing with anti-integrins. A retrospective study using the Simple Endoscopic Score for Crohn's Disease (SES_CD) to assess endoscopic severity in patients treated with NAT determined that mucosal healing (defined as decrease of SES-CD >70%) occurred in 42% of patients.[54] Patients who achieved mucosal healing had a lower risk of hospitalization than those who did not achieve this end point (RR, 0.17; 95% CI, 0.039–0.78). However, because this was a small retrospective study, larger prospective studies would be important to confirm these findings.

There also are few data on mucosal healing with VDZ. In one study, cumulative rates of mucosal healing after 6 and 12 months of maintenance therapy were 20% and 63%, respectively.[52] The median time to achieve mucosal healing was 33 weeks (21–14 weeks). Patients with severe disease activity and prior anti-TNF use were less likely to achieve mucosal healing.[52]

Long-Term Outcomes

Data on long-term outcomes of NAT-treated and VDZ-treated patients with CD are similarly limited. Use of NAT in a small cohort of patients with CD was the only factor that was found to modify the risk of surgery (hazard ratio [HR], 0.23; 95% CI, 0.06–0.98).[54] In a retrospective cohort study of patients with CD followed for 12 months, 51% of patients discontinued NAT, most commonly because of nonresponse.[55] In a prospective study of NAT, the cumulative probability of complete response within 1 year was 56% (28%–73%).[56]

In the US VICTORY study, the cumulative rates of surgery after 6 and 12 months of VDZ maintenance therapy were 10% and 23%, respectively.[52] Further prospective studies are required to determine the long-term outcomes of VDZ.

Safety

The major concern regarding NAT use has been the rare but serious occurrence of progressive multifocal leukoencephalopathy (PML), which is caused by the nonselective inhibition of $\alpha4\beta1$ integrin and lymphocyte tracking to the brain, thus causing reactivation of the John Cunningham (JC) virus.[50,57] The seroprevalence of JC virus in patients with CD is approximately 67.5%, similar to the general population (30%–70%). Previous use of thiopurines seems to increase the risk of a positive serology.[58] In NAT clinical trials, which included approximately 3000 patients, 3 cases of PML occurred. The mean latency from the start of NAT to the development of PML was 18 months.[59] As of June 2015, 566 cases of PML had been confirmed among more than 138,800 patients exposed to natalizumab (0.4%).[59]

In the ENCORE study, AEs with NAT treatment occurred in similar frequencies to placebo-treated patients; 9% of patients (23 of 260) in the natalizumab group and 13% of patients (32 of 250) in the placebo group discontinued treatment because of an AE.[45] The most common AEs were headache, nausea, abdominal pain, nasopharyngitis, fatigue, and CD exacerbation.

Given that VDZ is gut specific and, as opposed to NAT, does not affect leukocyte trafficking elsewhere, including the central nervous system, VDZ has a superior safety profile. Colombel and colleagues[59] recently published long-term safety data on 1723 patients exposed to VDZ for up to 5 years in previous clinical studies. Exposure-adjusted incidence rates for AEs and serious AEs (SAEs) were lower in VDZ-treated patients than in placebo-treated patients. Predictors of serious infection included the concomitant use of narcotics (HR, 2.72; 95% CI, 1.90–3.89) and corticosteroids (HR, 1.88; 95% CI, 1.35–2.63). Younger age was protective (HR, 0.97; 95% CI, 0.95–0.98). In a placebo controlled trial, 4 patients developed malignancies while on VDZ compared with 1 placebo-treated patient.[13] Including open-label studies, 9 VDZ-treated patients developed malignancies. Overall, VDZ was well tolerated in patients with moderate to severe CD. No cases of PML have been identified in this cohort or in any of the clinical trials of VDZ.

Similarly, Dulai and colleagues[52] found low rates of SAEs and serious infections in patients treated with VDZ. In a meta-analysis and systematic review, 8.8% of VDZ-treated patients developed SAEs, and there was no significant difference in the rate of AEs or serious infections between VDZ and NAT.[50] However, the rate of infusion reactions with NAT is higher than with VDZ ($P = .007$).

Quality of Life

Because VDZ was recently approved for treatment of CD, there are few data on HRQoL. In the GEMINI long-term safety study, an open-label phase 4 extension study, VDZ did have a positive effect on HRQoL in patients receiving maintenance therapy.[53]

The major RCTs of NAT therapy also found improvement in HRQoL.[45,48,60]

Comparative effectiveness

There are no head-to-head comparisons of NAT and VDZ, although a recent meta-analysis and systematic review compared outcomes of the 2 medications.[50] NAT and VDZ were superior to placebo for the induction of clinical remission in CD. There was no significant difference between the two medications in terms of failing to induce remission (NAT, RR 0.86 and 95% CI 0.8–0.93; and VDZ, RR 0.87 and 95% CI 0.79–0.95); the corresponding NNTs for NAT and VDZ for induction of remission were 9 and 10, respectively.[50] When patients were stratified by previous anti-TNF exposure, there still was no difference in efficacy of either NAT and VDZ for induction of remission.

In terms of maintenance therapy, ENACT-2 and GEMINI-2 were compared. At week 60, 55% of NAT-treated patients had sustained remission; at week 52, 39% of patients receiving VDZ had sustained remission.[50] These comparisons were not direct, and therefore differences in study design, unmeasured confounders, and population size cannot be directly controlled for. On meta-analysis, there was no significant difference in rates of treatment discontinuation between NAT and VDZ compared with placebo.[50]

INDIRECT COMPARISON OF ANTI–TUMOR NECROSIS FACTORS AND ANTI-INTEGRINS

A few studies have provided indirect comparisons between anti-TNFs and anti-integrins.[41,61] A network meta-analysis found that IFX and ADA (but not CZP) may be superior to NAT and VDZ in biologic-naive patients with CD.[41] IFX (RR, 6.11; 95% CrI, 2.49–18.29) and ADA (RR, 2.98; 95% CrI, 1.12–8.18) were more likely to induce remission than placebo; however, NAT (RR, 1.36; 95% CrI, 0.69–2.86) and VDZ (RR, 1.40; 95% CrI, 0.63–3.28) were not. Similar results were found for maintenance of remission.

When anti-TNFs and anti-integrins were compared by network meta-analysis, there was no significant difference for induction of clinical remission (OR, 1.13; 95% CI, 0.72–1.76) or maintenance of clinical remission (OR, 1.18; 95% CI, 0.55–2.50).[61] When RCTs of CZP were excluded from analysis, anti-TNFs did achieve significantly higher odds of clinical remission compared with anti-integrins (OR, 1.64; 95% CI, 1.10–2.44). However, exclusion of CZP RCTs from the maintenance of remission comparison did not reveal any significant difference between anti-TNFs and anti-integrins.

Another network meta-analysis studied the safety of anti-TNF and anti-integrin treatment of CD.[62] In induction studies, there were no significant differences in safety end points between ADA, VDZ, CZP, and placebo. However, based on a probability plot, VDZ may be the safest therapeutic option in terms of specific AEs such as arthralgias, headache, pyrexia, and nasopharyngitis.[62] In maintenance studies, there were no significant differences in safety assessments (SAEs or serious infections) in patients treated with IFX, ADA, or VDZ.[62]

Given the different mechanisms of actions between anti-TNFs and anti-integrins, CD phenotype and safety profile should be taken into account when deciding on a first-line agent. For example, as noted earlier, the data for fistula closure are currently more robust for anti-TNFs than for anti-integrins, so the former therapy may be preferred in patients with fistulizing disease. In contrast, for patients unwilling to accept anti-TNF therapy because of concerns about safety, VDZ therapy may be more acceptable.

SUMMARY

In patients with CD, anti-TNF therapy is efficacious for induction and maintenance of clinical remission, mucosal healing, reducing rates of surgery and hospitalizations, and improving HRQoL. Long-term data have shown that anti-TNFs are relatively safe medications and the benefits afforded by these medications outweigh their potential risks. Indirect comparisons suggest that IFX and ADA may be superior to CZP in the treatment of CD.

Anti-integrins, especially VDZ, are newer agents for CD treatment and therefore long-term efficacy and safety data are more limited. NAT and VDZ are efficacious for induction and maintenance of remission and improving HRQoL. VDZ is preferred to NAT because of its gut-specific selectivity and favorable side effect profile (particularly with regard to the risk of PML). Data on the efficacy of anti-integrins in patients with fistulizing disease are limited.

The decision between anti-TNFs or anti-integrins as first-line treatment in CD depends on disease severity, safety concerns, and prescription coverage. Given the existing data on long-term outcomes and safety, anti-TNFs are often preferred to anti-integrins. In particular, based on the gut-specific selectivity of VDZ, it may not be as effective as an anti-TNF in patients with perianal disease or extraintestinal manifestations, although further study is needed in these areas.

In contrast, in patients with milder disease who want to avoid the potential adverse effects of anti-TNFs, VDZ may be a reasonable alternative. At present, VDZ has been used most often as a second-line agent after anti-TNF failure. Additional clinical experience and preferably prospective, head-to-head studies will be important to determine whether VDZ should be considered more often for first-line therapy in CD.

REFERENCES

1. Abraham C, Cho JH. Inflammatory bowel disease. N Engl J Med 2009;361:2066–78.
2. Peyrin-Biroulet L, Deltenre P, de Suray N, et al. Efficacy and safety of tumor necrosis factor antagonists in Crohn's disease: meta-analysis of placebo-controlled trials. Clin Gastroenterol Hepatol 2008;6:644–53.
3. Sokol H, Seksik P, Cosnes J. Complications and surgery in the inflammatory bowel diseases biological era. Curr Opin Gastroenterol 2014;30:378–84.
4. Costa J, Magro F, Caldeira D, et al. Infliximab reduces hospitalizations and surgery interventions in patients with inflammatory bowel disease: a systematic review and meta-analysis. Inflamm Bowel Dis 2013;19:2098–110.
5. Singh S, Pardi DS. Update on anti-tumor necrosis factor agents in Crohn disease. Gastroenterol Clin North Am 2014;43:457–78.
6. Colombel JF, Sandborn WJ, Reinisch W, et al. Infliximab, azathioprine, or combination therapy for Crohn's disease. N Engl J Med 2010;362:1383–95.
7. Lemann M, Mary JY, Duclos B, et al. Infliximab plus azathioprine for steroid-dependent Crohn's disease patients: a randomized placebo-controlled trial. Gastroenterology 2006;130:1054–61.

8. Targan SR, Hanauer SB, van Deventer SJ, et al. A short-term study of chimeric monoclonal antibody cA2 to tumor necrosis factor alpha for Crohn's disease. Crohn's Disease cA2 Study Group. N Engl J Med 1997;337:1029–35.
9. Hanauer SB, Sandborn WJ, Rutgeerts P, et al. Human anti-tumor necrosis factor monoclonal antibody (adalimumab) in Crohn's disease: the CLASSIC-I trial. Gastroenterology 2006;130:323–33 [quiz: 591].
10. Sandborn WJ, Rutgeerts P, Enns R, et al. Adalimumab induction therapy for Crohn disease previously treated with infliximab: a randomized trial. Ann Intern Med 2007;146:829–38.
11. Watanabe M, Hibi T, Lomax KG, et al. Adalimumab for the induction and maintenance of clinical remission in Japanese patients with Crohn's disease. J Crohns Colitis 2012;6:160–73.
12. Sandborn WJ, Abreu MT, D'Haens G, et al. Certolizumab pegol in patients with moderate to severe Crohn's disease and secondary failure to infliximab. Clin Gastroenterol Hepatol 2010;8:688–95.e2.
13. Sandborn WJ, Feagan BG, Stoinov S, et al. Certolizumab pegol for the treatment of Crohn's disease. N Engl J Med 2007;357:228–38.
14. Schreiber S, Rutgeerts P, Fedorak RN, et al. A randomized, placebo-controlled trial of certolizumab pegol (CDP870) for treatment of Crohn's disease. Gastroenterology 2005;129:807–18.
15. Ford AC, Sandborn WJ, Khan KJ, et al. Efficacy of biological therapies in inflammatory bowel disease: systematic review and meta-analysis. Am J Gastroenterol 2011;106:644–59 [quiz: 660].
16. Present DH, Rutgeerts P, Targan S, et al. Infliximab for the treatment of fistulas in patients with Crohn's disease. N Engl J Med 1999;340:1398–405.
17. Sands BE, Anderson FH, Bernstein CN, et al. Infliximab maintenance therapy for fistulizing Crohn's disease. N Engl J Med 2004;350:876–85.
18. Colombel JF, Sandborn WJ, Rutgeerts P, et al. Adalimumab for maintenance of clinical response and remission in patients with Crohn's disease: the CHARM trial. Gastroenterology 2007;132:52–65.
19. Schreiber S, Khaliq-Kareemi M, Lawrance IC, et al. Maintenance therapy with certolizumab pegol for Crohn's disease. N Engl J Med 2007;357:239–50.
20. Rutgeerts P, Vermeire S, Van Assche G. Mucosal healing in inflammatory bowel disease: impossible ideal or therapeutic target? Gut 2007;56:453–5.
21. Cintolo M, Costantino G, Pallio S, et al. Mucosal healing in inflammatory bowel disease: maintain or de-escalate therapy. World J Gastrointest Pathophysiol 2016;7:1–16.
22. Shah SC, Colombel JF, Sands BE, et al. Systematic review with meta-analysis: mucosal healing is associated with improved long-term outcomes in Crohn's disease. Aliment Pharmacol Ther 2016;43:317–33.
23. Froslie KF, Jahnsen J, Moum BA, et al. Mucosal healing in inflammatory bowel disease: results from a Norwegian population-based cohort. Gastroenterology 2007;133:412–22.
24. Rutgeerts P, Van Assche G, Sandborn WJ, et al. Adalimumab induces and maintains mucosal healing in patients with Crohn's disease: data from the EXTEND trial. Gastroenterology 2012;142:1102–11.e2.
25. Hebuterne X, Lemann M, Bouhnik Y, et al. Endoscopic improvement of mucosal lesions in patients with moderate to severe ileocolonic Crohn's disease following treatment with certolizumab pegol. Gut 2013;62:201–8.
26. Munkholm P, Langholz E, Davidsen M, et al. Disease activity courses in a regional cohort of Crohn's disease patients. Scand J Gastroenterol 1995;30:699–706.

27. Solberg IC, Vatn MH, Hoie O, et al. Clinical course in Crohn's disease: results of a Norwegian population-based ten-year follow-up study. Clin Gastroenterol Hepatol 2007;5:1430–8.
28. Peyrin-Biroulet L, Harmsen WS, Tremaine WJ, et al. Surgery in a population-based cohort of Crohn's disease from Olmsted County, Minnesota (1970-2004). Am J Gastroenterol 2012;107:1693–701.
29. Shivashankar R, Tremaine W, Harmsen W, et al. Cumulative probability and outcomes of anti-tumor necrosis factor use in patients with Crohn's disease: a population-based study. Gastroenterology 2016;150(4 Suppl 1):S202–3.
30. Munkholm P. Crohn's disease–occurrence, course and prognosis. An epidemiologic cohort-study. Dan Med Bull 1997;44:287–302.
31. Rutgeerts P, Feagan BG, Lichtenstein GR, et al. Comparison of scheduled and episodic treatment strategies of infliximab in Crohn's disease. Gastroenterology 2004;126:402–13.
32. Lichtenstein GR, Yan S, Bala M, et al. Infliximab maintenance treatment reduces hospitalizations, surgeries, and procedures in fistulizing Crohn's disease. Gastroenterology 2005;128:862–9.
33. Feagan BG, Panaccione R, Sandborn WJ, et al. Effects of adalimumab therapy on incidence of hospitalization and surgery in Crohn's disease: results from the CHARM study. Gastroenterology 2008;135:1493–9.
34. Mao EJ, Hazlewood GS, Kaplan GG, et al. Systematic review with meta-analysis: comparative efficacy of immunosuppressants and biologics for reducing hospitalisation and surgery in Crohn's disease and ulcerative colitis. Aliment Pharmacol Ther 2017;45:3–13.
35. Singh S, Heien HC, Sangaralingham LR, et al. Comparative effectiveness and safety of anti-tumor necrosis factor agents in biologic-naive patients with Crohn's disease. Clin Gastroenterol Hepatol 2016;14:1120–9.e6.
36. Hanauer SB, Feagan BG, Lichtenstein GR, et al. Maintenance infliximab for Crohn's disease: the ACCENT I randomised trial. Lancet 2002;359:1541–9.
37. Feagan BG, Yan S, Bala M, et al. The effects of infliximab maintenance therapy on health-related quality of life. Am J Gastroenterol 2003;98:2232–8.
38. Loftus EV, Feagan BG, Colombel JF, et al. Effects of adalimumab maintenance therapy on health-related quality of life of patients with Crohn's disease: patient-reported outcomes of the CHARM trial. Am J Gastroenterol 2008;103:3132–41.
39. Feagan BG, Sandborn WJ, Wolf DC, et al. Randomised clinical trial: improvement in health outcomes with certolizumab pegol in patients with active Crohn's disease with prior loss of response to infliximab. Aliment Pharmacol Ther 2011;33:541–50.
40. Osterman MT, Haynes K, Delzell E, et al. Comparative effectiveness of infliximab and adalimumab for Crohn's disease. Clin Gastroenterol Hepatol 2014;12:811–7.e3.
41. Singh S, Garg SK, Pardi DS, et al. Comparative efficacy of biologic therapy in biologic-naive patients with Crohn disease: a systematic review and network meta-analysis. Mayo Clin Proc 2014;89:1621–35.
42. Stidham RW, Lee TC, Higgins PD, et al. Systematic review with network meta-analysis: the efficacy of anti-TNF agents for the treatment of Crohn's disease. Aliment Pharmacol Ther 2014;39:1349–62.
43. Hazlewood GS, Rezaie A, Borman M, et al. Comparative effectiveness of immunosuppressants and biologics for inducing and maintaining remission in Crohn's disease: a network meta-analysis. Gastroenterology 2015;148:344–54.e5 [quiz: e14–5].

44. Lin L, Liu X, Wang D, et al. Efficacy and safety of antiintegrin antibody for inflammatory bowel disease: a systematic review and meta-analysis. Medicine (Baltimore) 2015;94:e556.
45. Targan SR, Feagan BG, Fedorak RN, et al. Natalizumab for the treatment of active Crohn's disease: results of the ENCORE Trial. Gastroenterology 2007;132:1672–83.
46. Singh N, Deshpande R, Rabizadeh S, et al. Real world experience with natalizumab at a tertiary care pediatric IBD center. J Pediatr Gastroenterol Nutr 2016;62:863–6.
47. Sandborn WJ, Feagan BG, Rutgeerts P, et al. Vedolizumab as induction and maintenance therapy for Crohn's disease. N Engl J Med 2013;369:711–21.
48. Sandborn WJ, Colombel JF, Enns R, et al. Natalizumab induction and maintenance therapy for Crohn's disease. N Engl J Med 2005;353:1912–25.
49. Ghosh S, Goldin E, Gordon FH, et al. Natalizumab for active Crohn's disease. N Engl J Med 2003;348:24–32.
50. Chandar AK, Singh S, Murad MH, et al. Efficacy and safety of natalizumab and vedolizumab for the management of Crohn's disease: a systematic review and meta-analysis. Inflamm Bowel Dis 2015;21:1695–708.
51. Sands BE, Feagan BG, Rutgeerts P, et al. Effects of vedolizumab induction therapy for patients with Crohn's disease in whom tumor necrosis factor antagonist treatment failed. Gastroenterology 2014;147:618–27.e3.
52. Dulai PS, Singh S, Jiang X, et al. The real-world effectiveness and safety of vedolizumab for moderate-severe Crohn's disease: results from the US VICTORY consortium. Am J Gastroenterol 2016;111:1147–55.
53. Vermeire S, Loftus EV Jr, Colombel JF, et al. Long-term efficacy of vedolizumab for Crohn's disease. J Crohns Colitis 2017;11(4):412–24.
54. Sakuraba A, Annunziata ML, Cohen RD, et al. Mucosal healing is associated with improved long-term outcome of maintenance therapy with natalizumab in Crohn's disease. Inflamm Bowel Dis 2013;19:2577–83.
55. Sakuraba A, Keyashian K, Correia C, et al. Natalizumab in Crohn's disease: results from a US tertiary inflammatory bowel disease center. Inflamm Bowel Dis 2013;19:621–6.
56. Kane SV, Horst S, Sandborn WJ, et al. Natalizumab for moderate to severe Crohn's disease in clinical practice: the Mayo Clinic Rochester experience. Inflamm Bowel Dis 2012;18:2203–8.
57. Saruta M, Papadakis KA. Lymphocyte homing antagonists in the treatment of inflammatory bowel diseases. Gastroenterol Clin North Am 2014;43:581–601.
58. Bellaguarda E, Keyashian K, Pekow J, et al. Prevalence of antibodies against JC virus in patients with refractory Crohn's disease and effects of natalizumab therapy. Clin Gastroenterol Hepatol 2015;13:1919–25.
59. Colombel JF, Sands BE, Rutgeerts P, et al. The safety of vedolizumab for ulcerative colitis and Crohn's disease. Gut 2017;66(5):839–51.
60. Dudley-Brown S, Nag A, Cullinan C, et al. Health-related quality-of-life evaluation of Crohn disease patients after receiving natalizumab therapy. Gastroenterol Nurs 2009;32:327–39.
61. Miligkos M, Papamichael K, Casteele NV, et al. Efficacy and safety profile of anti-tumor necrosis factor-alpha versus anti-integrin agents for the treatment of Crohn's disease: a network meta-analysis of indirect comparisons. Clin Ther 2016;38:1342–58.e6.
62. Mocko P, Kawalec P, Pilc A. Safety profile of biologic drugs in the therapy of Crohn disease: a systematic review and network meta-analysis. Pharmacol Rep 2016;68:1237–43.

Ustekinumab and Anti-Interleukin-23 Agents in Crohn's Disease

Parakkal Deepak, MBBS, MS[a], William J. Sandborn, MD[b,*]

KEYWORDS

- Ustekinumab • Crohn's disease • Inflammatory bowel disease
- Interleukin-12/23 monoclonal antibody • Interleukin-12 • Interleukin-23

KEY POINTS

- Ustekinumab binds to the p40 subunit of interleukin (IL)-12 and IL-23 and prevents their interaction with the cell surface IL-12/23 receptors and downstream signaling and cytokine production.
- Approved dosing for induction regimen is weight based: 260 mg intravenous (IV) for less than 55 kg body weight, 390 mg IV for 55 to 85 kg, and 520 mg IV for greater than 85 kg followed by maintenance regimen, which is fixed dose: 90 mg subcutaneous every 8 weeks.
- Clinical response at week 6 was observed at 6 mg/kg induction dose in 33.7% of UNITI-I (prior exposure to TNF antagonists) and 55.5% in UNITI-II (naive to TNF antagonists) subjects.
- Ustekinumab is a Food and Drug Administration pregnancy category-B medication, with no signal for any infectious, cardiac, or malignancy-related adverse events seen in UNITI-I, II, or IM-UNITI trials.
- Specific IL-23 blockers are currently either in phase 2 trials (brazikumab [MEDI2070], risankizumab, and LY3074828) or are awaiting testing (tildrakizumab and guselkumab) in Crohn's disease.

INTRODUCTION

Crohn's disease (CD) is a chronic condition involving the entire gastrointestinal system, characterized by a transmural inflammatory reaction, likely as a result of the interaction between commensal flora in the gut and host microbial defenses in a

Disclosure Statement: See last page of article.

[a] Inflammatory Bowel Diseases Center, Division of Gastroenterology, John T. Milliken Department of Medicine, Washington University School of Medicine, 600 South Euclid Avenue, Campus Box 8124 Saint Louis, MO 63110, USA; [b] Inflammatory Bowel Diseases Center, Division of Gastroenterology, Department of Medicine, University of California San Diego, 9500 Gilman Drive, MC 0956, La Jolla, CA 92093, USA
* Corresponding author.
E-mail address: wsandborn@ucsd.edu

Gastroenterol Clin N Am 46 (2017) 603–626
http://dx.doi.org/10.1016/j.gtc.2017.05.013
0889-8553/17/

genetically predisposed individual.[1,2] Over the long term, the transmural inflammatory reaction leads to disease complications characterized by the development of strictures and/or fistulae that require surgeries and/or hospitalizations.

Given concerns regarding the adverse effects of the broader immunosuppression resulting from previously used therapies, recent drug development and treatment paradigm has since shifted toward targeting of specific pathways of inflammation. Dysregulation of both the innate and adaptive immunity responses have been described in CD. However, perturbations in adaptive immunity are more likely to result in tissue damage, with interleukin (IL)-12 and IL-23 acting as major drivers of the adaptive immune response.[2] Consequently, blockers of IL-12/23 as well as specific blockers of IL-23 have been developed as options for medical therapy in CD. This article briefly reviews the immunology of the IL-12/23 pathway; available data on the pharmacokinetics, efficacy, and safety of ustekinumab and its potential place in the treatment of CD; and the current status of specific IL-23 blockers in CD.

IMMUNOLOGY OF THE INTERLEUKIN-12/23 PATHWAY

A combination of resident and recruited cell populations regulate the adaptive immune responses, including mucosal B cells (immunoglobulin [Ig]A and IgG secretion), T cells (Th1, Th17, or Th2 phenotype), and regulatory T/B cells.[2] CD has been shown to have a predominant Th1 profile.[2] Phagocytic and dendritic cells produce IL-12 in response to microbial stimulation. IL-12 drives cell-mediated immunity by activating T-cell proliferation by Th1 cells.[3,4] This cytokine has a heterodimer structure composed of p40 and p35 protein subunits and these in turn bind to a heterodimeric receptor complex consisting of IL-12 receptor (IL-12R)β1 and IL-12Rβ2 chains expressed on the surface of T cells or natural killer (NK) cells.[5] IL-23 plays a major role in the expansion of committed Th17 cells.[6,7] This cytokine also is heterodimeric with p40 (common to both IL-12 and IL-23) and p19 protein subunits.[8] Preclinical studies have demonstrated the protective effect of neutralization of the p40 protein against the development of trinitrobenzene sulfonic acid (TNBS)-induced experimental colitis in mice.[9] Further studies in CD40-induced colitis in T-cell–deficient and B-cell–deficient mice and TNBS-induced colitis in LacZ knockin mice deficient for IL-23 p19 highlighted that both IL-12 and IL-23 might have a role in intestinal inflammation depending on the experimental mouse model.[10–13]

USTEKINUMAB

Ustekinumab (Stelara; Janssen Biotech, Horsham, PA) is a fully human IgG1 kappa monoclonal antibody that blocks IL-12 and IL-23.[14] The results of phase 2 and phase 3 trials led to its approval by the Food and Drug Administration for the treatment of moderately to severely active CD in adults (18 years or older) who have failed or were intolerant to treatment with immunomodulators or corticosteroids but never failed treatment with tumor necrosis factor (TNF) antagonists, or who failed or were intolerant to treatment with 1 or more TNF antagonists.[9,15–17]

Mechanism of Action

Ustekinumab binds to the p40 subunit of IL-12 and IL-23 and prevents their interaction with the cell surface IL-12 receptor β1 (IL-12Rβ1) receptor, subsequently inhibiting IL-12–mediated responses (intracellular phosphorylation of STAT4, cell surface marker expression, and interferon-γ cytokine production) and IL-23–mediated responses (intracellular STAT3 phosphorylation and IL-17A, IL-17F, and IL-22 cytokine protein production) (**Fig. 1**). The binding epitope for ustekinumab is located in the D1 domain of the p40 subunit, which is spatially distant from IL-12p35 and IL-23p19.[8]

Pharmacokinetics

The pharmacokinetic properties of ustekinumab are similar to those of human endogenous IgG1 with intravenous (IV) and subcutaneous (SC) administration with an extended elimination half-life of approximately 3 weeks, likely secondary to the salvage effect of the neonatal Fc receptor that protects antibody proteins from lysosomal degradation.[18] In patients with CD, following the recommended IV induction dose, mean peak serum ustekinumab concentration was 125.2 ± 33.6 μg/mL with steady-state concentration (mean trough concentration 2.51 ± 2.06 μg/mL) achieved by the start of the second maintenance dose.[19] The total volume of distribution at steady-state was 4.62 L, clearance 0.19 L/d (95% confidence interval [CI] 0.185–0.197) and an estimated median terminal half-life of approximately 19 days, in patients with CD. Metabolism of ustekinumab is expected to be similar to endogenous IgG with degradation into small peptides and amino acids via catabolic pathways.

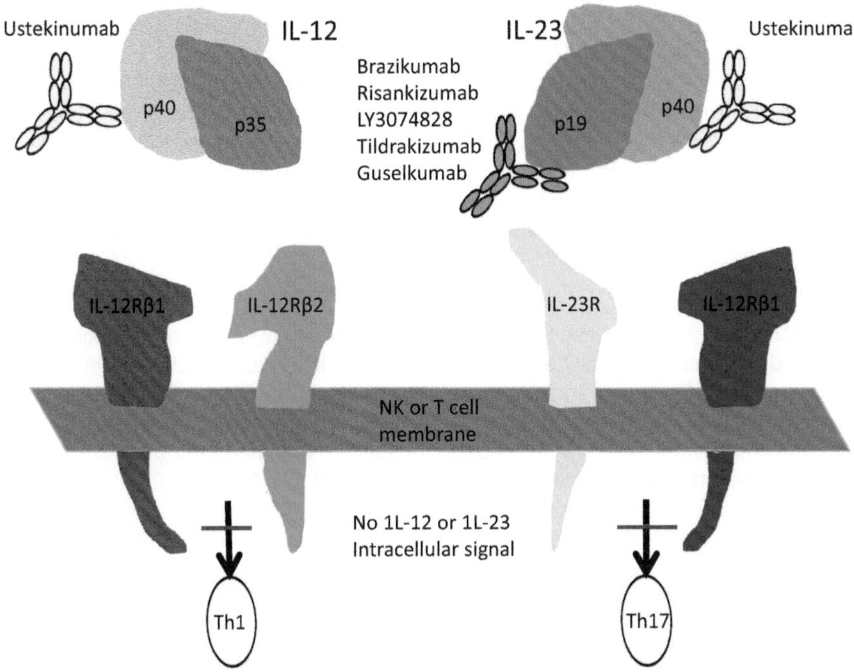

Fig. 1. Ustekinumab binds to the p40 subunit of IL-12 and IL-23, preventing binding with the NK or T-cell surface IL-12Rβ1, and inhibiting IL-12 signaling and further activation of Th1 subset of T cells as well as IL-23 signaling and further activation of Th17 subset of T cells. MEDI2070, risankizumab, LY3074828, tildrakizumab, and guselkumab bind to the p19 subunit of IL-23, preventing binding with the NK or T-cell surface IL-23 receptor-mediated signaling and further activation of Th17 subset of T cells (image not drawn to scale). (*Adapted from* Benson JM, Sachs CW, Treacy G, et al. Therapeutic targeting of the IL-12/23 pathways: generation and characterization of ustekinumab. Nat Biotechnol 2011;29(7):616; with permission.)

Differences in bioavailability depending on patient-specific characteristics, including body mass index, serum albumin concentration, concomitant immunosuppressive use, severity of inflammation and disease subtype, have been described with monoclonal antibodies.[20] Using population pharmacokinetic modeling, body weight, presence of diabetes mellitus, and antibodies to ustekinumab are the predominant determinants of ustekinumab clearance across 2 phase 3 trials in patients with moderate to severe plaque psoriasis (PHOENIX 1 and PHOENIX 2).[21] Concomitant medications, including amoxicillin and omeprazole, do not have a significant effect on the pharmacokinetics of ustekinumab.[22] The approved dosing for the induction regimen in CD is weight based: 260 mg IV for less than 55 kg body weight, 390 mg IV for 55 to 85 kg, and 520 mg IV for greater than 85 kg followed by the maintenance regimen, which is weight based: 90 mg SC every 8 weeks.

Efficacy

Psoriasis

PHOENIX 1 and PHOENIX 2 were phase III, multicenter, randomized, double-blind, placebo-controlled, parallel studies that were performed to evaluate the SC administration of ustekinumab in patients with moderate to severe chronic plaque psoriasis.[23,24] In PHOENIX 1, the primary endpoint of Psoriasis Area Severity Index (PASI) 75 at week 12 was achieved in 171 of those receiving 45 mg (255, 67.1%), and 170 of those receiving 90 mg of ustekinumab (256, 66.4%) compared with 8 placebo-treated patients (255, 3.1%).[23] In PHOENIX 2, the primary endpoint of PASI 75 at week 12 was met in 273 patients receiving 45 mg ustekinumab (66.7%), and 311 receiving 90 mg ustekinumab (75.7%), compared with 15 receiving placebo (3.7%).[24] Based on these studies, ustekinumab was approved for the treatment of chronic plaque psoriasis in the United States (October 2009) with a dosage regimen of 45 mg ustekinumab at baseline, 4 weeks, and every 12 weeks in those weighing 100 kg or less, and 90 mg ustekinumab at the same intervals for those heavier than 100 kg.[25]

Psoriatic arthritis

PSUMMIT 1 and 2 were phase III, multicenter, double-blind, placebo-controlled trials performed to evaluate the SC administration of ustekinumab in patients with active psoriatic arthritis (PsA).[26,27] In PSUMMIT1, a greater percentage of patients in both the 45-mg and 90-mg ustekinumab groups achieved the primary endpoint of 20% or greater improvement in the American College of Rheumatology (ACR20) criteria at week 24 compared with the placebo group (42.4%, 49.5%, and 22.8%, respectively, $P<.0001$ for both comparisons).[26] In PSUMMIT 2, comprising patients with active PsA despite treatment with conventional agents and/or TNF antagonists, the primary endpoint of ACR20 was achieved more often in the ustekinumab-treated (43.8% combined) than placebo-treated (20.2%) patients at week 24 ($P<.001$).[27]

Data from Crohn's disease

A phase IIa trial was conducted in TNF-antagonist–naive and agonist-experienced patients with CD (**Table 1**).[17] In the double-blind crossover component of this trial, 104 patients were randomized to 4 groups receiving either SC placebo or 90 mg ustekinumab at weeks 0 to 3, followed by 90 mg ustekinumab or SC placebo at weeks 8 to 11 or receiving either IV placebo or 4.5 mg/kg ustekinumab at week 0, followed by 4.5 mg/kg ustekinumab or IV placebo at week 8. The primary endpoint of clinical response at week 8 (70-point decrement and at least 25% reduction from the baseline in the CD activity index [CDAI] score) was achieved in 49% and 40% ($P = .34$) of those who received ustekinumab and placebo, respectively. In a subgroup of patients who

Table 1
Summary of randomized control trials (RCTs) on ustekinumab in Crohn's disease

Name of the Study	Type of RCT	Number of Patients	Primary Endpoint	Relevant Secondary Endpoints	Results	Serious Adverse Events[a]
Sandborn et al,[17]	Phase IIa, (crossover), moderate to severe Crohn's disease	104	Clinical response at week 8		UST[b]: 49% PBO: 40%	UST[b]: 4% PBO: 6%
				Clinical response at week 4 and 6	UST[b]: 53% PBO: 30%	
		49 (subgroup: previous exposure to IFX)		Clinical response at week 8	UST[b]: 59% PBO: 26%	
CERTIFI	Phase IIb, moderate to severe Crohn's disease: resistant to anti-TNF	526	Clinical response at week 6		UST: 39.7% (6 mg/kg dose IV) PBO: 23.5%	UST[c]: 5.8% PBO: 8.3%
		145 (subgroup: responders put on maintenance)		Clinical response at week 22	UST: 69.4% (90 mg SC) PBO: 42.5%	UST: 12.5%[d] PBO: 16.4%
				Clinical remission at week 22	UST: 41.7% (90 mg SC) PBO: 27.4%	
UNITI-1	Phase III, moderate to severe Crohn's disease: failed/ intolerant to anti-TNF	741	Clinical response at week 6		UST: 33.7% (6 mg/kg IV), 34.3% (130 mg IV) PBO: 21.5%	UST: 7.2% (6 mg/kg IV), 4.9% (130 mg IV) PBO: 6.1%
				Clinical remission at week 8	UST: 20.9% (6 mg/kg IV), 15.9% (130 mg IV) PBO: 7.3%	
				Clinical response at week 8	UST: 37.8% (6 mg/kg IV), 33.5% (130 mg IV) PBO: 20.2%	
UNITI-2	Phase III, moderate to severe Crohn's disease	628	Clinical response at 6 wk		UST: 55.5% (6-mg/kg IV), 51.7% (130 mg IV) PBO: 28.7%	UST: 2.9% (6 mg/kg IV), 4.7% (130 mg IV) PBO: 5.8%
				Clinical remission at week 8	UST: 40.2% (6 mg/kg IV), 30.6% (130 mg IV) PBO: 19.6%	
				Clinical response at week 8	UST: 57.9% (6 mg/kg IV), 47.4% (130 mg IV) PBO: 32.1%	

(*continued on next page*)

Table 1
(continued)

Name of the Study	Type of RCT	Number of Patients	Primary Endpoint	Relevant Secondary Endpoints	Results	Serious Adverse Events[a]
IM-UNITI	Phase III maintenance, UNITI-1 and UNITI-2 responders	397	Clinical remission at week 44		**UST: 53.1% (90 mg SC q 8w), 48.8% (90 mg SC q 12w)** PBO: 35.9%	UST: 9.9% (q8w), 12.2% (q12w) PBO: 15.0%
				Clinical response at week 44	**UST: 59.4% (90 mg SC q 8w), 58.1% (90 mg SC q 12w)** PBO: 44.3%	
				Corticosteroid-free remission at week 44	**UST: 46.9% (90 mg SC q 8w), 42.6% (90 mg SC q 12w)** PBO: 29.8%	
				Continued remission at week 44 among those in remission at inclusion	**UST: 66.7% (90 mg SC q 8w)**, 56.4% (90 mg SC q 12w) PBO: 45.6%	
				Clinical remission at 44 anti-TNF refractory/ intolerant	UST: 41.1% (90 mg SC q 8w), 38.6% (90 mg SC q 12w) PBO: 26.2%	
				Clinical remission at 44 conventional therapy failures	**UST: 62.5% (90 mg SC q 8w)**, 56.9% (90 mg SC q 12w) PBO: 44.2%	
				Clinical remission at 44 anti-TNF naive	UST: 65.4% (90 mg SC q 8w), 56.6% (90 mg SC q 12w) PBO: 49.0%	

Abbreviations: IFX, infliximab; IV, intravenous; PBO, placebo; q8w, every 8 weeks; q12w, every 12 weeks; SC, subcutaneous; TNF, tumor necrosis factor; UST, ustekinumab.

[a] Through week 8 unless specified.

[b] Combined subcutaneous and intravenous group.

[c] Combined data for 1 mg/kg, 3 mg/kg, and 6 mg/kg IV induction groups.

[d] Through week 22.

From Deepak P, Loftus EV Jr. Ustekinumab in treatment of Crohn's disease: design, development, and potential place in therapy. Drug Des Devel Ther 2016;10:3689; with permission.

were previously given infliximab (neither primary nor secondary nonresponders), clinical response at week 8 was significantly greater with ustekinumab compared with placebo (*P*<.05). Higher baseline serum C-reactive protein (CRP) values predicted larger treatment effects with ustekinumab, especially in infliximab-experienced patients, with a decrease in the CRP concentration paralleling clinic response observed with ustekinumab.[28]

In a subsequent double-blind, randomized, placebo-controlled phase IIb trial of patients with moderate to severe CD who had previously failed 1 or more TNF antagonists, clinical response (100-point decrease in CDAI score) at week 6 after a single dose of 1, 3, or 6 mg/kg of IV ustekinumab or placebo, was achieved in 36.6%, 34.1%, 39.7%, and 23.5%, respectively ($P = .005$), for the comparison with the 6 mg/kg group.[16] In the maintenance phase of this study of responders to ustekinumab at week 6, ustekinumab (90 mg SC) was superior to placebo for both clinical remission (CDAI <150 points, 41.7% vs 27.4%, $P = .03$), and response (69.4% vs 42.5%, $P<.001$) at 22 weeks.[16]

Subsequently, two 8-week phase III induction trials (UNITI-1 and 2) and one 44-week phase III maintenance trial (IM-UNITI) were conducted (**Fig. 2**).[29–32] In UNITI-1, 741 patients with moderate-severely active CD (CDAI 220–450), who previously failed or were intolerant to at least 1 TNF antagonist, were randomized (1:1:1) at week 0 to a single dose of IV placebo, ustekinumab 130 mg, or weight-based tiered ustekinumab dosing approximating 6 mg/kg (260 mg [weight ≤55 kg], 390 mg [weight >55 kg and ≤85 kg], or 520 mg [weight >85 kg]).[30] The primary endpoint of clinical response at week 6 (CDAI decrease of >100 points or if <150 in patients with baseline CDAI 220–248) was observed in 33.7% of those dosed at 6 mg/kg and 34.3% of the 130-mg dose versus 21.5% in placebo ($P = .003$ and 0.002, respectively). The secondary endpoint of clinical remission at week 8 (CDAI score <150

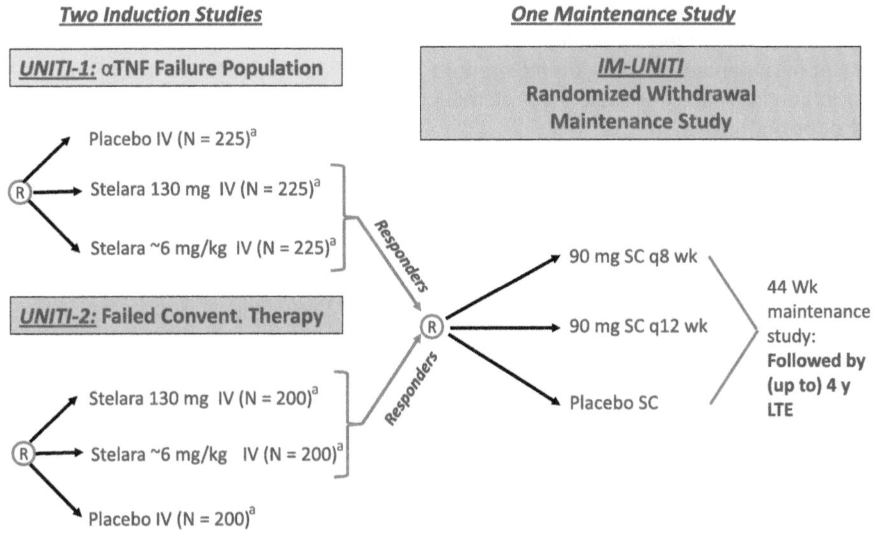

Fig. 2. Overall structure of UNITI phase III program. LTE, long-term extension. [a] Subjects randomized to placebo and subjects who are nonresponders to Stelara are eligible for nonrandomized maintenance dosing after completion of the induction study. (*From* Deepak P, Loftus EV Jr. Ustekinumab in treatment of Crohn's disease: design, development, and potential place in therapy. Drug Des Devel Ther 2016;10:3685–98; with permission.)

points) was observed in 20.9% of the 6-mg/kg group and 15.9% of the 130-mg group versus 7.3% on placebo ($P<.001$, $P = .003$, respectively). Clinical response at week 8 (CDAI 100-point response) was seen in 37.8% of the 6-mg/kg and 33.5% of the 130-mg ustekinumab groups, versus 20.2% on placebo (each $P\leq.001$).

UNITI-2 (n = 628) was another phase III induction trial of ustekinumab in patients with moderately to severely active CD, who had previously failed corticosteroids and/or immunomodulators and were either naive to or had been exposed to but not failed TNF antagonists.[31] The randomized dosing groups and endpoints were similar to UNITI-1. In UNITI-2, primary endpoint of clinical response at week 6 was achieved in 55.5% and 51.7% of the 6-mg/kg and 130-mg dosing groups, respectively, compared with 28.7% who received placebo ($P<.001$ for both comparisons). Secondary endpoint of clinical remission and response at week 8 were achieved in greater proportion of the 6-mg/kg and 130-mg ustekinumab dosing groups compared with placebo (see **Table 1**).

Patients with moderate-severe CD who achieved clinical response at week 8 (n = 397) in either UNITI-1 or UNITI-2 participated in IM-UNITI and were randomized (1:1:1) to maintenance SC injections of 90 mg ustekinumab every 8 weeks (q8w) or 12 weeks (q12w), or placebo.[32] The primary endpoint for the maintenance trial of remission (CDAI <150) at week 44 was achieved in a greater proportion of patients in the ustekinumab groups compared with placebo (53.1% and 48.8% in the q8w and q12w groups vs 35.9% on placebo; $P = .005$ and $P = .040$, respectively). Major secondary endpoints at week 44 (see **Table 1**) included clinical response, clinical remission among subjects in clinical remission after ustekinumab induction, corticosteroid-free remission, and clinical remission in patients refractory or intolerant to TNF antagonists (UNITI-1 subgroup). Significantly greater proportions of patients maintained clinical response at week 44 in the q8w (59.4%) and q12w (58.1%) ustekinumab groups versus placebo (44.3%; $P<.05$ for both). The proportions of patients in clinical remission and not receiving concomitant corticosteroids at week 44 were significantly higher in the q8w group (46.9%) and numerically higher in the q12w group (42.6%) versus placebo (29.8%; $P = .004$ and nominal $P = .035$, respectively). In the subset of patients refractory or intolerant to TNF antagonists (UNITI-1 subgroup), the proportion in clinical remission was numerically but not significantly greater than placebo for both dose groups.

Open-label studies

The open-label observational experience with ustekinumab before regulatory approval has been described in 7 studies (4 fully published articles and 3 abstracts) from tertiary inflammatory bowel disease (IBD) centers in North America and Europe (**Table 2**).[33–39] The experience from the IBD clinic at Mayo Clinic in Rochester, Minnesota, included 18 patients with refractory CD who had experienced failure of at least 2 TNF antagonists in 89% of patients, methotrexate in 83%, and thiopurines in 89%. The cumulative probability of clinical response is listed in **Table 2**. The cumulative probability of loss of response among patients with partial or complete response was 25% at 1, 3, and 6 months. The ustekinumab experience at McGill University, Montreal, included 38 patients with CD, all of whom had previously failed at least 1 TNF antagonist.[34] The induction dose varied from 45 mg (weeks 0 and 4) to 90 mg (weeks 0, 1, 2, or 0, 4) while maintenance doses varied between 45 mg every 12 weeks or 90 mg every 4, 8, or 12 weeks. Initial clinical response (at week 12 or first follow-up visit) and during maintenance is listed in **Table 2**. Dose escalation was required in 18 patients (47.7%) by either interval reduction (17/18) or with both dose escalation and interval reduction (1/18) and was successful in 61.1% of them.

The ustekinumab experience across tertiary French and Swiss IBD centers that are part of the Groupe d'Etude Thérapeutique des Affections Inflammatoires du tube Digestif (GETAID) included 122 consecutive patients with CD, all of whom had failed at least 1, 92% failed 2, 37% failed 3, and 2% all 4 TNF antagonists.[35] Initial clinical benefit (at 3 months) and during maintenance therapy with ustekinumab is listed in **Table 2**. Additionally, concomitant immunosuppressant therapy at study inclusion increased the odds for a clinical benefit from ustekinumab (odds ratio [OR] 5.43, 95% CI 1.14–25.77, $P = .03$).

The open-label experience across 42 Spanish tertiary IBD centers included 116 consecutive patients with CD who failed at least 1 immunomodulator and 1 TNF antagonist and received treatment with ustekinumab for at least 2 months.[36] Clinical response (decrease in Harvey-Bradshaw index [HBI] score by 3 points or more from the baseline) after induction and during maintenance dosing of ustekinumab is listed in **Table 2**. Dose escalation by interval reduction was required in 10% of the patients and effective in most (73%) of those patients. Perianal disease also improved in 11 (61%) of 18 patients with active perianal disease.

The ustekinumab experience at Vanderbilt University and the University of Maryland was reported in 45 patients with refractory CD, 100% of whom had failed at least 1 prior TNF antagonist and 98% failed at least 2 prior TNF antagonist therapies.[37] Clinical response (decrease in HBI score of 3 or more points) and clinical remission (HBI $\leq$3) is depicted in **Table 2**.

A retrospective multicenter cohort study at the Universities of Calgary and Alberta, in the Canadian province of Alberta, reported 82 patients with CD who received ustekinumab[38]; 91.4% had previously failed 1 TNF antagonist and 74.4% had failed more than 1 biologic. Clinical response (HBI reduction >2 points and tapering off corticosteroids) at 3 months, 6 months, and 12 months is depicted in **Table 2**. Another retrospective cohort of 53 patients was reported from the University of British Columbia, Canada, of which 45 had follow-up response assessment.[39] Induction regimens varied between 90 mg SC at wk 0, 1, and 2 versus a higher-dose induction with 270 mg SC at wk 0 and 180 mg SC at wks 1 and 2. Maintenance dosing was 90 mg SC every 8 weeks for both regimens. Symptomatic response assessment based on physician documentation is detailed in **Table 2**. Endoscopic or radiologic response or improvement was achieved in 62% (16/26) assessed.

Endoscopic response as treatment endpoint

Mucosal healing was demonstrated in 19.5% in the ustekinumab group (8/41) in the CERTIFI study.[16] In an endoscopic substudy of IM-UNITI, patients had colonoscopies at baseline (approximately UNITI week 0), then 8 and 52 weeks later (IM-UNITI week 44), all of which were scored for simplified endoscopic activity score for CD (SES-CD) by a single blinded central reader.[40] Patients with SES-CD $\geq$3 (ie, ulceration in $\geq$1 segment) at induction week 0 were eligible for analysis. Primary endpoint was change in SES-CD at induction week 8 ([6 mg/kg and 130 mg ustekinumab dosing UNITI-I and II combined] vs placebo). Efficacy at maintenance week 44 was evaluated in the primary randomized maintenance population and the post hoc pooled maintenance population (randomized and nonrandomized populations combined). The results are shown in **Table 3**. A total of 252 patients were eligible for the endoscopic substudy. Ustekinumab induced significantly greater reduction in SES-CD at week 8 compared with placebo, with similar results by induction study and dose. Additionally, a clinically meaningful (SES-CD reduction $\geq$3 from week 0 colonoscopy) and statistically significant endoscopic improvement was seen in 47.7% of the ustekinumab group compared with 29.9% with placebo. In the larger post hoc pooled maintenance

Table 2
Real-world experience with ustekinumab in refractory Crohn's disease

S. No.	References	Center	Study Period	No. of Patients	Prior Exposure to ≥2 Anti-TNFs	UST Induction SC Dosing[a]	UST Maintenance SC Dosing[a]	Clinical Response	Endoscopic Response
1.	Batista et al,[33] 2014	Mayo Clinic, Rochester, NY	1/2008–8/2013	18	89%	45–270 mg SC at wk 0	90 mg SC q 8 wk	Initial response: 11.1% and 38.9% at 1 and 2 mo Maintenance response: 44.4%, at 6 mo	MH: 38%
2.	Kopylov et al,[34] 2014	McGill University, Canada	3/2011–11/2013	38	95%	90 mg at wk 0, 1 & 2	45 mg q 12 wk or 90 mg q 4, 8 or 12 wk	Initial response: 73.7% Maintenance response: 80% and 88.9% at 6 and 12 mo	ER: 779% MH: 15%
3.	Wils et al,[35] 2016	GETAID group, France and Switzerland	3/2011–12/2014	122	92%	90 mg at wk 0 and 4	90 mg q 8 wk	Initial response: 65% at 3 mo Maintenance response: 93% and 68% at 6 and 12 mo	ER: 77% MH: 9%
4.	Khorrami et al,[36] 2016	Spanish multicenter	3/2010–12/2014	116	87%	90 mg at wk 0, 1, 2, and 3	90 mg q 8 wk	Initial response: 84% Maintenance response: 74% and 64% at 6 and 12 mo	ER: 69% MH: 31%

5.	Harris et al,[37] 2016	Vanderbilt University and University of Maryland, USA	6/2011–6/2014	45	98%	90 mg at wk 0, 4, and 12; 270 mg booster at wk 8 no or limited clinical response	90 mg q 8 wk	Clinical response: 46% Clinical remission: 35%	ER: 76% MH: 24%
6.	Ma et al,[38] 2016	University of Calgary and University of Alberta, Canada	2011–2015	82	74%	Weight-adjusted induction (3 vs 6 mg/kg)	90 mg SC q 8 or q 12 wk	Initial response: 67.1% at 3 mo Maintenance response: 67.9% and 49.3% at 6 and 12 mo	—
7.	Greenup et al,[39] 2016	University of British Columbia	9/2012–1/2016	45	54%	90 mg SC wk 0, 1, and 2	90 mg SC q 8 wk	Initial response: 53% Maintenance response: 67% and 65% at 6 and 12 mo	—

Abbreviations: ER, endoscopic response; GETAID, Groupe d'Etude Thérapeutique des Affections Inflammatoires du tube Digestif; MH, mucosal healing; q, every; SC, subcutaneous; TNF, tumor necrosis factor-alpha; UST, ustekinumab.

[a] Most common dosing regimen.

Data from Refs.[33–39]

Table 3
Objective assessment of response to ustekinumab in UNITI-I, UNITI-II, and IM-UNITI with colonoscopy

		Induction Week 8 (UNITI-I and UNITI-II)		Maintenance Week 44 (IM-UNITI)		
Characteristic	**Endpoint**	**PBO (n = 97)**	**UST (n = 155)**	**PBO (n = 51)**	**90 mg UST q12w (n = 47)**	**90 mg UST q8w (n = 74)**
SES-CD Change from BL, mean (SD)	Primary endpoint	−0.7 (4.97)	−2.8 (8.10)[a]	−2.0 (5.35)	−1.5 (4.22)	−3.8 (6.02)
Clinically meaningful endoscopic improvement, %	SES-CD reduction ≥3 from induction BL	29.9	47.7[a]	27.5	29.8	48.6[a]
Endoscopic response, %	SES-CD reduction ≥50% from induction BL	13.4	20.6	4.2	5.9	24.1[a]
Endoscopic remission, %	SES-CD total score ≤2	4.1	7.7	9.8	12.8	20.3
Mucosal healing, %	Complete absence of ulcers	4.1	9.0	9.8	12.8	21.6

Abbreviations: BL, baseline; PBO, placebo; q8w, every 8 weeks; q12w, every 12 weeks; SES-CD, simplified endoscopic activity score for Crohn's disease; UST, ustekinumab.

[a] $P<.05$.

Data from Sandborn WJ, Gasink C, Chan D, et al. Endoscopic healing in induction and maintenance with ustekinumab in the phase 3 UNITI Crohn's disease program [abstract]. Am J Gastroenterol 2016;111(1):S278–9.

population (see **Table 3**), consistent trends supporting ustekinumab maintenance, again especially ustekinumab 90 mg q8w compared with placebo, across endoscopic endpoints at week 44. In real-world studies, mucosal healing has varied from 9% up to 38% using SC induction and maintenance dosing regimens (see **Table 2**).[33–37]

Immunogenicity and role of therapeutic drug monitoring

Antibodies to ustekinumab have been reported only in an exceedingly low percentage of patients, varying from 0.2% in the induction period of UNITI-I and II, 0.7% in the CERTIFI trial (through week 36), and up to 2.3% through week 44 in IM-UNITI.[16,41,42] In a real-world experience at McGill University, none of the 49 patients tested had detectable antibodies to ustekinumab at more than 6 months' usage.[43]

Across the 3 phase III trials, serum ustekinumab trough concentrations were dose-proportional at the end of induction (week 8 trough of 2.1 μg/mL and 6.4 μg/mL for the 130-mg and 6-mg/kg dose groups, respectively) and during maintenance phase (median steady-state trough range of 0.61–0.76 μg/mL and 1.97–2.24 μg/mL and for the q12w and q8w groups respectively).[42] Additionally, a positive association was seen between clinical remission at week 8 (UNITI-1 and UNITI-2) and week 24 (IM-UNITI) and trough ustekinumab concentrations. A serum ustekinumab level greater than 4.5 μg/mL was associated with endoscopic response (72.2% sensitivity, 83.3% specificity; $P = .0006$; area under the curve 0.782) and a composite outcome of steroid-free clinical remission and endoscopic response (50% vs 15%, $P = .024$), in real-world data published from McGill University.[43] Additionally, a ustekinumab level greater than 5 μg/mL, compared with lower levels, was associated with normal serum CRP (63.6% vs 33%, $P = .024$).

The efficacy and safety of dose adjustment of ustekinumab was evaluated during phase III trials in patients who underwent dose adjustment following loss of response, defined as a CDAI score of ≥220 and a ≥100 point increase from the maintenance baseline CDAI score, between weeks 8 and 32.[44] They underwent a single dose adjustment as follows: placebo→q8w, q12w→q8w, and q8w→q8w (no dose adjustment). Twenty-three percent of the patients in the q12w underwent dose adjustment, with clinical remission (CDAI <150) and clinical response (≥100-point decrease in CDAI) observed in 41% and 55% in the q12w→q8w group when assessed 16 weeks later. No increases or changes in patterns of adverse events were seen among patients who dose adjusted. The dose escalation data in addition to the association between trough concentrations and clinical response/remission shows the promise of therapeutic drug monitoring to optimize ustekinumab response in clinical practice.

Comparative efficacy

The comparative effectiveness of ustekinumab was tested head-to-head with etanercept in patients with moderate to severe psoriasis in a phase III trial with adaptive randomization design with study investigators (but not the patient) blinded to treatment allocation.[45] The superiority of ustekinumab over etanercept was demonstrated at week 12, with those receiving ustekinumab 45 mg or 90 mg (week 0 and 4) achieving PASI 75 in 67.5% and 73.8% of patients, respectively, compared with 56.8% of those receiving etanercept at 50 mg SC twice weekly ($P = .01$ and $P = .001$ respectively).

In the absence of head-head trials in CD, a systematic review with pairwise and network meta-analysis has compared the efficacy of ustekinumab in comparison with TNF antagonists and vedolizumab and relative ranking (using the surface under the cumulative ranking curve or SUCRA method).[46] On network meta-analysis, compared with placebo, ustekinumab (OR 2.51; 95% CI 1.4–4.6; SUCRA rank 0.71) and adalimumab (OR 2.2; 95% CI 1.1–4.7; SUCRA rank 0.91), but not vedolizumab

(OR 1.63; 95% CI 0.9–3.2; SUCRA rank 0.35) were superior to placebo and ranked higher than vedolizumab for induction of clinical remission in patients with prior exposure to TNF antagonists.

Safety Data

Data from psoriasis

In PHOENIX 1, the most common adverse events (AEs) were reported as upper respiratory tract infections, nasopharyngitis, headache, and arthralgia.[23] Comparable rates of all AEs and serious AEs were reported in the ustekinumab and placebo groups. These were most commonly infections and cardiac events. No malignancies were reported except during the crossover phase (1 case each of prostate cancer and thyroid cancer) and the withdrawal phase (1 case of colon cancer). In PHOENIX 2, during the placebo-controlled phase, AEs were comparable between the ustekinumab and placebo groups and were similar to PHOENIX 1.[24] Through the 3 phases, 1 case each of basal cell skin cancer and squamous cell cancer of the tongue was reported in the ustekinumab group.

At year 5 of follow-up, event rates per 100 patient-years (45 mg, 90 mg, respectively) were comparable for overall AEs (242.6, 225.3), serious AEs (7.0, 7.2), serious infections (0.98, 1.19), nonmelanoma skin cancers (0.64, 0.44), other malignancies (0.59, 0.61), and major cardiovascular events (0.56, 0.36) among 3117 patients from the 4 randomized, blinded, phase II and III ustekinumab studies in psoriasis.[47] The rates of malignancies (excluding nonmelanoma skin cancers) were reassuringly comparable with those expected in the general US population (standardized incidence ratio [SIR] 0.98; 95% CI 0.74–1.29). The cumulative incidence rates for malignancy, major cardiovascular events, serious infection, or mortality with ustekinumab were also comparable to or lower than other biologics in the Psoriasis Longitudinal Assessment and Registry (PSOLAR) containing data on 4364 patients who had received ustekinumab for psoriasis.[48]

Data from Crohn's disease

In the phase IIa study, the rate of serious AEs was similar between the ustekinumab and placebo groups, with 1 case of prostate cancer (with increased prostate-specific antigen levels before study entry) and 2 cases of serious infections (viral gastroenteritis and disseminated histoplasmosis) recorded in patients receiving ustekinumab.[17] In the phase IIb study, common nongastrointestinal AEs included headache, arthralgia, and nasopharyngitis.[16] The rates of serious infections were similar between the ustekinumab and placebo groups.

In the UNITI-I and UNITI-II studies, the proportion of patients with AEs, serious AEs, and infections were similar in the ustekinumab and placebo groups.[30,31] One significant opportunistic infection (*Listeria* meningitis) was reported in the group receiving 6 mg/kg ustekinumab in UNITI-I. No malignancies, deaths, major adverse cardiovascular events, or tuberculosis (TB) occurred in ustekinumab-treated patients in either induction trial through week 20. In the 44-week IM-UNITI trial, similar proportions of patients with any AEs, serious AEs and serious infections were seen among the q8w (81.7%, 9.9%, and 2.3%), q12w (80.3%, 12.2%, and 5.3%) and placebo (83.5%, 15.0%, and 2.3%) groups.[32] Two patients reported malignancies (1 basal cell carcinoma in each of the placebo and q8w groups) in the randomized population, and a single case of active TB and a case of metastatic small bowel adenocarcinoma were reported in the nonrandomized population. There was no relationship between serum ustekinumab concentrations and the incidence of infections, serious infections, or serious AEs following induction or maintenance treatment with ustekinumab in UNITI-1, UNITI-2, and IM-UNITI.[42]

Despite the cardiac events reported in the psoriasis trials, meta-analysis of randomized controlled clinical trials concluded that there was no significant difference in the rate of major cardiac events observed in patients receiving anti–IL-12/IL-23 antibodies or TNF antagonists.[49] Reversible posterior leukoencephalopathy syndrome (RPLS) is a rare, generally reversible neurologic syndrome that can present with acute onset of headache, visual disturbances, altered mental status, and seizures.[50] Transient cerebral edema without infarction is usually seen on computed tomography or MRI in the parietal and/or occipital lobes of the brain. A single case has been reported in a 65-year-old woman who developed RPLS after 12 doses over 2 years; the relationship of RPLS with ustekinumab is unclear.[51] Although no exacerbation of demyelinating events was reported in a phase II trial of ustekinumab in multiple sclerosis, there has been 1 case report of central demyelination diagnosed 1 year after ustekinumab treatment in a 63-year-old patient with CD previously exposed to 3 other TNF antagonists.[52,53]

Data in pregnancy

Based on animal studies in cynomolgus monkeys and with limited human data, ustekinumab has been classified as a Food and Drug Administration (FDA) class B medication.[25,54,55] Across 4 psoriasis studies and 29 pregnancies with maternal exposure to at least 1 dose of ustekinumab, no congenital anomalies have been reported.[56] The rate of spontaneous abortion is comparable to the general population (15%–20%), and no association has been reported between a longer duration of ustekinumab exposure before the reported pregnancy and adverse outcomes. Transplacental transfer has been reported in the PIANO registry (n = 3) with ratios (to maternal serum levels) in the infant at birth similar to infliximab and adalimumab.[57] However, no association has been seen between detectable drug levels of biologics in the infant and the risk of infections, and breastfeeding is not contraindicated while on biologics.[57] It would appear prudent to avoid live-virus vaccines for the first 6 months in infants born to mothers exposed to ustekinumab, given the detectable drug levels.[58]

POTENTIAL PLACE OF USTEKINUMAB IN THE THERAPY OF CROHN'S DISEASE

Current options for biologics with regulatory approval in the management of CD include the TNF antagonists (infliximab, adalimumab, and certolizumab pegol) and the anti-integrins, vedolizumab and natalizumab.[59] From a practical standpoint, TNF antagonists are currently positioned as first-line biologics in the management of moderate-severe CD, although this is largely based on physician experience and reimbursement policies, because both vedolizumab and ustekinumab are more effective in anti-TNF naive patients than anti-TNF experienced patients, they both have safety profiles that appear more favorable than anti-TNF drugs, and their efficacy appears generally comparable to anti-TNF drugs.[60] However, even in circumstances in which first-line therapy with TNF antagonists is preferred, primary nonresponse to TNF antagonists occurs in approximately 13% to 40% of patients and a secondary loss of response is estimated to occur at a rate of 13% per year.[61–63]

In the group of patients intolerant or refractory to TNF antagonists (UNITI-1), ustekinumab achieved clinical response at week 6 (34.3% with 130 mg vs 21.5% with placebo) similar to that shown with vedolizumab in GEMINI 3 (39.2% vs 22.3% with placebo, P = .001).[30,64] Clinical remission (CDAI <150) at week 8 with ustekinumab (15.9%–20.9%) was also similar to the rates shown with vedolizumab at weeks 6 and 10 (15.2% and 26.6%) in this group of patients. Compared with maintenance phase of GEMINI 2 among initial responders to vedolizumab, ustekinumab demonstrated a higher rate of clinical remission at week 44 in this group of patients, ranging from 38.6% (90 mg q12w) to 41.1% (90 mg q8w).[32,65] A recent network meta-analysis suggests that ustekinumab may be ranked higher than vedolizumab as a second-line option in patients with prior exposure to TNF antagonists.[46] However, head-head trials are needed to shed more light on relative positioning of ustekinumab and vedolizumab as second-line options in this group of patients.

As noted previously, the UNITI-2 data show that it potentially also may have a role among TNF-antagonist–naive patients considering its favorable safety profile, potentially as a first-line biologic. In some jurisdictions, this may be limited by reimbursement considerations, especially with the introduction of biosimilars that are either FDA approved (infliximab biosimilar, CT-P13) or pending approval (adalimumab biosimilar, ABP 501).[66,67]

Specific subsets of patients with CD may be ideal candidates for ustekinumab therapy. These include patients with psoriasis and CD as well as those who develop TNF-antagonist–induced psoriasis.[68] In a cohort of 434 patients with IBD, all 9 patients with CD and severe psoriasiform lesions and/or TNF-antagonist–induced alopecia were successfully treated with ustekinumab. IL-17A expression was identified as a predictor of the need for ustekinumab over topical therapy ($P = .001$).[68] Pyoderma gangrenosum (PG), especially in those recalcitrant to TNF antagonists and located in the peristomal area, also have been treated with ustekinumab.[69–71] Although the effects of the blockade of the IL-12/23 pathway on extraintestinal manifestations (EIMs) are currently unknown, studies have shown elevated serum IL-23 in patients with CD with associated arthritis and sacroiliitis and lesional IL-23 expression in PG.[71,72] Additionally, recently published results of a post hoc analysis of the GEMINI 2 study did not show statistically significant benefit of vedolizumab over placebo for the treatment of EIMs in CD.[73] This suggests another subset in which ustekinumab may be preferred over vedolizumab in those with prominent EIMs. An algorithm for the use of ustekinumab based on current available literature is proposed in **Fig. 3**.

SPECIFIC INTERLEUKIN-23 INHIBITION

Efficacy of blocking of the IL-12/23 axis has been shown in mouse models of psoriasis and multiple sclerosis.[74] There are emerging data in psoriasis that selective blockade of IL-23 may be critical in the pathogenesis of psoriasis more so than combined IL-12/23 blockade.[75] The idea behind specifically targeting the p19 subunit of IL-23 is to also increase safety by allowing for normal IL-12–mediated Th1 response required in the immune response to intracellular pathogens (interferon-gamma release from T and NK cells) while conferring the same efficacy as with p40 antibodies.[74,76] IL-12 mediated Th1 response has been postulated to play a role in susceptibility to mycobacterial disease more so than IL-23 mediated Th17 response.[77] Other pathogens have been explored showing similar relationship, including *Pneumocystis jirovecii*, *Cryptococcus neoformans*, and *Toxoplasmosis gondii*.[78–80] By leaving IL-12 intact and targeting only IL-23p19, host immunity to a variety of pathogens could be preserved, as discussed previously.

Drugs specifically targeting the p19 subunit of IL-23 that are currently being tested include brazikumab, risankizumab and LY3074828.[81–86]

Brazikumab (MEDI2070)

Brazikumab (MEDI2070, AMG-139; Amgen, Thousand Oaks, CA, and MedImmune, Gaithersburg, MD) is a fully human IgG2 monoclonal antibody, which selectively binds p19 (see **Fig. 1**), which is another subunit of IL-23 that has no impact on IL-12, resulting in a more selective inhibition of the IL-23 axis than ustekinumab. A phase IIa trial

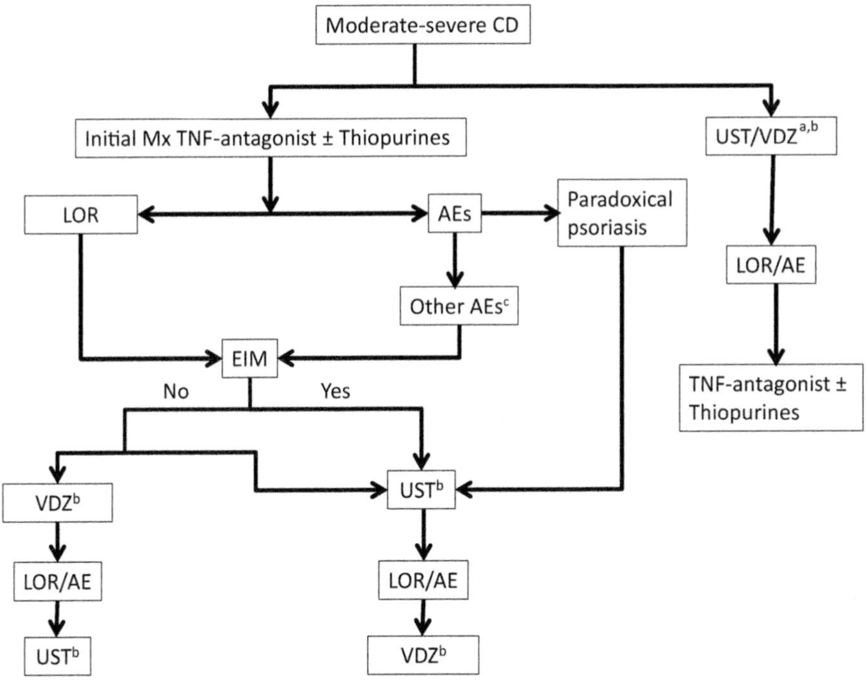

Fig. 3. Proposed algorithm for use of ustekinumab in moderate-severe CD. [a] Safety profiles may favor vedolizumab and ustekinumab, whereas reimbursement considerations, more data regarding mucosal healing, and more extensive experience may favor TNF antagonists. [b] With or without concomitant immunomodulatory. LOR, loss of response; UST, ustekinumab; VDZ, vedolizumab. [c] including neurological adverse events.

(NCT01714726) has been conducted in 121 patients with moderate to severe CD who have failed or were intolerant to prior TNF antagonist therapy (68.9% had ≥2, 38.7% had primary TNF-antagonist failure).[81] Patients were randomized to receive brazikumab 700 mg infusions or placebo at weeks 0 and 4, and at week 8, with 112 completing the study until week 8. Clinical effect at week 8 (defined as >100-point improvement from baseline CDAI or clinical remission with CDAI <150) was observed in 49.2% of brazikumab-treated patients compared with 26.7% of patients receiving placebo (P = .010). Additional prespecified composite outcome of clinical effect AND ≥50% reduction from baseline CRP or fecal calprotectin was achieved in 42.4% treated with brazikumab versus 10.0% with placebo (P<.001). No increased rate of AEs with active treatment was observed over 12 weeks as compared with placebo. A phase IIb double-blind, multidose, placebo-controlled trial of brazikumab is currently recruiting (NCT02574637).[83]

Risankizumab

Recently, results from a phase II trial with risankizumab (BI-655066; Boehringer Ingelheim, Ingelheim am Rhein, Germany, and Abbvie, North Chicago, IL) in patients with moderate to severe CD (n = 121) were reported with 94.2% of patients having previously been exposed to ≥1 TNF antagonist.[82,86] In this trial, patients were randomly assigned to receive 200 or 600 mg BI-655066 IV or placebo at weeks 0, 4, and 8. At week 12 (primary endpoint), clinical remission (defined as CDAI <150) was achieved by 24.4% and 36.6% of patients with 200 mg and 600 mg compared with 15.4% of patients with placebo (P = .308 and P = .025). Compared with placebo, 600 mg BI-655066 dose achieved significantly higher clinical response (41.5% vs 20.5%, P = .037), endoscopic remission (19.5% vs 2.6%, P = .017), and endoscopic response (36.6% vs 12.8%, P = .014), but not deep remission (12.2% vs 0.0%, P = .062). AEs were similar between BI 655066 and placebo with no dose-related increase in AEs. An open-label, single-group, long-term safety extension trial for subjects who responded to treatment with risankizumab in a preceding trial is currently active (NCT02513459).[84]

Mirikizumab (LY3074828, Eli Lilly, Indianapolis, IN) is currently recruiting in a phase II trial titled SERENITY (NCT02891226).[85] Primary outcome measure will be the proportion of participants achieving 50% reduction from baseline at week 12 on the SES-CD. Other drugs specifically targeting the p19 subunit of IL-23: tildrakizumab (MK-3222; Sun Pharma, Mumbai, India, and Merck, Kenilworth, NJ) and guselkumab (Janssen Biotech, Horsham, PA) in CD, will likely be entering clinical trials in the near future.[87,88]

Data from psoriasis, including head-head comparisons, have even suggested the superiority of IL-23 alone blockade over 12/23 blockade. In a phase II head-to-head psoriasis study, after 9 months, 69% of patients with moderate to severe plaque psoriasis maintained clear or almost clear skin (PASI 90) with risankizumab in the higher-dose group compared with 30% of patients on ustekinumab.[89,90] The NAVIGATE clinical trial comparing the relative efficacy of ustekinumab with guselkumab in patients with moderate to severe plaque-type psoriasis has been completed and results are awaited.[91]

FUTURE DIRECTIONS

The effects of ustekinumab on healing of perianal disease and treating extraintestinal manifestations are currently unknown. Additionally, threshold ustekinumab trough concentrations measured on the FDA-approved regimen that correlate with clinical, endoscopic, and radiological response is unknown.[92] Development of predictive biomarkers for selecting patients likely to respond to ustekinumab may be the next step toward precision medicine in CD by using, instead of a stepwise approach, starting with TNF antagonists followed by ustekinumab or vedolizumab or vice-versa. Serum-soluble IL-2 receptor may be one such molecule.[93]

DISCLOSURE STATEMENT

P. Deepak has no conflicts of interest to disclose. Dr W.J. Sandborn reports grants and personal fees from Pfizer, Prometheus Laboratories, AbbVie, Boehringer Ingelheim, Takeda, Atlantic Pharmaceuticals, Janssen, Bristol-Myers Squibb, Genentech, Nutrition Science Partners, and personal fees from Kyowa Hakko Kirin, Millennium Pharmaceuticals, Celgene Cellular Therapeutics, Santarus, Salix Pharmaceuticals, Catabasis Pharmaceuticals, Vertex Pharmaceuticals, Warner Chilcott, Gilead Sciences, Cosmo Pharmaceuticals, Ferring Pharmaceuticals, Sigmoid Biotechnologies, Tillotts Pharma, Am Pharma BV, Dr. August Wolff, Avaxia Biologics, Zyngenia, Ironwood Pharmaceuticals, Index Pharmaceuticals, Nestle, Lexicon Pharmaceuticals, UCB Pharma, Orexigen, Luitpold Pharmaceuticals, Baxter Healthcare, Ferring Research Institute, Amgen, Novo Nordisk, Mesoblast Inc, Shire, Ardelyx Inc, Actavis, Seattle Genetics, MedImmune (AstraZeneca), Actogenix NV, Lipid Therapeutics Gmbh, Eisai, Qu Biologics, Toray Industries Inc, Teva Pharmaceuticals, Eli Lilly, Chiasma, TiGenix, Adherion Therapeutics, Immune Pharmaceuticals, Celgene, Arena

Pharmaceuticals, Ambrx Inc, Akros Pharma, Vascular Biogenics, Theradiag, Forward Pharma, Regeneron, Galapagos, Seres Health, Ritter Pharmaceuticals, Theravance, Palatin, Biogen, and personal fees from the University of Western Ontario (owner of Robarts Clinical Trials).

REFERENCES

1. Abraham C, Cho JH. Inflammatory bowel disease. N Engl J Med 2009;361(21): 2066–78.
2. Xavier RJ, Podolsky DK. Unravelling the pathogenesis of inflammatory bowel disease. Nature 2007;448(7152):427–34.
3. Trinchieri G. Interleukin-12 and the regulation of innate resistance and adaptive immunity. Nat Rev Immunol 2003;3(2):133–46.
4. Kobayashi M, Fitz L, Ryan M, et al. Identification and purification of natural killer cell stimulatory factor (NKSF), a cytokine with multiple biologic effects on human lymphocytes. J Exp Med 1989;170(3):827–45.
5. Presky DH, Yang H, Minetti LJ, et al. A functional interleukin 12 receptor complex is composed of two beta-type cytokine receptor subunits. Proc Natl Acad Sci U S A 1996;93(24):14002–7.
6. Parham C, Chirica M, Timans J, et al. A receptor for the heterodimeric cytokine IL-23 is composed of IL-12Rbeta1 and a novel cytokine receptor subunit, IL-23R. J Immunol 2002;168(11):5699–708.
7. Aggarwal S, Ghilardi N, Xie MH, et al. Interleukin-23 promotes a distinct CD4 T cell activation state characterized by the production of interleukin-17. J Biol Chem 2003;278(3):1910–4.
8. Benson JM, Sachs CW, Treacy G, et al. Therapeutic targeting of the IL-12/23 pathways: generation and characterization of ustekinumab. Nat Biotechnol 2011;29(7):615–24.
9. Neurath MF, Fuss I, Kelsall BL, et al. Antibodies to interleukin 12 abrogate established experimental colitis in mice. J Exp Med 1995;182(5):1281–90.
10. Uhlig HH, McKenzie BS, Hue S, et al. Differential activity of IL-12 and IL-23 in mucosal and systemic innate immune pathology. Immunity 2006;25(2):309–18.
11. Becker C, Dornhoff H, Neufert C, et al. Cutting edge: IL-23 cross-regulates IL-12 production in T cell-dependent experimental colitis. J Immunol 2006;177(5): 2760–4.
12. Strober W, Fuss IJ. Proinflammatory cytokines in the pathogenesis of inflammatory bowel diseases. Gastroenterology 2011;140(6):1756–67.
13. Niederreiter L, Adolph TE, Kaser A. Anti-IL-12/23 in Crohn's disease: bench and bedside. Curr Drug Targets 2013;14(12):1379–84.
14. Deepak P, Loftus EV Jr. Ustekinumab in treatment of Crohn's disease: design, development, and potential place in therapy. Drug Des Devel Ther 2016;10: 3685–98.
15. Mannon PJ, Fuss IJ, Mayer L, et al. Anti-interleukin-12 antibody for active Crohn's disease. N Engl J Med 2004;351(20):2069–79.
16. Sandborn WJ, Gasink C, Gao LL, et al. Ustekinumab induction and maintenance therapy in refractory Crohn's disease. N Engl J Med 2012;367(16):1519–28.
17. Sandborn WJ, Feagan BG, Fedorak RN, et al. A randomized trial of Ustekinumab, a human interleukin-12/23 monoclonal antibody, in patients with moderate-to-severe Crohn's disease. Gastroenterology 2008;135(4):1130–41.
18. Wang W, Wang EQ, Balthasar JP. Monoclonal antibody pharmacokinetics and pharmacodynamics. Clin Pharmacol Ther 2008;84(5):548–58.

19. Stelara(R) [package insert]. Horsham (PA): Janssen Biotech, Inc; 2016. Available at: http://www.stelarahcp.com/pdf/PrescribingInformation.pdf. Accessed February 20, 2017.
20. Ordas I, Mould DR, Feagan BG, et al. Anti-TNF monoclonal antibodies in inflammatory bowel disease: pharmacokinetics-based dosing paradigms. Clin Pharmacol Ther 2012;91(4):635–46.
21. Zhu Y, Hu C, Lu M, et al. Population pharmacokinetic modeling of ustekinumab, a human monoclonal antibody targeting IL-12/23p40, in patients with moderate to severe plaque psoriasis. J Clin Pharmacol 2009;49(2):162–75.
22. Zhou H, Davis HM. Risk-based strategy for the assessment of pharmacokinetic drug-drug interactions for therapeutic monoclonal antibodies. Drug Discov Today 2009;14(17–18):891–8.
23. Leonardi CL, Kimball AB, Papp KA, et al. Efficacy and safety of ustekinumab, a human interleukin-12/23 monoclonal antibody, in patients with psoriasis: 76-week results from a randomised, double-blind, placebo-controlled trial (PHOENIX 1). Lancet 2008;371(9625):1665–74.
24. Papp KA, Langley RG, Lebwohl M, et al. Efficacy and safety of ustekinumab, a human interleukin-12/23 monoclonal antibody, in patients with psoriasis: 52-week results from a randomised, double-blind, placebo-controlled trial (PHOENIX 2). Lancet 2008;371(9625):1675–84.
25. Ryan C, Thrash B, Warren RB, et al. The use of ustekinumab in autoimmune disease. Expert Opin Biol Ther 2010;10(4):587–604.
26. McInnes IB, Kavanaugh A, Gottlieb AB, et al. Efficacy and safety of ustekinumab in patients with active psoriatic arthritis: 1 year results of the phase 3, multicentre, double-blind, placebo-controlled PSUMMIT 1 trial. Lancet 2013;382(9894): 780–9.
27. Ritchlin C, Rahman P, Kavanaugh A, et al. Efficacy and safety of the anti-IL-12/23 p40 monoclonal antibody, ustekinumab, in patients with active psoriatic arthritis despite conventional non-biological and biological anti-tumour necrosis factor therapy: 6-month and 1-year results of the phase 3, multicentre, double-blind, placebo-controlled, randomised PSUMMIT 2 trial. Ann Rheum Dis 2014;73(6): 990–9.
28. Toedter GP, Blank M, Lang Y, et al. Relationship of C-reactive protein with clinical response after therapy with ustekinumab in Crohn's disease. Am J Gastroenterol 2009;104(11):2768–73.
29. Feagan BG, Sandborn WJ, Gasink C, et al. Ustekinumab as induction and maintenance therapy for Crohn's disease. N Engl J Med 2016;375(20):1946–60.
30. Sandborn W, Gasink C, Blank M, et al. O-001 a multicenter, double-blind, placebo-controlled phase3 study of ustekinumab, a human IL-12/23P40 mAB, in moderate-service Crohn's disease refractory to anti-TFNalpha: UNITI-1 [abstract]. Inflamm Bowel Dis 2016;22(Suppl 1):S1.
31. Feagan B, Gasink C, Lang Y, et al. OP054-LB4 A multicenter, double-blind, placebo-controlled Ph3 study of ustekinumab, a human monoclonal antibody to IL-12/23p40, in patients with moderately-severely active Crohn's disease who are naïve or not refractory to anti-TNFa: UNITI-2 [abstract]. United European Gastroenterol J 2015;3(6):2.
32. Sandborn W, Feagan BG, Gasink C, et al. 768 a phase 3 randomized, multicenter, double-blind, placebo-controlled study of ustekinumab maintenance therapy in moderate-severe Crohn's disease patients: results from IM-UNITI [abstract]. Gastroenterology 2016;150(4):S157–8.

33. Batista DD, Yadav S, Harmsen WS, et al. Su1420 ustekinumab treatment for Crohn's disease in clinical practice: experience at a tertiary medical center [abstract]. Gastroenterology 2014;146(5). S-464–5.
34. Kopylov U, Afif W, Cohen A, et al. Subcutaneous ustekinumab for the treatment of anti-TNF resistant Crohn's disease–the McGill experience. J Crohns Colitis 2014; 8(11):1516–22.
35. Wils P, Bouhnik Y, Michetti P, et al. Subcutaneous ustekinumab provides clinical benefit for two-thirds of patients with Crohn's disease refractory to anti-tumor necrosis factor agents. Clin Gastroenterol Hepatol 2016;14(2):242–50.e1-2.
36. Khorrami S, Ginard D, Marin-Jimenez I, et al. Ustekinumab for the treatment of refractory Crohn's disease: the Spanish experience in a large multicentre open-label cohort. Inflamm Bowel Dis 2016;22(7):1662–9.
37. Harris KA, Horst S, Gadani A, et al. Patients with refractory Crohn's disease successfully treated with ustekinumab. Inflamm Bowel Dis 2016;22(2):397–401.
38. Ma C, Fedorak R, Kaplan G, et al. Ustekinumab is effective for the induction and maintenance of response in Crohn's disease: a multi-center cohort study [abstract]. Am J Gastroenterol 2016;111(1):S294.
39. Greenup AJ, Rosenfeld G, Bressler B. Ustekinumab use in Crohn's disease: real-life Canadian experience [abstract]. Am J Gastroenterol 2016;111(1):S334–5.
40. Sandborn WJ, Gasink C, Chan D, et al. Endoscopic healing in induction and maintenance with ustekinumab in the phase 3 UNITI Crohn's disease program [abstract]. Am J Gastroenterol 2016;111(1):S278–9.
41. Adedokun O, Xu Z, Gasink C, et al. Pharmacokinetics and exposure-response relationships of intravenously administered ustekinumab during induction treatment in patients with Crohn's disease: results from the UNITI-1 and UNITI-2 studies [abstract]. J Crohns Colitis 2016;10:S23–4.
42. Adedokun OJ, Xu Z, Gasink C, et al. Sa1934 pharmacokinetics and exposure-response relationships of ustekinumab during IV induction and SC maintenance treatment of patients with Crohn's disease with ustekinumab: results from the UNITI-1, UNITI-2, and IM-UNITI studies [abstract]. Gastroenterology 2016; 150(4):S408.
43. Battat R, Kopylov U, Bessissow T, et al. Association of ustekinumab trough concentrations with clinical, biochemical, and endoscopic outcomes [abstract]. J Crohns Colitis 2016;10:S74.
44. Sands B, Gasink C, Jacobstein D, et al. Efficacy and safety of dose adjustment and delayed response to ustekinumab in moderate-severe Crohn's disease patients: results from the IM-UNITI maintenance study [abstract]. Am J Gastroenterol 2016;111(1):S302–3.
45. Griffiths CE, Strober BE, van de Kerkhof P, et al. Comparison of ustekinumab and etanercept for moderate-to-severe psoriasis. N Engl J Med 2010;362(2):118–28.
46. Singh S, Fumery M, Dulai PS, et al. P-122 comparative efficacy of pharmacological agents for moderate-severe Crohn's disease in patients with prior exposure to anti-TNF agents: a network meta-analysis [abstract]. Inflamm Bowel Dis 2017; 23(2):S44.
47. Papp KA, Griffiths CE, Gordon K, et al. Long-term safety of ustekinumab in patients with moderate-to-severe psoriasis: final results from 5 years of follow-up. Br J Dermatol 2013;168(4):844–54.
48. Papp K, Gottlieb AB, Naldi L, et al. Safety surveillance for ustekinumab and other psoriasis treatments from the psoriasis longitudinal assessment and registry (PSOLAR). J Drugs Dermatol 2015;14(7):706–14.

49. Ryan C, Leonardi CL, Krueger JG, et al. Association between biologic therapies for chronic plaque psoriasis and cardiovascular events: a meta-analysis of randomized controlled trials. JAMA 2011;306(8):864–71.
50. Hinchey J, Chaves C, Appignani B, et al. A reversible posterior leukoencephalopathy syndrome. N Engl J Med 1996;334(8):494–500.
51. Gratton D, Szapary P, Goyal K, et al. Reversible posterior leukoencephalopathy syndrome in a patient treated with ustekinumab: case report and review of the literature. Arch Dermatol 2011;147(10):1197–202.
52. Segal BM, Constantinescu CS, Raychaudhuri A, et al. Repeated subcutaneous injections of IL12/23 p40 neutralising antibody, ustekinumab, in patients with relapsing-remitting multiple sclerosis: a phase II, double-blind, placebo-controlled, randomised, dose-ranging study. Lancet Neurol 2008;7(9):796–804.
53. Badat Y, Meissner WG, Laharie D. Demyelination in a patient receiving ustekinumab for refractory Crohn's disease. J Crohns Colitis 2014;8(9):1138–9.
54. McConnell RA, Mahadevan U. Use of immunomodulators and biologics before, during, and after pregnancy. Inflamm Bowel Dis 2016;22(1):213–23.
55. Martin PL, Sachs C, Imai N, et al. Development in the cynomolgus macaque following administration of ustekinumab, a human anti-IL-12/23p40 monoclonal antibody, during pregnancy and lactation. Birth Defects Res B Dev Reprod Toxicol 2010;89(5):351–63.
56. Schaufelberg BW, Horn E, Cather JC, et al. Pregnancy outcomes in women exposed to ustekinumab in the psoriasis clinical development program [abstract]. J Am Acad Dermatol 2014;70(5):AB178.
57. Mahadevan U, Martin C, Kane SV, et al. 437 Do infant serum levels of biologic agents at birth correlate with risk of adverse outcomes? Results from the PIANO registry [abstract]. Gastroenterology 2016;150(4):S91–2.
58. Nguyen GC, Seow CH, Maxwell C, et al. The Toronto consensus statements for the management of inflammatory bowel disease in pregnancy. Gastroenterology 2016;150(3):734–57.e1.
59. Deepak P, Bruining DH. Update on the medical management of Crohn's disease. Curr Gastroenterol Rep 2015;17(11):41.
60. Terdiman JP, Gruss CB, Heidelbaugh JJ, et al. American Gastroenterological Association Institute guideline on the use of thiopurines, methotrexate, and anti-TNF-alpha biologic drugs for the induction and maintenance of remission in inflammatory Crohn's disease. Gastroenterology 2013;145(6):1459–63.
61. Ding NS, Hart A, De Cruz P. Systematic review: predicting and optimising response to anti-TNF therapy in Crohn's disease—algorithm for practical management. Aliment Pharmacol Ther 2016;43(1):30–51.
62. Ben-Horin S, Chowers Y. Review article: loss of response to anti-TNF treatments in Crohn's disease. Aliment Pharmacol Ther 2011;33(9):987–95.
63. Billioud V, Sandborn WJ, Peyrin-Biroulet L. Loss of response and need for adalimumab dose intensification in Crohn's disease: a systematic review. Am J Gastroenterol 2011;106(4):674–84.
64. Sands BE, Feagan BG, Rutgeerts P, et al. Effects of vedolizumab induction therapy for patients with Crohn's disease in whom tumor necrosis factor antagonist treatment failed. Gastroenterology 2014;147(3):618–27.e3.
65. Sandborn WJ, Feagan BG, Rutgeerts P, et al. Vedolizumab as induction and maintenance therapy for Crohn's disease. N Engl J Med 2013;369(8):711–21.
66. Ben-Horin S, Casteele NV, Schreiber S, et al. Biosimilars in inflammatory bowel disease: facts and fears of extrapolation. Clin Gastroenterol Hepatol 2016;14(12):1685–96.

67. Papamichael K, Van Stappen T, Jairath V, et al. Review article: pharmacological aspects of anti-TNF biosimilars in inflammatory bowel diseases. Aliment Pharmacol Ther 2015;42(10):1158–69.
68. Tillack C, Ehmann LM, Friedrich M, et al. Anti-TNF antibody-induced psoriasiform skin lesions in patients with inflammatory bowel disease are characterised by interferon-gamma-expressing Th1 cells and IL-17A/IL-22-expressing Th17 cells and respond to anti-IL-12/IL-23 antibody treatment. Gut 2014;63(4):567–77.
69. Fahmy M, Ramamoorthy S, Hata T, et al. Ustekinumab for peristomal pyoderma gangrenosum. Am J Gastroenterol 2012;107(5):794–5.
70. Goldminz AM, Botto NC, Gottlieb AB. Severely recalcitrant pyoderma gangrenosum successfully treated with ustekinumab. J Am Acad Dermatol 2012;67(5): e237–8.
71. Guenova E, Teske A, Fehrenbacher B, et al. Interleukin 23 expression in pyoderma gangrenosum and targeted therapy with ustekinumab. Arch Dermatol 2011;147(10):1203–5.
72. Gheita TA, El G II, El-Fishawy HS, et al. Involvement of IL-23 in enteropathic arthritis patients with inflammatory bowel disease: preliminary results. Clin Rheumatol 2014;33(5):713–7.
73. Rubin D, Feagan B, Dryden G, et al. The effect of vedolizumab on extraintestinal manifestations in patients with Crohn's disease in GEMINI 2 [abstract]. Inflamm Bowel Dis 2016;22:S42–3.
74. Levin AA, Gottlieb AB. Specific targeting of interleukin-23p19 as effective treatment for psoriasis. J Am Acad Dermatol 2014;70(3):555–61.
75. Campa M, Mansouri B, Warren R, et al. A review of biologic therapies targeting IL-23 and IL-17 for use in moderate-to-severe plaque psoriasis. Dermatol Ther (Heidelb) 2016;6(1):1–12.
76. Croxford AL, Kulig P, Becher B. IL-12-and IL-23 in health and disease. Cytokine Growth Factor Rev 2014;25(4):415–21.
77. Chackerian AA, Chen SJ, Brodie SJ, et al. Neutralization or absence of the interleukin-23 pathway does not compromise immunity to mycobacterial infection. Infect Immun 2006;74(11):6092–9.
78. Rudner XL, Happel KI, Young EA, et al. Interleukin-23 (IL-23)-IL-17 cytokine axis in murine *Pneumocystis carinii* infection. Infect Immun 2007;75(6):3055–61.
79. Kleinschek MA, Muller U, Brodie SJ, et al. IL-23 enhances the inflammatory cell response in *Cryptococcus neoformans* infection and induces a cytokine pattern distinct from IL-12. J Immunol 2006;176(2):1098–106.
80. Lieberman LA, Cardillo F, Owyang AM, et al. IL-23 provides a limited mechanism of resistance to acute toxoplasmosis in the absence of IL-12. J Immunol 2004; 173(3):1887–93.
81. Sands BE, Chen J, Penney M, et al. 830 Initial evaluation of MEDI2070 (specific Anti-IL-23 antibody) in patients with active Crohn's disease who have failed anti-TNF antibody therapy: a randomized, double-blind placebo-controlled phase 2A induction study [abstract]. Gastroenterology 2015;148(4). S-163–4.
82. Feagan BG, Sandborn W, Panés J, et al. 812a Efficacy and safety of induction therapy with the selective IL-23 inhibitor BI 655066, in patients with moderate-to-severe Crohn's disease: results of a randomized, double-blind, placebo-controlled phase II study [abstract]. Gastroenterology 2016;150(4):S1266.
83. MedImmune LLC. A phase 2b double-blind, multi-dose, placebo-controlled study to evaluate the efficacy and safety of MEDI2070 in subjects with moderate to severe Crohn's disease who have failed or are intolerant to anti tumor necrosis factor-alpha therapy. Bethesda (MD): National Library of Medicine (US); 2000.

NLM Identifier: NCT02574637. Available at: https://clinicaltrials.gov/show/NCT02574637. Accessed January 2, 2017.
84. AbbVie Inc. An open label, single group, long term safety extension trial of BI 655066/ABBV-066 (Risankizumab), in patients with moderately to severely active Crohn's disease. Bethesda (MD): National Library of Medicine (US); 2000. NLM Identifier: NCT02513459. Available at: https://clinicaltrials.gov/show/NCT02513459. Accessed January 2, 2017.
85. Eli Lilly and Company. A phase 2, multicenter, randomized, parallel-arm, placebo-controlled study of LY3074828 in subjects with active Crohn's disease (SERENITY). Bethesda (MD): National Library of Medicine (US); 2000. NLM Identifier: NCT02891226. Available at: https://clinicaltrials.gov/show/NCT02891226. Accessed January 2, 2017.
86. Feagan BG, Sandborn WJ, D'Haens G, et al. Efficacy and safety of induction therapy with the selective IL-23 inhibitor risankizumab (BI 655066) in patients with moderate-to-severe Crohn's disease: a randomised, double-blind, placebo-controlled phase 2 study. Lancet 2017;389(10080):1699–709.
87. Sun Pharma and Merck & Co. Inc. Enter into licensing agreement for tildrakizumab MC, Inc [press release]. Merck Sharp & Dohme Corp; 2014. Available at: http://www.merck.com/licensing/our-partnership/sunpharma_partnership.html. Accessed October 7, 2016.
88. Sandborn WJ. The present and future of inflammatory bowel disease treatment. Gastroenterol Hepatol 2016;12(7):438–41.
89. Boehringer Ingelheim, Inc. Boehringer Ingelheim's investigational biologic cleared skin better, faster and for longer than ustekinumab in phase II psoriasis study [press release]. Boehringer Ingelheim, Inc; 2015. Available at: https://www.boehringer-ingelheim.com/press-release/boehringer-ingelheim-s-investigational-biologic-cleared-skin-better-faster-and-longer. Accessed October 7, 2016.
90. Papp K, Menter A, Sofen H, et al. Efficacy and safety of different dose regimens of a selective IL-23p19 inhibitor (BI 655066) compared with ustekinumab in patients with moderate-to-severe plaque psoriasis with and without psoriatic arthritis [abstract]. Arthritis Rheumatol 2015;67(Suppl 10). Available at: http://acrabstracts.org/abstract/efficacy-and-safety-of-different-dose-regimens-of-a-selective-il-23p19-inhibitor-bi-655066-compared-with-ustekinumab-in-patients-with-moderate-to-severe-plaque-psoriasis-with-and-without-psoriatic-a/. Accessed October 9, 2016.
91. Janssen Research & Development LLC. A study of guselkumab in participants with moderate to severe plaque-type psoriasis and an inadequate response to ustekinumab (NAVIGATE). Bethesda (MD): National Library of Medicine (US); 2000. NLM Identifier: NCT02203032. Available at: https://www.clinicaltrials.gov/ct2/show/NCT02203032. Accessed October 7, 2016.
92. Deepak P, Fletcher JG, Fidler JL, et al. Long-term maintenance of radiological response is associated with decreased probability of surgeries, hospitalizations, and corticosteroids usage in Crohn's disease patients. Gastroenterology 2016;150(4):S130.
93. Kuehbacher T, Nikolaus S, Schreiber S. Serum soluble IL2-receptor is increased in a subpopulation of Crohn's disease patients, who respond to open label use of ustekinumab, a human monoclonal antibody to IL-12/23p40. Gastroenterology 2011;140(5):S-589.

Janus Kinase Antagonists and Other Novel Small Molecules for the Treatment of Crohn's Disease

Brigid S. Boland, MD[a,*], Séverine Vermeire, MD, PhD[b]

KEYWORDS

- Crohn's disease • Jak inhibitor • Filgotinib • TGF-β • SMAD7 • Mongersen
- Sphingosine-1-phosphate receptor • Ozanimod

KEY POINTS

- Small molecule therapies for Crohn's disease offer potential benefits over biologics, including shorter half-lives, lack of immunogenicity, and oral route of administration.
- Janus kinase inhibitors block multiple cytokine pathways simultaneously and will likely be an effective oral therapy for Crohn's disease and ulcerative colitis.
- Filgotinib, a Janus kinase 1-specific inhibitor, was recently shown to be effective in inducing clinical remission in Crohn's disease.
- Mongersen inhibits Smad7 and thereby restores transforming growth factor-β signaling and may be an effective oral targeted therapy.
- Sphingosine-1 phosphate receptor modulators impair B-cell and T-cell lymphocyte trafficking by downregulating receptors that facilitate egress from lymph nodes.

INTRODUCTION

Current management of moderate to severe Crohn's disease typically includes thiopurines (azathioprine, 6-mercaptopurine), methotrexate, tumor necrosis factor (TNF) inhibitors (infliximab, adalimumab, and certolizumab pegol), integrin inhibitors (natalizumab

Disclosures: B.S. Boland has received consulting fees from Abbvie and has received grant support from Takeda and Janssen. S. Vermeire has received grant support from AbbVie, MSD, and Takeda; received speaker fees from AbbVie, MSD, Takeda, Ferring, Dr. Falk Pharma, Hospira, Pfizer, and Tillots; and served as a consultant for AbbVie, MSD, Takeda, Ferring, Genentech/Roche, Shire, Pfizer Inc, Galapagos, Mundipharma, Hospira, Celgene, Second Genome, and Janssen.

[a] Division of Gastroenterology, Department of Medicine, Inflammatory Bowel Disease Center, ACTRI, University of California San Diego, 9452 Medical Center Drive, La Jolla, CA 92093, USA; [b] Department of Gastroenterology, University Hospitals Leuven, Herestraat 49,3000 Leuven, Belgium

* Corresponding author.

E-mail address: bboland@ucsd.edu

Gastroenterol Clin N Am 46 (2017) 627–644

http://dx.doi.org/10.1016/j.gtc.2017.05.015

and vedolizumab), and most recently IL-12/23 inhibitors (ustekinumab). Although these therapies are effective for a proportion of patients with Crohn's disease, approximately two-thirds of patients are primary or secondary failures to TNF inhibitors.[1,2] These patients who fail TNF inhibitors are less likely to respond to vedolizumab as well as to ustekinumab.[3,4] Therefore, there is a great need for therapies that are easier to tolerate and work through novel mechanisms of action. More specifically, small molecules that act on different pathways have emerged as an appealing alternative to biologics based on their oral route of administration, minimal risk of immunogenicity, and less interpatient pharmacokinetic variability. Small molecule therapies are emerging as future therapies for Crohn's disease.

SMALL MOLECULE THERAPIES: ADVANTAGE OVER BIOLOGICS

Oral Administration

Many of the current effective therapies for the induction and maintenance of moderate to severely active Crohn's disease are biologics, which are complex proteins made by living cells, weighing up to 150 kDa (**Table 1**).[5] The complex structure of biologics necessitates an intravenous or subcutaneous route of administration and contributes to variability in pharmacokinetics and immunogenicity. In contrast, small molecules are defined by a molecular weight of less than 900 Da, which allows diffusion across cell membranes.[6] The most clear benefit of small molecules is the ability to be administered as oral medications, which is appealing to patients as a convenient route of administration, and small molecules importantly have less pharmacokinetic variability. Ultimately, oral medications increase patient satisfaction and treatment adherence, which leads to improved efficacy.[7]

Shorter Half-Life

In contrast with the longer half-life of biologics, small molecules typically have much shorter half-lives with once or twice daily dosing of medications. Although the more frequent dosing may be inconvenient in some instances, the shorter half-life enables faster withdrawal of medication, particularly in cases of infection, pregnancy, or surgery, where one would like to stop an immune-suppressing medication.

Less Immunogenicity

One of the major limitations in the practical use of biologics is immunogenicity, which leads to the development of antibodies that may lead to loss of response to a medication as well as potentially adverse reactions. Immune modulators are frequently used in combination with biologics to reduce the risk of antibody formation, but are associated with potential side effects. Antibodies are the consequence of immunologic antigenic responses to large molecules; however, small molecules have

Table 1
Comparison of biologics and small molecules

	Biologics	Small Molecules
Weight (Daltons)	Large (>1000)	Small (<1000)
Route of administration	Parenteral	Oral
Half-life	Short	Long
Immunogenicity	Potential risk	Low risk
Drug–drug interactions	Rare	Potential

significantly less antigenic potential based on their size. In effect, the minimal risk of immunogenicity may improve the durability of response to small molecules as compared with biologics.

Although small molecules may have different side effects, such as more drug–drug interactions, as compared with biologics, they offer unique benefits, including the oral route of administration and minimal immunogenicity.

PATHOPHYSIOLOGY OF JANUS KINASE INHIBITION

The Janus Kinase Family

The JAK family are nonreceptor tyrosine kinases with a conserved kinase that is enzymatically active and consist of JAK1, JAK2, JAK3, and tyrosine kinase 2 (TYK2). The JAK family play a central role in signaling transduction for multiple growth factors as well as cytokines, including ones that have been implicated in the pathogenesis of autoimmune diseases based on genome wide association studies, as well as mouse models of inflammation.[8,9]

Type I and II cytokines

JAK proteins mediate intracellular signaling from type I and type II transmembrane receptors upon binding of the associated cytokine. Type I cytokines play a role in many bodily processes, including inflammation as well as normal growth and maturation of myeloid cells. Receptors for type I cytokines contain a common subunit, such as γ-chain (γc, or IL-2 receptor γ subunit), β-chain (CD131), and glycoprotein 130 (gp130 or CD130). The γc-receptors include IL-2, IL-4, IL-7, IL-9, and IL-15, with intracellular signaling mediated by JAK1 and JAK3. Common β-chain receptors include IL-3, IL-5, and granulocyte macrophage colony stimulating factor, with signaling dependent on JAK2. IL-6, IL-11, and IL-27 are part of the common gp130 chain receptors and signal via JAK1, JAK2, and TYK2.[9,10] The dimeric receptor family includes IL-12 and IL-23, which signal through JAK2 and TYK2 as well as IL-35, which uses JAK1 and JAK2. The hormone-like family consists of erythropoietin, thrombopoietin, growth hormone, granulocyte-CSF, and leptin, which use JAK2 for intracellular signaling (**Table 2**).[8,9]

Type II cytokines include the interferon (IFN) and IL-10 family. IFN-α and IFN-β signal via JAK1 and TYK2, whereas IFN-γ uses JAK1 and JAK2. The IL-10–related cytokines are associated with regulatory T-cell activity and include IL-10, IL-19, IL-20, and IL-22, which signal through JAK1, JAK2, and TYK2.[8,9]

Mechanisms of Janus Kinase Signaling

JAK proteins associate with the intracellular portion of cytokine and hormone receptors that lack intrinsic catalytic activity and propagate intracellular signaling that eventually leads to transcriptional changes (**Fig. 1**). Upon binding of a cytokine or hormone to its receptor, the subunits of receptors form multimers, enabling JAK proteins to phosphorylate the associated cytokine receptor. The phosphorylated intracellular cytokine receptor facilitates recruitment of signaling transducers and activators of transcription (STATs). JAK proteins phosphorylate STAT proteins, leading to STAT homodimerization. The STAT homodimer localizes to the nucleus and activates downstream transcription that plays a critical role in inflammation and many other cellular processes.[10,11] Unique combinations of JAKs and STAT proteins lead to unique transcriptional changes associated with different cytokines or hormones.

Janus Kinase Signaling and the Pathogenesis of Inflammatory Bowel Disease

The pathophysiology of IBD is a complex process related to dysbiotic microbiota and environmental factors in a genetically susceptible individual that leads to an abnormal

Table 2
Summary of type I and type II cytokine signaling

	Cytokine	Associated JAK	Associated STAT
Type I cytokine receptors			
Common γ-chain	IL-2	JAK1, JAK3	3, 5
	IL-4	JAK1, JAK3	6
	IL-7	JAK1, JAK3	3, 5
	IL-9	JAK1, JAK3	1, 3, 5
	IL-13	JAK1, JAK3, TYK2	1, 3, 5
	IL-15	JAK1, JAK3	3, 5
	IL-21	JAK1, JAK3	1, 3, 5
Common β-chain	GM-CSF	JAK2	3, 5
	IL-3	JAK2	3, 5, 6
	IL-5	JAK2	3, 5, 6
gp130 chain	IL-6	JAK1, JAK2, TYK2	1, 3
	IL-11	JAK1, JAK2, TYK2	3
	IL-27	JAK1, JAK2, TYK2	1, 2, 3, 4, 5
Dimers	IL-12	JAK2, TYK2	4
	IL-23	JAK2, TYK2	3, 4
	IL-27	JAK1, JAK2	1, 3
	IL-35	JAK1, JAK2	1, 4
Hormone	EPO	JAK2	5
	TPO	JAK2	1, 3, 5
	G-CSF	JAK2	5
	Growth hormone	JAK2	3, 5
	Leptin	JAK2	3, 5
Type II cytokine receptors			
IFN family	IFN-α/β	JAK1, TYK2	1, 2, 3, 4, 5
	IFN-γ	JAK1, JAK2	1
	IL-28	JAK1, TYK2	1, 2, 3, 4, 5
	IL-29	JAK1, TYK2	1, 2, 3, 4, 5
IL-10 family	IL-10	JAK1, JAK2, TYK2	1, 3, 5
	IL-19	JAK1, JAK2, TYK2	3
	IL-20	JAK1, JAK2, TYK2	3
	IL-22	JAK1, JAK2, TYK2	1, 3, 5

Abbreviations: EPO, erythropoietin; GM-CSF, granulocyte macrophage colony stimulating factor; IFN, interferon; IL, interleukin; JAK, Janus kinase; STAT, signaling transducers and activators of transcription; TPO, thrombopoietin; TYK, tyrosine kinase.

Adapted from Boland BS, Sandborn WJ, Chang JT. Update on Janus kinase antagonists in inflammatory bowel disease. Gastroenterol Clin North Am 2014;43(3):603–17; with permission.

innate and adaptive immune response. The inflammatory response in IBD is related to activation of the innate and adaptive immune response that is characterized by an excess in inflammatory T cells, typically type 1 helper T cells (Th1) and type 17 helper T cells (Th17) in Crohn's disease with insufficient activity of regulatory T cells, and JAK proteins are known to play a critical role in inflammation signaling.[12] Key pathways involved in the pathogenesis of IBD include IL-12 and IL-23, which drive differentiation of CD4 T cells into Th1 and Th17 cell, respectively, via JAK2 and TYK2,[13] and common γc cytokines, including IL-2, IL-4, IL-7, IL-9, IL-14, and IL-21, use JAK1 and JAK3 to regulate the adaptive immune response.[14] Genome-wide association studies have underscored the importance of the JAK signaling pathway, identifying polymorphisms in JAK2, TYK2, STAT3, IL-23 receptor, and IL-12 that increase the risk of IBD.[15] Based on the role of JAK signaling in inflammation, JAK inhibition is an appealing target for

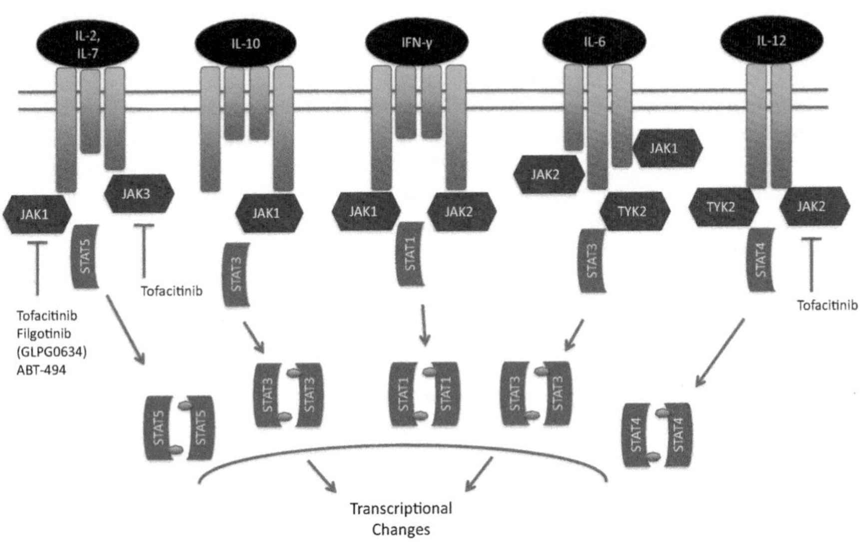

Fig. 1. Janus kinase (JAK) signaling pathways related to inflammatory bowel disease and therapeutic targets of JAK inhibitors. Upon cytokine binding to its receptor, JAKs phosphorylate its associated cytokine receptor and creates a docking site for signaling transducers and activators of transcription (STAT) signaling molecules. JAKs then phosphorylate STAT proteins to facilitate STAT dimerization, followed by translocation to the nucleus and transcriptional activation of downstream target genes. For simplicity, some nonessential JAK family members have been omitted. IFN, interferon. (*Adapted from* Boland BS, Sandborn WJ, Chang JT. Update on Janus kinase antagonists in inflammatory bowel disease. Gastroenterol Clin North Am 2014;43(3):603–17; with permission.)

the treatment of IBD; however, JAK signaling is complex and plays a critical role in multiple cellular pathways, regulating normal cellular growth and development, which may lead to dose-limiting side effects.

TOFACITINIB: A PAN JANUS KINASE INHIBITOR

Tofacitinib (CP-690550) is the first oral, small molecule JAK inhibitor used in clinical trials and has been approved for rheumatoid arthritis (RA). Tofacitinib has a short half-life of 3 hours and specifically inhibits JAK1, JAK2, and JAK3; however, in vitro studies show preferential inhibition of JAK1 and JAK3 over JAK2.[16] As a consequence of JAK1 inhibition, tofacitinib blocks gp130 family cytokines, such as IL-6 and IL-11, as well as type II cytokines including IFN-α, IFN-β, and IL-10. In addition, tofacitinib inhibits IL-2, IL-4, IL-6, IL-7, IL-9, IL-15, and IL-21, which signal through JAK3. Tofacitinib has less effect on JAK2 signaling, but there is mild inhibition of β-chain signaling, including IL-3, IL-5, granulocyte macrophage colony stimulating factor, erythropoietin, and IFN-γ signaling.[17] Through these effects, tofacitinib interferes with the development of pathogenic Th1 and Th17 cells as well as with B-cell function.[18,19] Preclinical studies confirmed that tofacitinib had a potential dampening effect on both adaptive and innate immunity that contribute to the pathogenesis of IBD as well as other autoimmune diseases, such as RA and psoriasis.[16]

Tofacitinib in Ulcerative Colitis

In an 8-week dose-finding, phase II, randomized, placebo-controlled trial, tofacitinib showed a robust dose-dependent effect in patients with moderate to severely active ulcerative colitis (UC) (NCT00787202). There was a significant improvement in terms of the clinical response (32%, 48%, 61%, and 78% in the 0.5-, 3-, 10-, and 15-mg tofacitinib arms, respectively, vs 42% on placebo), clinical remission (13%, 33%, 48%, and 41% in the 0.5-, 3-, 10-, and 15-mg tofacitinib arms, respectively, vs 10% on placebo), and endoscopic remission (10%, 18%, 30%, and 27% in the 0.5-, 3-, 10-, and 15-mg tofacitinib arms, respectively, vs 2% on placebo) on tofacitinib as compared with placebo. Furthermore, reductions in objective markers of inflammation, including C-reactive protein (CRP) and fecal calprotectin provided additional support for the clinical efficacy of tofacitinib.[20] As a consequence, 2 phase III studies of tofacitinib 10 mg twice daily were conducted in more than 1000 patients with UC, OCTAVE 1 (NCT01465763) and OCTAVE 2 (NCT01458951). Clinical remission rates after an 8-week induction were higher in tofacitinib as compared with placebo (18.5% vs 8.2% in OCTAVE 1 [*P* = .007]; 16.6% and 3.6% in OCTAVE 2 [*P* = .005]), and rates of mucosal healing were greater in the tofacinib groups as compared with placebo.[21] The patients who had responded clinically to induction therapy in the OCTAVE 1 and 2 trials were then randomized to receive placebo, 5 mg twice daily or 10 mg twice daily in the OCTAVE Sustain trial.[21] Remission at week 52 occurred in 34%-40% of the tofacitinib-treated patients compared to 11.1% of placebo treated patients (p<0.001 for both comparisons).[21] Overall infection rates were higher in the tofacitinib-treated patients, but overall serious infections were not significantly different.[21] A total of 5.1% of the patients treated with tofacitinib 10 mg twice daily experienced an episode of herpes zoster compared with 0.5% of placebo-treated patients.[21]

Tofacitinib in Crohn's Disease

Although tofacitinib showed early promise in phase II trials for UC, the Crohn's disease trial failed to meet its primary endpoint of clinical response defined as a reduction in the Crohn's Disease Activity Index (CDAI) by 70 or more points from baseline at week 4. The phase II, placebo-controlled clinical trial (NCT00615199) enrolled a total of 138 patients who were randomized to 4 weeks of tofacitinib 1 mg, 5 mg, 15 mg, or placebo twice daily. At week 4, the clinical response rates were 36%, 58%, and 46% in the 1-mg, 5-mg, and 15-mg tofacitinib arms, respectively, but were not different from the high placebo response rate of 47%. Clinical remission rates were not significantly different (31%, 24%, and 14% in the 1-, 5-, and 15-mg tofacitinib arms, respectively, vs 21% in the placebo arm). Although the primary and secondary endpoints were not met in the setting of high placebo response rates, there were modest dose-related reductions in week 4 CRP and fecal calprotectin concentrations with the higher doses, suggesting a reduction in objective inflammation and a probable biologic effect. The phase II study included patients with active Crohn's disease defined based on CDAI scores between 250 and 450, but endoscopic confirmation of disease activity was not mandatory.[22] There were high placebo rates based on reduction in CDAI, which may have potentially obscured the ability to detect clinically meaningful differences in a short study.

A second phase IIB study of tofacitinib in moderately to severely active Crohn's disease was conducted that aimed to address some of the weaknesses from the first phase II trial. The study was an 8-week treatment study where baseline disease activity was confirmed with endoscopy. Although the clinical remission rates of 43.5% and 43% on tofacinitib 5 mg and 10 mg, respectively, were not higher than the placebo rate of 36.7%, there were notable improvements in objective markers of inflammation with reduction in mean CRP concentrations in the tofacintinib 5-mg and 10-mg doses (−2.2 and −7 mg/L, respectively) as compared with placebo (−0.4 mg/L). In stark contrast with results from most clinical trials in Crohn's disease, the response and remission rates were not lower in anti-TNF experienced as compared with anti-TNF–naïve patients, which, if clinically relevant, would make tofacitinib an ideal second-line therapy.[23] To date, tofacitinib has not been shown to be an effective therapy for Crohn's disease, although there are some objective markers to suggest potential efficacy.

Safety and Tolerability of Tofacitinib

Tofacinitib has been well-tolerated in the clinical trials that have been conducted in UC and Crohn's disease; however, the safety profile has primarily been derived from the phase III clinical trials in patients with RA, where doses of 5 or 10 mg twice daily were initially studied leading to its approval and frequent use. In a meta_analysis of 8 randomized, controlled induction trials with tofacitinib in RA, there were no differences in adverse events, including infections, or study withdrawal as a consequence of side effects in the tofacitinib groups as compared with the placebo group.[24] In a pooled analysis of the phase II, phase III, and long-term extension studies of tofacitinib in RA, the rate of serious infections was 3.09 per 100 patient-years (95% CI, 2.73–3.95). The most common infections were bronchitis, herpes zoster (HZ), influenza, upper respiratory infections, and urinary tract infections, and age, corticosteroid dose, and tofacitinib dose were independent risk factors for infection. Overall, the risk of infection and mortality on tofacitinib was comparable with that of patients with RA being treated with biologics; however, there was an increase in the relative risk of HZ that was specific to tofacitinib.[25]

As a consequence of JAK2 inhibition, tofacitinib has the potential to cause bone marrow suppression. In the phase III RA clinical trials, neutrophil counts decreased modestly with low rates of neutropenia (1.2% from months 0 to 3; 0.8% from months 3 to 6), but without an increase in associated infections. Interestingly, hemoglobin concentrations did not change significantly.[26] In addition, there have been consistent dose-related increases in high-density lipoprotein cholesterol and low-density lipoprotein cholesterol by an average of 10% to 20%, which reverses after cessation of therapy.[20,22,26,27] The lipid changes, however, have not translated into a significant increase in cardiovascular events, although larger studies are needed to assess the magnitude and significance of any cardiovascular signal.[27]

Herpes Zoster Risk with Janus Kinase Inhibitors

Reactivation of varicella zoster virus, called HZ, seems to be an infectious risk that may be relevant to JAK inhibitors.[25] The risk seems to be related to the suppressive effect on natural killer cells through JAK1 and JAK3 inhibition. Based on the phase II, phase III, and extension studies with tofacitinib in RA, 239 of 4789 participants were diagnosed with HZ with an incidence rate of 4.4 per 100 patient-years (95% CI, 3.8–4.9). Age, but not tofacitinib dose, was associated independently with risk of zoster. Overall, there were no cases of disseminated or visceral zoster, nor mortatlity associated with HZ.[28] Based on the evolving experience in RA, varicella zoster virus vaccination before the initiation of JAK inhibitors may become a routine practice, particularly with the introduction of a non-live, highly effective vaccine.[29]

Risk of Malignancy with Janus Kinase Inhibitors

Natural killer cells and IFN play critical roles in immune surveillance, and there is concern that disrupting these pathways through the inhibition of JAK1 and/or JAK3 may lead to an increased risk of malignancy. Understanding the risk of malignancy with medications will require long-term extension trials and extensive clinical experience, and to date the longest experience and greatest number of patients have been treated with tofacitinib in RA. In a pooled analysis of 14 phase II, phase III, and long-term extension studies in RA, the incidence rate for all malignancies (excluding nonmelanoma skin cancers) was 0.85

per 100 patient-years and was not different from the age-adjusted rates from the US National Cancer Institute Surveillance and Epidemiology and End Results database. Specifically, the incidence rate for lymphoma was 0.08 events per 100 patient-years without a time- or dose-dependent association with therapy, and the rates were not significantly different than rates in RA patients, although ongoing surveillance will further define the potential malignancy risk.[30] The early clinical data do not show a signal for malignancy, but long-term extension studies are critical in defining this risk with tofacinitib and other JAK inhibitors.

Filgotinib: novel selective Janus kinase 1 inhibitor

Selective JAK1 inhibitors have been developed in an effort to improve both efficacy and minimize side effects from JAK2 and JAK3 inhibition. Filgotinib (formerly called GLPG0634, GS-6034) is an oral selective JAK1 inhibitor with a 6-hour half-life with maximal pharmacodynamics effects achieved with once daily dosing. Filgotinib shows 50-fold selectivity for JAK1 over JAK3 inhibition and 30-fold selectivity for JAK1 over JAK2 inhibition in human blood. The small molecule inhibited differentiation of Th1 and Th2 cells with less of an effect on Th17 cells and showed a dose-dependent effect against a rodent model of collagen-induced arthritis.[31] In a phase IIB clinical trial in RA, filgotinib showed a dose-dependent response in combination with methotrexate.[32]

FITZROY: Phase II Filgotinib Study in Crohn's Disease

The first phase II clinical trial showed early but robust evidence supporting the efficacy and safety of filgotinib for moderate to severely active Crohn's disease. The FITZROY study (NCT02048618) was a randomized, placebo-controlled, phase II clinical trial of filgotinib 200 mg/d for 10 weeks with an exploratory extension phase in 174 Crohn's disease patients. The study was carefully designed to include patients with not only active symptoms (CDAI 220–450 inclusive), but also endoscopically active Crohn's disease as defined by the Simple Endoscopic Score for Crohn's Disease (SES-CD) of 7 or greater, or 4 or greater in cases of isolated ileitis and confirmed by central endoscopic reading, leading to a high screening failure rate of 44%. The primary outcome, clinical remission with a CDAI of less than 150, was achieved in 47% of patients on filgotinib 200 mg/d as compared with 23% of patients on placebo (P = .0077). The clinical remission rates increased throughout the duration of the study and may continue to increase with ongoing therapy. In addition, there were significantly higher rates of CDAI-100 response, biological remission defined as normalization of CRP, and improvement in quality of life scores in the treatment arm, supporting the clinical efficacy of filgotinib.[33]

With the use of centralized reading, the overall endoscopic response and remission rates in the FITZROY study were low at week 10; however, 25% of patients on filgotinib as compared with 14% on placebo had a 50% reduction the SES-CD score with similar but less robust trends in endoscopic remission.[33] Although the phase II study was not powered for endoscopic outcomes, the endoscopic results confirm a meaningful effect from JAK1 inhibition beyond clinical response and remission; however, the low absolute endoscopic response at week 10 may raise mechanistic questions about the timing and potential for JAK inhibitors to heal the transmural inflammatory process in Crohn's disease completely. Alternatively, our endoscopic scoring systems have been developed for assessing active disease and may not be the best tools for assessing healing.

Filgotinib in Anti-tumor Necrosis Factor–Exposed Patients with Crohn's Disease

The next-generation biologics have consistently had lower clinical response and remission rates in anti-TNF–exposed as compared with anti-TNF–naive patients, creating an increasing need for effective therapies for anti-TNF–experienced patients.[3,34] Similarly, in the FITZROY study, the difference in remission rates between filgotinib and placebo were much greater in anti-TNF–naive patients (60% vs 13% in filgotinib vs placebo) as compared with anti-TNF–exposed patients (37% vs 29% in filgotinib vs placebo).[33] Consistent with other studies, anti-TNF exposure seems to be a surrogate for refractory Crohn's disease that may be associated with lower rates of response to filgotinib.

Safety and Tolerability of Filgotinib

Overall, filgotinib has been well-tolerated in the small studies of Crohn's disease, although larger phase III studies are necessary to detect safety signals. The safety analysis from the phase IIB clinical trial pooled the different filgotinib dosing regimens over 20 weeks, and serious infections were reported in 3% of the filgotinib group (4 of 152), whereas none were reported in the placebo arm. In contrast with tofacitinib, there were no significant changes in lymphocyte or neutrophil counts. The higher dose of filgotinib had an effect on lipids with a mean increase of 11% in high-density lipoprotein cholesterol and 12% in low-density lipoprotein cholesterol at week 20; however, there was a mean increase of 4% in high-density lipoprotein cholesterol and 13% in low-density lipoprotein cholesterol in the placebo arm, raising some questions about the presence and magnitude of an effect of filgotinib on lipids. Overall, the selectivity of filgotinib seems to have significantly improved the tolerability and potentially efficacy in Crohn's disease as compared with tofacitinib.[33]

Janus Kinase Inhibitors: An Evolving Pipeline

Other JAK inhibitors are undergoing development and clinical trials for Crohn's disease. Upadacitinib (ABT-494), a specific JAK1 inhibitor, is being evaluated in Crohn's disease in a phase II clinical trial (NCT0236549) that has completed enrollment.[35] Co-primary endpoints in this highly refractory population of 220 patients with moderately to severely active Crohn's disease were clinical remission (stool frequency </=1.5 and abdominal pain </=1) at week 16 and endoscopic remission (SES-CD </=4 with >/=2 decrease) at week 12 or 16. Clinical remission was achieved in 27% of patients receiving upadacitinib 6 mg twice daily compared to 11% in the placebo group ($p<0.10$). Endoscopic remission occurred in 22% of patients on upadacitinib 24 mg twice daily and 14% of those on 24 mg once daily compared to 0% of the placebo group ($p<0.05$).[36] With an increasing understanding of the benefits of selective JAK inhibition, additional JAK inhibitors are being developed with specificities designed to maximize clinical effect and minimize side effects.

TARGETING NOVEL INFLAMMATORY PATHWAYS

Transforming Growth Factor-β1 and Inflammation

Transforming growth factor-β1 (TGF-β1) is a cytokine with pleiotropic effects that is expressed in the gut and serves a critical role in regulating inflammatory pathways. Upon TGF-β1 binding to its receptor, a heterodimer consisting of type I (TGF-βRI) and type II (TGF-βRII) subunits, TGF-βRI is phosphorylated and activated, which leads to phosphorylation of downstream signaling molecules, Smad2 and Smad3. Upon phosphorylation, Smad2 and Smad3 form a complex with Smad4, translocating to the nucleus to initiate transcriptional changes that suppress inflammatory gene expression.[37–39] A counterregulatory member of the Smad family, Smad7, attenuates TGF-β1 signaling through binding to the ligand-bound TGF-β1–receptor inhibitor complex that leads to degradation of the receptor and effectively prevents Smad2 and Smad3 phosphorylation as well as its downstream effects (**Fig. 2**).[38,40]

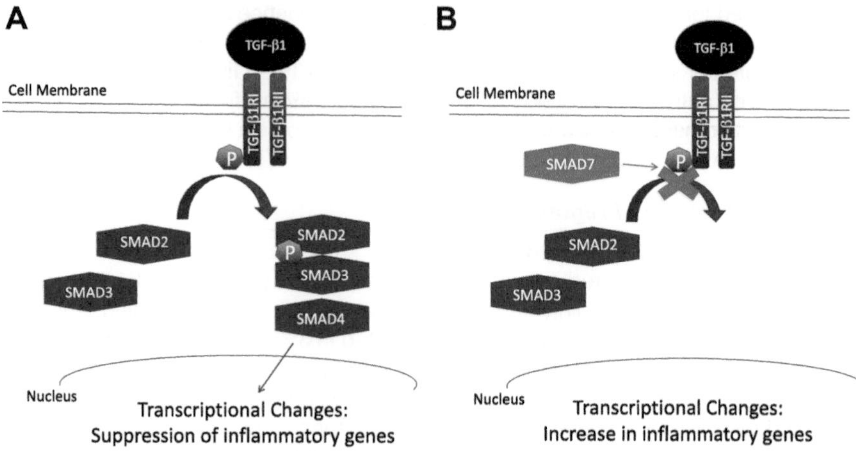

Fig. 2. Transforming growth factor (TGF)-β1 signaling pathway and Smad7. (*A*) TGF-β1 binds to the TGF-β1 receptor, which leads to phosphorylation of the intracellular portion of the TGF-β1 RI. TGF-β1 receptor inhibitor (RI) in turn phosphorylates Smad2 and Smad3, which then complex with Smad4. The complex of Smad2, Smad3, and Smad4 translocate to the nucleus of the cell and suppress inflammatory gene expression. (*B*) Overexpression Smad7 interferes with this pathway whereby Smad7 binds to TGF-β1 RI and inhibits Smad2 and Smad3 phosphorylation. Smad7 interferes with the antiinflammatory effects of TGF-β1, leading to an increase in inflammatory gene expression.

Transforming Growth Factor-β1 and Smad7 in Crohn's Disease

TGF-β1 plays a critical role in suppressing inflammation, and dysregulation of TGF-β1 plays an important role in the pathophysiology of Crohn's disease. Although TGF-β1 RNA is overexpressed in inflamed as compared with noninflamed intestinal tissue from patients with Crohn's disease, Smad7 is simultaneously overexpressed and inhibits TGF-β1–dependent Smad signaling and its antiinflammatory effects.[41,42] Inhibition of Smad7 in lamina propria mononuclear cells from patients with UC and Crohn's disease restored TGF-β1–dependent signaling with Smad3 phosphorylation and reduced inflammatory cytokine production.[42] Moreover, Smad7 inhibition with an antisense oligonucleotide restored TGF-β1–dependent signaling with reduction in inflammatory cytokine expression and ameliorated the oxazolone- and TNBS-induced mouse models of colitis, although this could not be confirmed in the T-cell transfer model of colitis.[43] Together, these findings provided a strong rationale for Smad7 as a therapeutic target in IBD.

Mongersen: Smad7 antisense oligonucleotide

Based on successful use in mouse colitis models and homology between human and mouse SMAD7, mongersen (formerly GED0301), a 21-based single-strand antisense oligonucleotide, was developed to inhibit Smad7. The oligonucleotide is a complementary sequence that binds to Smad7 messenger RNA and causes RNase H-mediated degradation, decreasing Smad7 expression. The oligonucleotide is coated by methacrylic acid–ethyl acrylate copolymers that facilitate pH-dependent delivery of the antisense oligonucleotide directly to the terminal ileum and right colon.[44] Based on mouse colitis models, Smad7 antisense oligonucleotides seem to undergo endocytosis by epithelial and lamina propria mononuclear cells in the gastrointestinal tract with minimal systemic absorption.[43] Furthermore, in the phase I dose-finding study of mongersen in 15 patients with Crohn's disease, the study drug was only detected at a low concentration in a single blood sample from 1 patient, providing significant support for its lack of systemic delivery and distribution.[44]

In a phase II, randomized clinical trial, a 2-week course of mongersen had a dose-dependent effect on clinical remission in participants with terminal ileum and/or right sided colonic Crohn's disease. One hundred sixty-six participants with active Crohn's disease based on CDAI scores were randomized to 10 mg, 40 mg, or 160 mg/d of mongersen or placebo for 2 weeks, and the primary outcome was clinical remission, defined as a CDAI of less than 150 for 2 weeks after completing treatment. Clinical remission rates were 65% in the 160-mg group and 55% in the 40-mg group, which were significantly higher than rates of 12% in the 10-mg group and 10% in the placebo group. Clinical response, CDAI reduction by 100, was achieved in significantly more patients in the 160 mg group (72%), 40-mg group (58%), and 10-mg group (37%) as compared with placebo (17%), suggesting a dose-dependent effect. Of the patients with elevated baseline CRP (>3 mg/L), mongersen did not, however, reduce CRP at multiple times points, although there was a reduction in serum concentrations of IL-8 and TNF-α in the higher doses.[45]

Although the response and remission rates were markedly high, particularly given the short study duration, there remain significant concerns about the reproducibility of the study given the reliance on clinical scores in the absence of endoscopy as part of both the inclusion criteria and secondary endpoints, and the disconnect between clinical response and CRP response. Based on the initial study, the results were not generalizable to all patients with Crohn's disease because the study excluded a significant proportion of patients with Crohn's disease, including those with lesions in the upper gastrointestinal tract or left colon, as well as those with fistulas or perianal disease. Although the short duration of the study treatment raises some additional questions about the optimal duration of treatment and duration of effect, a local delivery system and a lasting clinical benefit beyond its use would be ideal characteristics of a new therapy.

In an effort to address the limitations of the phase II study, an exploratory open-label trial randomized 163 participants with active Crohn's disease confirmed by endoscopy with central reading to mongersen 160 mg/d for 4, 8, or 12 weeks. Results show evidence that mongersen has an effect on endoscopic disease activity. At week 12, 37% of all participants had 25% or greater reduction, and 15% had 50% or greater reduction in SES-CD scores. Specifically, in patients with baseline SES-CD score over 12, 63% and 31% had 25% or greater and 50% or greater reduction in SES-CD, respectively. There was a decrease in mean concentrations of CRP and fecal calprotectin in participants with elevated concentrations at baseline, but it is unclear what proportion of patients normalized their CRP.[46] Phase III clinical trials of mongersen are ongoing and will provide a better understanding about its efficacy in Crohn's disease.

Effect of Smad7 Inhibition on Fibrosis

Based on its counterregulatory effects on inflammation, TGF-β1 has been identified as a potential therapeutic target in Crohn's disease; however, TGF-β1 is a pleiotropic cytokine with profibrotic effects, stimulating fibroblasts to produce collagen.[47] Given the potential complications associated with fibrosis in Crohn's disease, there is concern about potential profibrotic effects of SMAD7 inhibition. Although limited data are available to address this concern, a phase I extension study of Crohn's disease patients who were treated with mongersen for 1 week monitored for stricture development over 6 months using small intestine contrast ultrasound imaging as well as serum biomarkers for intestinal fibrosis (basic fibroblast growth factors, human chitinase 3-like1, matrix metalloproteinases, and tissue inhibitor 1 of matrix metalloproteinase). In this study with a short treatment duration with mongersen, there was no increase in development of bowel obstructions or strictures, or changes in biomarkers for fibrosis in 14 participants.[48] Although there was no evidence of fibrosis in this phase I extension study, further assessments for strictures with a longer duration of treatment with mongersen are needed.

Safety and Tolerability of Mongersen

Mongersen was well-tolerated in the phase I and phase II studies in Crohn's disease. The majority of the serious adverse events were Crohn's disease-related symptoms or complications, occurring in the placebo and mongersen arms with similar frequencies, and the majority of other adverse events were mild. There was no signal suggesting an increase in infections or opportunistic infections. Although antisense toxicity has been reported to cause complement activation, complement concentrations were monitored and were unchanged during therapy.[45]

TARGETING LYMPHOCYTE TRAFFICKING: OTHER SMALL MOLECULES FOR CROHN'S DISEASE

Lymphocyte trafficking plays a central role in the innate and adaptive immune response, and inhibition of lymphocyte trafficking using monoclonal antibodies to α4, such as natalizumab, and α4β7, such as vedolizumab, is an effective mechanism of action for treatment of Crohn's disease.[4] Sphingosine-1-phosphate (S1P) receptor 1 agonists are an alternative mechanism to interfere with lymphocyte trafficking.

Sphingosine-1-Phosphate Receptors

There are 5 receptors in the S1P G-coupled receptor family ($S1P_{1\text{-}5}$) that, upon binding of S1P, help to regulate a variety of cellular functions, including lymphocyte trafficking, vascular tone, heart rate, and many others. Although the 5 receptors play roles in multiple cellular processes, $S1P_1$ receptors are expressed in unique anatomic locations and regulate lymphocyte egress from the lymph nodes with S1P concentration gradients (**Fig. 3**).[49] S1P expression is typically low in the lymph nodes and drives $S1P_1$

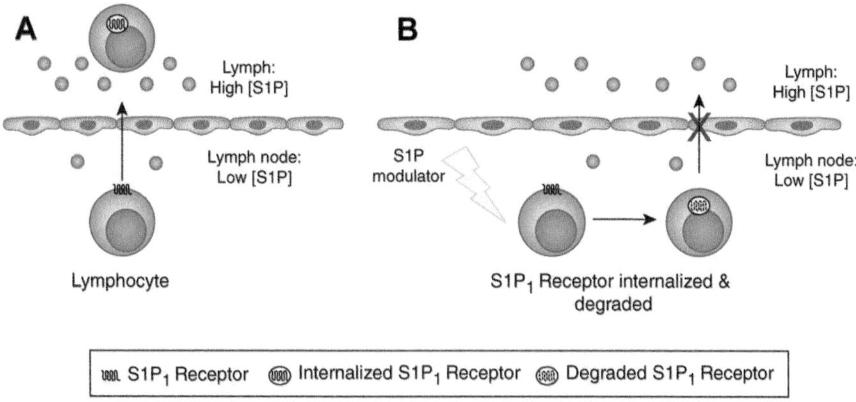

Fig. 3. Lymphocyte trafficking and sphingosine-1-phosphate 1 ($S1P_1$) receptor modulation. (*A*) In areas of low S1P concentration, $S1P_1$ receptors are expressed on lymphocytes, which facilitate egress from areas of low to high S1P concentration. After egress out of the lymph node, $S1P_1$ receptor expression is downregulated. (*B*) In the setting of an S1P modulator, the $S1P_1$ receptor is internalized and degraded, preventing lymphocyte egress from the lymph node.

receptor expression on lymphocytes to facilitate migration to areas of higher S1P concentrations. S1P modulators bind to $S1P_1$ receptors, initiate internalization, and lead to reversible degradation of the $S1P_1R$. As a consequence, lymphocytes lacking $S1P_1R$ expression cannot migrate out of the lymph nodes and into the blood to perform effector functions. Successful modulation of this pathway leads to a reduction in the number of effector T cells circulating in the peripheral blood and in the target organs, such as the gastrointestinal tract.[50]

Fingolimod: Sphingosine-1-Phosphate Modulator for Multiple Sclerosis

The first nonselective S1P receptor modulator used in clinical trials and approved for use in multiple sclerosis was fingolimod (FTY720). Fingolimod, a prodrug, undergoes phosphorylation and activation as an agonist of $S1P_{1\text{-}5}$ receptors.[51] In patients with multiple sclerosis treated with FTY720, there was an 80% and 60% reduction in peripheral $CD4^+$ and $CD8^+$ T cells, respectively, with a selective reduction in naïve T cells and central memory T cells, while effector memory T cells that maintain immune surveillance were preserved.[52] The half-life of fingolimod was relatively long, translating into prolonged periods of lymphopenia. Although modulation of the $S1P_1$ pathway drove the immune suppression, the $S1P_3$-mediated effects led to limiting cardiac side effects, including bradycardia, QT prolongation, and atrioventricular blockade.[53]

Ozanimod: Sphingosine-1-phosphate 1 receptor modulator

Ozanimod (RPC-1063) is a small molecule developed with $S1P_1$ and $S1P_5$ receptor specificity and has a greater than 10,000-fold selectivity for $S1P_1$ over $S1P_{2\text{-}4}$, which minimizes potential cardiac side effects. Like fingolimod, ozanimod induces sustained $S1P_1$ receptor internalization and degradation with a dose-dependent reduction in peripheral lymphocytes, specifically $CCR7^+$ T and B lymphocytes. The half-life of ozanimod is shorter (5 hours in mice) than fingolimod in animal models, leading to shorter periods of lymphopenia. In the TNBS-induced and naïve T-cell adoptive transfer colitis mouse model, ozanimod was associated with a dose-dependent reduction in weight loss and other indices of inflammation, providing rationale for use in humans with IBD.[54]

Ozanimod in Ulcerative Colitis: Phase II Study Results

A phase II, double-blind, placebo-controlled phase II study of ozanimod (NCT01647516) examining the safety and efficacy in patients with moderately to severely active UC showed a positive clinical effect. One hundred ninety-seven adults with moderately to severely active UC with a Mayo Clinic Score of 6 to 12 were randomized to ozanimod 0.5 mg, 1 mg, or placebo for 32 weeks. The primary outcome, clinical remission with a Mayo Clinic score of 2 or less at week 8 with centralized endoscopy reading, was achieved in 14% and 16% in the ozanimod 0.5 mg and 1 mg groups, respectively, as compared with 6% in placebo; however, the differences were only statistically significant between the ozanimod 1 mg group and placebo ($P = .0048$). Clinical response rates at week 8 were higher at 54% and 57% in the 0.5 mg and 1 mg ozanimod arms, respectively, as compared with 37% in the placebo arm. Furthermore, the rates of mucosal healing rates were higher at 28% and 34% in the 0.5 mg and 1 mg ozanimod groups, respectively, as compared with 12% in the placebo arm ($P = .06$ and .02, respectively). Although the primary outcome was measured at week 8, the rates of clinical remission at week 32 were higher, with larger differences between the treatment group and placebo: 26% and 21% in the 0.5 mg group and 1 mg group, respectively, as compared with 6% in the placebo group.[55] The increasing rates of remission from week 8 to week 32 suggest that a longer duration of treatment improves the efficacy of ozanimod, mirroring the evolving experience with leukocyte trafficking inhibitors with a relatively slow onset of action with response rates that increase with duration of therapy.[34,55] Furthermore, the low placebo response rates were likely related to the use of blinded central reading of endoscopy at baseline, week 8, and week 32 with strict criteria for clinical remission.[55] Overall, the study suggests that ozanimod is likely to be effective in UC; however, the phase III study is ongoing.

Safety and Tolerability of Ozanimod in Ulcerative Colitis

Although the phase II ozanimod study in UC was not powered for safety, the study drug was well-tolerated. There was a single patient with preexisting bradycardia who experienced a transient, asymptomatic episode of first-degree atrioventricular block; however, there were no additional cardiovascular side effects, in contrast with fingolimod. Four patients on ozanimod developed elevated alanine aminotransferase blood concentrations that were more than 3 times the upper limit of normal without additional sequelae; however, the mechanism underlying this abnormality is not understood.[55]

Ozanimod: Effect on Lymphocyte Count

In the phase II study of ozanimod in UC, the mean absolute lymphocyte count from blood decreased by 32% and 49% in patients in the 0.5 mg and 1 mg ozanimod arms, respectively, at week 8. In the ozanimod 1 mg group, approximately 50% of patients had absolute lymphocyte counts below the normal range with a dose-dependent effect; however, there were no incidences of grade 4 lymphopenia (absolute lymphocyte count of $<0.2 \times 10^9$/L) or infectious complications.[56]

Ozanimod in Crohn's Disease

Although there are no data currently available to assess the efficacy of ozanimod in Crohn's disease, a phase II open-label study of ozanimod in moderately to severely active Crohn's disease is being conducted to assess the efficacy.[35] Based on the efficacy of lymphocyte trafficking inhibitors in Crohn's disease, ozanimod has a high likelihood of being an effective therapy for Crohn's disease, although it may have a slow onset of action. Although it is difficult to predict in the absence of any clinical trials in Crohn's disease, ozanimod may be an appealing alternative to leukocyte trafficking inhibitors, particularly if rapid drug clearance in biologics were a concern. In comparison with vedolizumab, ozanimod may have additional immune-suppressing effects that may provide some additional clinical benefit in Crohn's disease. Further studies will help to elucidate the potential role of ozanimod in Crohn's disease.

SUMMARY

There are a number of innovative small molecule, oral medications for Crohn's disease that act through unique mechanisms of action, including JAK-cytokine signaling inhibition, Smad7 inhibition on the TGF-β pathway, and S1P receptor modulation that interferes with lymphocyte trafficking (**Table 3**). The phase II study of filgotinib (FITZROY) in Crohn's disease showed a promising signal suggesting clinical efficacy with significantly fewer side effects as compared with nonspecific JAK inhibitors. JAK inhibitors may, therefore, become the medication of choice in patients who developed antibodies to other biologics. Although mongersen has limited clinical data at this time, its mode of local delivery to the areas of inflammation without systemic absorption may represent the next generation of treatments for Crohn's disease. Similarly,

Table 3
Summary of small molecules for Crohn disease

Medication	Mechanism of Action	Clinical Trial Status	Safety Concerns	Approved Conditions
Tofacitinib	Pan JAK inhibitor	Phase II completed	Effects of JAK2 inhibition	Rheumatoid arthritis
Filgotinib (GLPG0634)	JAK1 inhibitor	Phase II completed Phase III recruiting	VZV reactivation	None
Upadacitinib (ABT-494)	JAK1 inhibitor	Phase II ongoing	VZV reactivation	None
Mongersen (GED0301)	Smad7 inhibitor	Phase II completed Phase III recruiting	Complement activation	None
Ozanimod	$S1P_1R$ modulator	Phase II recruiting	Lymphopenia	None

Abbreviations: JAK, Janus kinase; $S1P_1R$, sphingosine-1-phosphate; VZV, varicella zoster virus.

ozanimod is a potential therapy for Crohn's disease based on its efficacy in an early trial in UC and may become an oral alternative to lymphocyte trafficking agents. Small molecules offer unique benefits as compared with biologics in terms of the oral route of administration, minimal risk of immunogenicity, and shorter half-lives, and represent the next era of therapies for Crohn's disease.

REFERENCES

1. Hanauer SB, Feagan BG, Lichtenstein GR, et al. Maintenance infliximab for Crohn's disease: the ACCENT I randomised trial. Lancet 2002;359(9317):1541–9.
2. Colombel JF, Sandborn WJ, Rutgeerts P, et al. Adalimumab for maintenance of clinical response and remission in patients with Crohn's disease: the CHARM trial. Gastroenterology 2007;132(1):52–65.
3. Sandborn WJ, Gasink C, Gao LL, et al. Ustekinumab induction and maintenance therapy in refractory Crohn's disease. N Engl J Med 2012;367(16):1519–28.
4. Sandborn WJ, Feagan BG, Rutgeerts P, et al. Vedolizumab as induction and maintenance therapy for Crohn's disease. N Engl J Med 2013;369(8):711–21.
5. Remicade [package insert]. Horsham, PA: Janssen Biotech, Inc; 2013.
6. Leeson PD, Springthorpe B. The influence of drug-like concepts on decision-making in medicinal chemistry. Nat Rev Drug Discov 2007;6(11):881–90.
7. Cramer JA, Roy A, Burrell A, et al. Medication compliance and persistence: terminology and definitions. Value Health 2008;11(1):44–7.
8. O'Shea JJ, Kontzias A, Yamaoka K, et al. Janus kinase inhibitors in autoimmune diseases. Ann Rheum Dis 2013;72(Suppl 2):ii111–5.
9. Gadina M, Hilton D, Johnston JA, et al. Signaling by type I and II cytokine receptors: ten years after. Curr Opin Immunol 2001;13(3):363–73.
10. Darnell JE Jr. STATs and gene regulation. Science 1997;277(5332):1630–5.
11. Darnell JE Jr, Kerr IM, Stark GR. Jak-STAT pathways and transcriptional activation in response to IFNs and other extracellular signaling proteins. Science 1994; 264(5164):1415–21.

12. Atreya R, Neurath MF. IBD pathogenesis in 2014: molecular pathways controlling barrier function in IBD. Nat Rev Gastroenterol Hepatol 2015;12(2):67–8.
13. Langrish CL, McKenzie BS, Wilson NJ, et al. IL-12 and IL-23: master regulators of innate and adaptive immunity. Immunol Rev 2004;202:96–105.
14. Hofmann SR, Ettinger R, Zhou YJ, et al. Cytokines and their role in lymphoid development, differentiation and homeostasis. Curr Opin Allergy Clin Immunol 2002;2(6):495–506.
15. Jostins L, Ripke S, Weersma RK, et al. Host-microbe interactions have shaped the genetic architecture of inflammatory bowel disease. Nature 2012; 491(7422):119–24.
16. Ghoreschi K, Jesson MI, Li X, et al. Modulation of innate and adaptive immune responses by tofacitinib (CP-690,550). J Immunol 2011;186(7):4234–43.
17. Leonard WJ, O'Shea JJ. Jaks and STATs: biological implications. Annu Rev Immunol 1998;16:293–322.
18. Maeshima K, Yamaoka K, Kubo S, et al. The JAK inhibitor tofacitinib regulates synovitis through inhibition of interferon-gamma and interleukin-17 production by human CD4+ T cells. Arthritis Rheum 2012;64(6):1790–8.
19. Rosengren S, Corr M, Firestein GS, et al. The JAK inhibitor CP-690,550 (tofacitinib) inhibits TNF-induced chemokine expression in fibroblast-like synoviocytes: autocrine role of type I interferon. Ann Rheum Dis 2012;71(3):440–7.
20. Sandborn WJ, Ghosh S, Panes J, et al. Tofacitinib, an oral Janus kinase inhibitor, in active ulcerative colitis. N Engl J Med 2012;367(7):616–24.
21. Sandborn WJ, Su C, Sands BE, et al. Tofacitinib as induction and maintenance therapy for ulcerative colitis. N Engl J Med 2017;376:1723–36.
22. Sandborn WJ, Ghosh S, Panes J, et al. A phase 2 study of tofacitinib, an oral Janus kinase inhibitor, in patients with Crohn's disease. Clin Gastroenterol Hepatol 2014;12(9):1485–93.e2.
23. Panés J, SW, Schreiber S, et al. Efficacy and safety of oral tofacitinib for induction therapy in patients with moderate-to-severe Crohns disease: results of a Phase 2b randomised placebo-controlled trial. ECCO Congress 2016.
24. He Y, Wong AY, Chan EW, et al. Efficacy and safety of tofacitinib in the treatment of rheumatoid arthritis: a systematic review and meta-analysis. BMC Musculoskelet Disord 2013;14:298.
25. Cohen S, Radominski SC, Gomez-Reino JJ, et al. Analysis of infections and all-cause mortality in phase II, phase III, and long-term extension studies of tofacitinib in patients with rheumatoid arthritis. Arthritis Rheumatol 2014;66(11): 2924–37.
26. Fleischmann R, Kremer J, Cush J, et al. Placebo-controlled trial of tofacitinib monotherapy in rheumatoid arthritis. N Engl J Med 2012;367(6):495–507.
27. Charles-Schoeman C, Wicker P, Gonzalez-Gay MA, et al. Cardiovascular safety findings in patients with rheumatoid arthritis treated with tofacitinib, an oral Janus kinase inhibitor. Semin Arthritis Rheum 2016;46(3):261–71.
28. Winthrop KL, Yamanaka H, Valdez H, et al. Herpes zoster and tofacitinib therapy in patients with rheumatoid arthritis. Arthritis Rheumatol 2014;66(10):2675–84.
29. Cunningham AL, Lal H, Kovac M, et al. Efficacy of the herpes zoster subunit vaccine in adults 70 years of age or older. N Engl J Med 2016;375(11):1019–32.
30. Curtis JR, Lee EB, Kaplan IV, et al. Tofacitinib, an oral Janus kinase inhibitor: analysis of malignancies across the rheumatoid arthritis clinical development programme. Ann Rheum Dis 2016;75(5):831–41.

31. Van Rompaey L, Galien R, van der Aar EM, et al. Preclinical characterization of GLPG0634, a selective inhibitor of JAK1, for the treatment of inflammatory diseases. J Immunol 2013;191(7):3568–77.
32. Westhovens R, Taylor PC, Alten R, et al. Filgotinib (GLPG0634/GS-6034), an oral JAK1 selective inhibitor, is effective in combination with methotrexate (MTX) in patients with active rheumatoid arthritis and insufficient response to MTX: results from a randomised, dose-finding study (DARWIN 1). Ann Rheum Dis 2016; 76(6):998–1008.
33. Vermeire S, Schreiber S, Petryka R, et al. Clinical remission in patients with moderate-to-severe Crohn's disease treated with filgotinib (the FITZROY study): results from a phase 2, double-blind, randomised, placebo-controlled trial. Lancet 2016;389(10066):266–75.
34. Sands BE, Feagan BG, Rutgeerts P, et al. Effects of vedolizumab induction therapy for patients with Crohn's disease in whom tumor necrosis factor antagonist treatment failed. Gastroenterology 2014;147(3):618–27.e3.
35. Available at: clinicaltrials.gov. Accessed December 29, 2016.
36. Sandborn WJ, Feagan BG, Panes J, et al. Safety and efficacy of upadacitinib (ABT-494), an oral JAK1 inhibitor, as induction therapy in patients with Crohn's disease: results from CELEST (abstract). Gastroenterology 2017;152:S1308–9.
37. Heldin CH, Miyazono K, ten Dijke P. TGF-beta signalling from cell membrane to nucleus through SMAD proteins. Nature 1997;390(6659):465–71.
38. Nakao A, Imamura T, Souchelnytskyi S, et al. TGF-beta receptor-mediated signalling through Smad2, Smad3 and Smad4. EMBO J 1997;16(17):5353–62.
39. Fantini MC, Becker C, Monteleone G, et al. Cutting edge: TGF-beta induces a regulatory phenotype in CD4+CD25- T cells through Foxp3 induction and down-regulation of Smad7. J Immunol 2004;172(9):5149–53.
40. Nakao A, Afrakhte M, Moren A, et al. Identification of Smad7, a TGFbeta-inducible antagonist of TGF-beta signalling. Nature 1997;389(6651):631–5.
41. Babyatsky MW, Rossiter G, Podolsky DK. Expression of transforming growth factors alpha and beta in colonic mucosa in inflammatory bowel disease. Gastroenterology 1996;110(4):975–84.
42. Monteleone G, Kumberova A, Croft NM, et al. Blocking Smad7 restores TGF-beta1 signaling in chronic inflammatory bowel disease. J Clin Invest 2001; 108(4):601–9.
43. Boirivant M, Pallone F, Di Giacinto C, et al. Inhibition of Smad7 with a specific antisense oligonucleotide facilitates TGF-beta1-mediated suppression of colitis. Gastroenterology 2006;131(6):1786–98.
44. Monteleone G, Fantini MC, Onali S, et al. Phase I clinical trial of Smad7 knockdown using antisense oligonucleotide in patients with active Crohn's disease. Mol Ther 2012;20(4):870–6.
45. Monteleone G, Neurath MF, Ardizzone S, et al. Mongersen, an oral SMAD7 antisense oligonucleotide, and Crohn's disease. N Engl J Med 2015;372(12): 1104–13.
46. Feagan B, Sands BE, Rossiter G, et al. A Randomized, Double-blind, Multicenter Study to Explore the Efficacy of Oral GED-0301 (Mongersen) on Endoscopic Activity and Clinical Effects in Both TNF-Naive and TNF-Experienced Subjects with Active Crohn's Disease. United European Gastroenterology Week 2016.
47. Border WA, Noble NA. Transforming growth factor beta in tissue fibrosis. N Engl J Med 1994;331(19):1286–92.

48. Zorzi F, Calabrese E, Monteleone I, et al. A phase 1 open-label trial shows that smad7 antisense oligonucleotide (GED0301) does not increase the risk of small bowel strictures in Crohn's disease. Aliment Pharmacol Ther 2012;36(9):850–7.
49. Rosen H, Gonzalez-Cabrera PJ, Sanna MG, et al. Sphingosine 1-phosphate receptor signaling. Annu Rev Biochem 2009;78:743–68.
50. Marsolais D, Rosen H. Chemical modulators of sphingosine-1-phosphate receptors as barrier-oriented therapeutic molecules. Nat Rev Drug Discov 2009;8(4): 297–307.
51. Mandala S, Hajdu R, Bergstrom J, et al. Alteration of lymphocyte trafficking by sphingosine-1-phosphate receptor agonists. Science 2002;296(5566):346–9.
52. Mehling M, Brinkmann V, Antel J, et al. FTY720 therapy exerts differential effects on T cell subsets in multiple sclerosis. Neurology 2008;71(16):1261–7.
53. Kappos L, Radue EW, O'Connor P, et al. A placebo-controlled trial of oral fingolimod in relapsing multiple sclerosis. N Engl J Med 2010;362(5):387–401.
54. Scott FL, Clemons B, Brooks J, et al. Ozanimod (RPC1063) is a potent sphingosine-1-phosphate receptor-1 (S1P1) and receptor-5 (S1P5) agonist with autoimmune disease-modifying activity. Br J Pharmacol 2016;173(11): 1778–92.
55. Sandborn WJ, Feagan BG, Wolf DC, et al. Ozanimod induction and maintenance treatment for ulcerative colitis. N Engl J Med 2016;374(18):1754–62.
56. Sandborn WJ, Feagan BG. Ozanimod treatment for ulcerative colitis. N Engl J Med 2016;375(8):e17.

Update on Therapeutic Drug Monitoring in Crohn's Disease

Valérie Heron, MD, FRCPC, Waqqas Afif, MD, MSc, FRCPC*

KEYWORDS

- Therapeutic drug monitoring • Biologics • Anti-tumor necrosis factor
- Drug concentrations • Anti-drug antibodies • Crohn's disease
- Inflammatory bowel disease

KEY POINTS

- Therapeutic drug monitoring involves measuring drug concentrations and anti–drug antibodies, which are associated with clinical and endoscopic outcomes.
- In patients with a loss of response to anti–tumor necrosis factor therapy, therapeutic drug monitoring is clinically useful and likely cost-effective.
- There is evidence for the use of therapeutic drug monitoring in the withdrawal of immunosuppression in combination therapy, dose deescalation, post–drug holiday, and perhaps post-induction monitoring.
- Therapeutic drug monitoring in routine maintenance therapy has not yet been shown to improve treatment efficacy.
- There is interassay variability, and optimal therapeutic drug and antibody thresholds remain to be firmly established.

INTRODUCTION

Therapeutic drug monitoring (TDM) is one of the cornerstones of personalized medicine and has been widely used to improve the treatment of various diseases. In the setting of infectious disease and transplant medicine, measuring serum concentrations of antibiotics and immunosuppressive medications has dramatically improved patient outcomes. The understanding of the pharmacokinetic and pharmacodynamic

Disclosures: W. Afif has consulted for Janssen, Abbvie, Takeda, Pfizer, Merck, and Shire and has obtained research funding from Janssen, Abbvie, Prometheus Labs, and Theradiag.
Division of Gastroenterology, McGill University Health Center, Montreal General Hospital, McGill University, 1650 Cedar Avenue, Montreal, Quebec H3G 1A4, Canada
* Corresponding author. McGill University Health Center, Montreal General Hospital, 1650 Cedar Avenue, Room C7-200, Montreal, Quebec H3G 1A4, Canada.
E-mail address: waqqas.afif@mcgill.ca

Gastroenterol Clin N Am 46 (2017) 645–659
http://dx.doi.org/10.1016/j.gtc.2017.05.014
gastro.theclinics.com

properties of these medications has aided in achieving therapeutic targets, thereby optimizing efficacy while limiting potential drug-related toxicity.

The introduction of biologic therapies in the treatment of Crohn's disease (CD) has ushered in a new era of treatment. These drugs have the potential to alter the natural history of this progressive disease. Unfortunately, remission rates with these biologic medications are only approximately 40%,[1] and in those who do achieve remission, the rate of loss of response (LOR) is more than 10% per year.[2] There is evidence to suggest that the use of TDM may help to guide and optimize therapy in CD patients on biologic medications. In clinical practice, measuring drug and anti–drug antibody (ADA) concentrations has already been used to adapt treatment strategies in a variety of situations.

In this review, we examine the available data on TDM, with both anti–tumor necrosis factor (anti-TNF) agents and newer biologic medications, in the treatment of patients with CD.

MEASURING BIOLOGIC CONCENTRATIONS AND ANTI–DRUG ANTIBODIES

Before any discussion on the use of TDM, there must be a clear understanding of the various techniques available to measure drug and ADA concentrations. Depending on the technique used, the thresholds to alter therapy can vary significantly from assay to assay as well as between different laboratories. This lack of a standardized testing method therefore limits the ability to reliably compare drug and antibody thresholds with patient outcomes in clinical studies. Therefore, an understanding of TDM assays is important to help accurately interpret the results of available data. Commercialized assays include various techniques such as enzyme-linked immunosorbent assay (ELISA), electro-chemiluminescence immunoassay (ECLIA), radioimmunoassay (RIA), and a high mobility shift assay (HMSA).

Most studies to date were performed using a conventional solid phase ELISA. In this technique, TNF is plated, which binds anti-TNF from a serum sample. Labeled anti–immunoglobulin G is then added, which binds the anti-TNF to allow for measurement of drug concentration. Drug concentrations generated by ELISA assays are thought to be congruent between different laboratories, as demonstrated by a recent trial comparing 3 European assays.[3] Measurement of ADAs, using ELISA, is performed by plating anti-TNF. However, an important limitation of this method is that it is a drug-sensitive assay. Therefore, ADAs can only be detected in the absence of circulating anti-TNF, because serum anti-TNF renders ADAs undetectable.[4] An alternative "sandwiched" ELISA technique uses a monoclonal antibody in the detection phase, which limits the problem of serum anti-TNF interfering with ADA measurement and is therefore considered a drug-tolerant assay.[5] RIA yields a higher sensitivity and specificity than ELISA and is less prone to drug interference. However, it involves the use of radioisotopes rendering the technique more complex.[6] The homogenous mobility shift assay (Prometheus Laboratories, San Diego, CA, USA) was developed to allow both drug levels and antibodies to be detected simultaneously.[7] This method uses fluorescent-labeled anti-TNF for the detection of ADA and fluorescent-labeled TNF-alpha for the measurement of drug levels. Resulting labeled immune complexes are subsequently detected based on their specific molecular weight.[8] Similarly, ECLIA (LabCorp, Calabasas Hills, CA, USA) detects anti–drug antibodies even in the presence of anti-TNF.[6] Although this technique has been shown to detect IFX with higher sensitivity (lower limit of detection) than ELISA-based assays, its use has not yet been validated in clinical trials.[6] Cost, availability, and accessibility are major factors that influence the routine use of these diagnostic tests. In general, regardless of the assay, drug concentrations are relatively well correlated and reported in micrograms per milliliter.[9] The titer of ADAs and the units of measurement can vary widely depending on the type of assay and whether it is drug sensitive or drug tolerant.[10]

The timing of TDM is also important to accurately interpret the results. Most studies measure anti-TNF concentrations at dosing trough, just before the infusion. However, some data suggest there may also be a role for the measurement of non-trough levels, so as to not delay TDM-based treatment decisions. A small prospective observational study of 17 CD patients showed a correlation between nontrough IFX levels $\geq$15 μg/mL (ELISA) at week 4 or $\geq$6.5 μg/mL at week 6 and therapeutic trough levels $\geq$ 3 μg/mL (correlation coefficient of 0.95 and 0.96, respectively).[11] For adalimumab (ADAL), one small study of 7 patients tested drug concentrations 6 times during a 2-week period and found minimal variation of drug concentrations during the dosing interval.[12] These results suggest that for subcutaneous medications, testing at dosing trough may not be needed.

ASSOCIATION BETWEEN THERAPEUTIC DRUG MONITORING AND CLINICAL AND ENDOSCOPIC OUTCOMES

The effect of anti-TNF drug concentrations and of anti–drug antibodies on clinical outcomes has been well established.[4,13–15] The first landmark study that demonstrated a relationship between drug and antibody concentrations and clinical outcomes was published in 2003.[4] This cohort study of 125 CD patients on IFX found a correlation between IFX levels at 4 weeks and IFX trough levels. In this study, IFX levels greater than 12 μg/mL (ELISA) at week 4 were associated with a longer duration of clinical response (81.5 days, 95% confidence interval [CI] 68–98 vs 68.5 days, 95% CI 52–77, P<.01).[4] In a retrospective analysis of the landmark ACCENT 1 trial, IFX levels greater than 3.5 μg/mL (ELISA) at week 14 were associated with sustained clinical response at week 54 (P = .0042).[16] Likewise, a recent observational study of 1487 trough serum samples from 483 patients with CD, who participated in 4 clinical studies on maintenance therapy, showed that IFX levels greater than 2.79 μg/mL and undetectable anti-IFX antibodies (HMSA, <3.15 U/mL) were predictive of remission during maintenance therapy for CD (P<.001 and P = .002, respectively).[17]

Similar effects of drug concentrations and antibodies have been found with ADAL. In one observational study of 168 patients with CD, early ADAL trough levels greater than 0.33 μg/mL (ELISA) predicted a sustained clinical response (P = .01). In this same study, lower trough levels were observed among patients who discontinued ADAL than in those who continued maintenance treatment (2.5 μg/mL vs 5.9 μg/mL, P = .012).[18] A cross-sectional study of 71 CD patients on ADAL identified a threshold of 5.85 μg/mL (ELISA) as being predictive of clinical remission (positive likelihood ratio [LR] 2.3).[19] The presence of ADAs was positively correlated with active disease (P<.001).[19]

Mucosal healing (MH) has become widely accepted as a key treatment target in inflammatory bowel disease (IBD).[20] Unfortunately, data regarding endoscopic outcomes of TDM remain somewhat limited. Nevertheless, available studies suggest a positive effect of higher drug concentration and a deleterious effect of anti–drug antibodies on MH.

A prospective study including both patients with ulcerative colitis (UC) and patients with CD showed an association between IFX levels and MH.[21] In this study, UC patients underwent proctosigmoidoscopy 8 weeks after IFX optimization, whereas MH in CD patients was assessed using fecal calprotectin levels less than 250 μg/g at week 8 as a surrogate for MH. An incremental increase in IFX level by greater than

0.5 μg/mL (ELISA) was associated with MH (LR 2.02, 95% CI 1.01–4.08, $P = .048$).[21] In a cross-sectional study of 40 patients on ADAL maintenance therapy for either CD or UC, MH was associated with higher ADAL levels (ELISA) than those with endoscopically active disease (6.5 μg/mL vs 4.2 μg/mL, $P < .005$).[22] In a more recent study of 60 patients with CD, even higher ADAL trough concentrations of 14.7 μg/mL (HMSA) were significantly associated with MH, compared with 3.4 μg/mL in those without ($P = 6.25 \times 10^{-5}$).[23]

One study proposed a therapeutic target of 6 to 10 μg/mL for IFX and 8 to 12 μg/mL for ADAL for a targeted outcome of MH.[24] In a retrospective study, these investigators demonstrated that IFX concentrations greater than 5 μg/mL and ADAL concentrations greater than 7.1 μg/mL (ELISA) had an 85% specificity for predicting MH in patients with IBD. They also showed that for equivalent IFX concentrations, patients with detectable levels of anti-IFX antibodies were less likely to achieve MH (16% vs 50%, $P = .003$).[24] Although TDM is not widely available for certolizumab, in clinical studies, higher drug concentrations have been associated with increased rates of MH.[25]

THERAPEUTIC DRUG MONITORING IN COMBINATION THERAPY

Several studies and meta-analyses have demonstrated the potential of combination therapy with an immunomodulator to increase anti-TNF concentrations and suppress antibody formation.[26,27] The SONIC study showed that combination therapy with azathioprine was associated with higher levels of IFX, decreased antibody formation, and a higher rate of steroid-free clinical remission, when compared with IFX monotherapy.[28] The COMMIT trial also showed less antibody formation and higher drug levels, with combination therapy for IFX and methotrexate, but this did not translate to significant clinical benefit during maintenance therapy.[29] In the rheumatoid arthritis literature, the use of low-dose methotrexate to protect against the development of ADAs has been demonstrated,[30,31] and recommendations for its use in IBD are derived mainly from these data.[32]

LOSS OF RESPONSE

Patients who fail to respond to anti-TNF agents are classified as having a primary nonresponse (PNR) or secondary LOR. PNR refers to those who do not achieve a clinical response to the induction phase of treatment. Current literature does not support the routine use of TDM in the context of PNR in CD. However, it should be noted that in patients with a high inflammatory load, such as in severe UC where there is an antigen sink with increased TNF and increased elimination, it is difficult to differentiate PNR from the possibility of inadequate drug concentrations, without the use of TDM.[33–35]

Secondary LOR typically refers to those who lose response after an initial therapeutic benefit. The mechanisms surrounding LOR are not always clear. Multiple factors impact on anti-TNF pharmacokinetics and can increase the clearance of anti-TNF medications: male gender, increased body mass index, decreased serum albumin, increased C-reactive protein (CRP), presence of ADAs, and the lack concomitant immunomodulator therapy.[8] Non-inflammatory causes should always be considered in the setting of clinical symptoms of LOR, particularly in the setting of adequate drug levels. Appropriate testing to confirm active inflammation, including biomarker testing (CRP and fecal calprotectin), imaging, or endoscopy, may be warranted, because symptoms may in fact be related to other processes such as strictures, irritable bowel syndrome, or infections. If one of these conditions is identified, patients should be treated accordingly and may not require adjustment of their anti-TNF therapy. Traditionally, LOR would prompt an empiric dose escalation and typically recaptures 60% to 70% of patients.[36] However, the use of TDM now allows for personalized strategies to optimize patient care. In a retrospective study of 155 IBD patients on IFX, the measurement of drug levels and of ADA influenced management in 73% of cases.[37]

Anti–tumor Necrosis Factor Concentrations

In one of the first studies looking at the clinical utility of TDM, patients with an LOR and undetectable IFX trough concentrations (ELISA) had a partial or complete response 86% of the time with dose escalation, whereas only 33% responded to switching to another anti-TNF (P<.016).[37] This study highlighted the importance of TDM, particularly with regards to optimizing therapy with the first anti-TNF therapy used before changing to another anti-TNF.

Similarly, in a retrospective study of 247 IBD patients with LOR to IFX or ADAL, patients with low levels of anti-TNF concentrations (ELISA, <4.5 μg/mL for ADAL and <3.8 μg/mL for IFX) had a longer duration of response with dose intensification than with switching to a different anti-TNF (P = .02).[38] In this same study, patients with LOR in the setting of adequate drug levels responded better to switching out of class than to optimization of the anti-TNF (P = .002).[38]

It is clear that patients with inadequate drug concentrations, however they are defined, benefit from dose intensification. However, the upper threshold above which clinical benefit would no longer be expected is still unclear. Although a concentration of 3 to 7 μg/mL has been suggested with the data presented above, it is unclear whether higher doses may be needed in certain clinical situations. Indeed, in a recent cross-sectional study of 117 patients with active perianal fistulas, higher IFX levels were associated with a significantly higher rate of fistula healing versus those who had continued active fistulas (18.5 vs 6.5 μg/mL, P<.0001).[39]

Anti–drug Antibodies

It is well established that ADAs are associated with a current or impending LOR.[27,40,41] A meta-analysis of 13 studies, that utilized either ELISA or RIA assays, showed that the presence of ADAs significantly increased the risk of a clinical LOR in patients with CD on IFX (risk ratio 3.2, 95% CI 2.0–4.9, P<.0001).[42] Similarly, antibodies to ADAL were associated with a clinical LOR (odds ratio [OR] 10.15, 95% CI 3.90–26.40, P<.0001) in another meta-analysis of 13 studies.[43] In this clinical situation, one strategy is to switch to another anti-TNF agent. In one study, when antibodies to IFX were detected, 92% of patients responded partially or completely when they were switched to a different anti-TNF agent, whereas only 17% responded to a dose escalation (P<.004).[37] However, there are new data to suggest that the simple presence of antibodies does not preclude optimizing with the same anti-TNF medication. It has been demonstrated that in patients with low ADAs (<9 μg/mL with IFX and <4 μg/mL with ADAL), drug optimization was more effective than changing to a different anti-TNF (P = .02).[38] Alternatively, patients with high levels of anti–drug antibodies experienced a longer duration of response when they were switched to another anti-TNF agent than with dose intensification (P = .03).[38] As mentioned earlier, the titers and units of measurement for antibodies can vary widely between assays, and individual laboratories should have thresholds to classify low- versus high-titer antibodies. For example, in parts of Canada, the assay used is an ELISA (Gamma Dynacare, Laval, QC, Canada) that reports antibodies as arbitrary units per milliliter (AU/mL), and one study showed a correlation of 8 μg/mL to be equivalent to 130 AU/mL.[44]

When faced with LOR in the context of antibody formation, another potential strategy to salvage anti-TNF response is the addition of an immunomodulator. A small retrospective study of IBD patients with LOR to anti-TNF therapy, in the setting of anti–drug antibodies (RIA for ADA detection), demonstrated that the addition of methotrexate or of a thiopurine resulted in the loss of ADAs with an increase in drug concentrations in 86% (n = 7) and 70% (n = 10), respectively.[45] Optimization of the immunomodulator in patients on combination therapy yielded the same outcome in 100% of patients (n = 2).[45] Dose intensification of anti-TNF alone suppressed antibodies in 36% of patients (n = 22).[45] Likewise, another small study showed that in patients with an LOR to IFX in the presence of ADAs, the addition of azathioprine or methotrexate was associated with increased clinical response and the disappearance of antibodies.[46]

Based on the evidence presented in this section and a recent expert panel publication (using the RAND/UCLA Appropriateness Method of Analysis), the authors have proposed an algorithm to guide the management of patients experiencing LOR to anti-TNF therapy based on anti-TNF levels and ADAs (**Fig. 1**).[47] The exact thresholds for drug concentrations and ADAs are still not clear, but the concentrations listed are based on available literature and expert opinion. The clinical context of TDM results must always be taken into account. For example, a patient with symptoms and minimal inflammation, but at the upper limit of the threshold, could still conceivably benefit from dose escalation. On the other hand, a patient with a drug concentration at the upper limit, but with severe inflammation, would likely not benefit from further dose escalation. The mechanisms and pharmacokinetics in partial response are thought to be similar to that of LOR, and TDM is likely clinically useful in this clinical context as well. Recommendations with regards to further proposed indications for TDM (**Table 1**) are examined in later discussion.

THERAPEUTIC DRUG MONITORING AFTER INDUCTION

There is evidence to suggest that early trough concentrations can predict response at a later time point. In a post hoc analysis of the ACCENT I data, median week 14 trough concentrations were higher in patients that responded at week 54.[16] A week 14, trough IFX concentration of $\geq$3.5 μg/mL (ELISA) predicted an increased durable

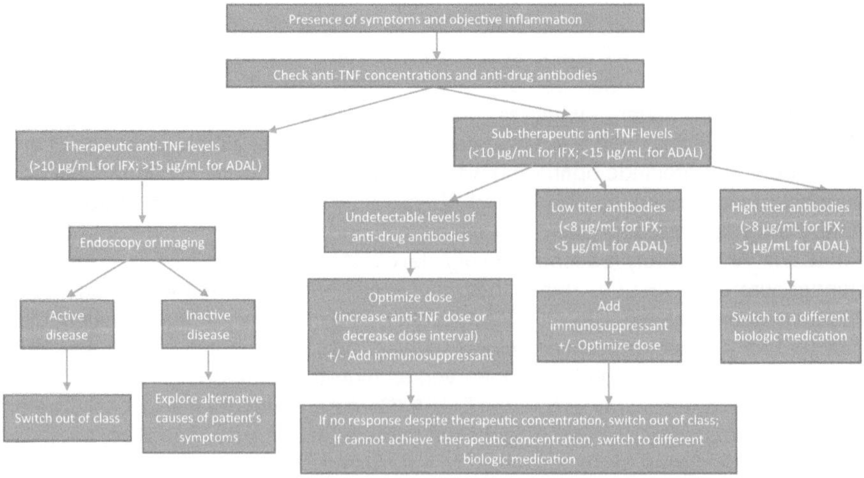

Fig. 1. Algorithm to guide the management of patients experiencing LOR to anti-TNF therapy based on TDM.

Table 1
Indications for therapeutic drug monitoring in Crohn's disease patients on biologic therapy

Indication	Recommendation
Secondary LOR/partial response	Yes
Post-induction, PNR	No
Post-induction, before maintenance therapy	Maybe
Maintenance therapy in patients in remission	No
Withdrawal of immunosuppression in combination therapy	Yes
Dose de-escalation	Yes
After a drug holiday (during reinduction treatment)	Yes

response (OR 3.5, 95% CI 1.1–11.4).[16] In addition, in a pediatric IBD study, a week 14 trough level of greater than 7 μg/mL (ELISA) had a positive predictive value of 100% for clinical remission.[48] Similar studies demonstrating this association between early trough concentration and clinical outcomes exist for ADAL as well.[49,50] In a retrospective study, IFX trough levels less than 2.2 μg/mL (HMSA) at week 14 predicted the formation of anti-IFX antibodies with 94% specificity and 79% sensitivity.[51] Furthermore, these low trough levels had 74% specificity and 82% sensitivity (LR 3.1, $P = .0026$) for LOR or hypersensitivity reaction, resulting in discontinuation of IFX. Although data are limited, based on these findings, the authors recommended the measurement of IFX levels at week 14.[51]

However, this indication for TDM remains controversial, and further studies are needed to support this practice. Although a clear association exists between post-induction trough and clinical outcomes, there are no data to suggest that early intervention by increasing the dose will lead to improved clinical outcomes. In fact, a recent expert panel review of this evidence reported there was significant uncertainty about routine assessment of drug concentrations after induction therapy.[47]

THERAPEUTIC DRUG MONITORING AND MAINTENANCE THERAPY

Given the lack of benefit in recent studies, TDM is not routinely recommended during maintenance anti-TNF therapy. The TAXIT trial assessed outcomes of 263 IBD patients on IFX maintenance therapy for at least 14 weeks who had been optimized to a target trough level of 3 to 7 μg/mL (ELISA).[52] After this optimization period, patients were randomized to dose adjustments based on either trough levels or clinical parameters. The study did not show any significant difference in remission, defined by clinical and biochemical features, between the 2 groups (68.8% vs 65.9%, $P = .686$) at 1 year.[52] Of note, however, during the follow-up period, fewer flares occurred in the group that was monitored with trough levels (7% vs 17%, $P = .18$), and there was a significantly decreased need for rescue therapy in the level-based arm compared with the clinical-based arm (5.5% vs 17.3%, $P<.0038$).[52]

The TAILORIX trial randomized active CD patients after IFX and thiopurine induction to dose optimization based on IFX concentrations as well as clinical and biochemical features, versus dose optimization based solely on clinical symptoms.[53] At 1 year, the rates of steroid-free clinical remission and endoscopic remission were not significantly different between the groups.[53] However, there were significant weaknesses with this study. Most importantly, only 47% and 46% of patients in the 2 TDM arms of the study were able to achieve a therapeutic concentration of greater than 3 μg/mL during the study period.[53] This lack of adequate drug exposure, likely secondary to delays in increasing the drug dose, could certainly have contributed to the lack of benefit observed.

The positive secondary endpoints in the TAXIT study and the weaknesses of the TAILORIX trial indicate that there still may be a benefit of routine TDM in patients in clinical remission. Therefore, although the clinical data do not yet support the use of TDM in routine maintenance, further larger studies with adequate therapeutic drug exposure are still needed to further clarify the utility of TDM in this setting. A recent expert panel review suggested the TDM "at least once during the first year of maintenance therapy" was appropriate, although the evidence for this recommendation is limited.[47]

DOSE DE-ESCALATION

There is evidence to suggest that patients in clinical remission on an anti-TNF medication can be dose de-escalated. As mentioned previously, during the dose optimization phase of the TAXIT study, all patients were optimized to concentrations of 3 to 7 μg/mL.[52] Before randomization, 26% of patients underwent IFX dose reduction to achieve this therapeutic range. Among these patients, rates of clinical remission and mean CRP levels did not vary significantly after dose reduction.[52] These results indicate that patients in clinical remission can safely be dose deescalated. In clinical practice, dose deescalation should likely be reserved for patients in both clinical and endoscopic remission.

THERAPEUTIC DRUG MONITORING AND WITHDRAWAL OF COMBINATION THERAPY

TDM can also help guide the decision to withdraw an immunomodulator from patients on combination therapy. Withdrawal of immunosuppressive therapy was first assessed in a randomized trial of 80 patients in remission for greater than 6 months.[54] Patients were randomized to withdrawal of the immunosuppressive therapy versus continuing combination therapy. Although there was no difference in the primary outcome, defined as the need to decrease IFX dosing interval or cessation of IFX therapy, patients that discontinued immunosuppressive therapy had a higher mean CRP and lower trough IFX concentrations (1.65 μg/mL, interquartile range [IQR] 0.54–3.68 vs 2.87 μg/mL, IQR 1.35–4.72, $P<.0001$, ELISA).[54] In another study, patients treated with an immunomodulator and IFX, trough concentrations greater than 5 μg/mL (ELISA) at withdrawal of the immunomodulator predicted an ongoing response with a positive predictive value of 100%.[55] These higher IFX levels were also associated with a lower risk of dose increase (hazard ratio [HR] 0.36, 95% CI 0.14 to 0.91, $P = .03$), surgical intervention (HR 0.10, 95% CI 0.01–0.76, $P = .03$), and LOR resulting in discontinuation of IFX (HR 0.16, 95% CI 0.03–0.74, $P = .02$).[55] In contrast, LOR occurred in 86% of patients on combination therapy in whom IFX levels were undetectable at the time of immunomodulator withdrawal ($n = 7$).[55] A recent non-randomized, prospective study compared outcomes of patients in deep remission for at least 6 months on azathioprine and IFX, who were assigned to either unchanged combination therapy (cohort A), decrease of azathioprine by half (minimum dose 50 mg/d; cohort B), or IFX monotherapy (cohort C).[56] Dose reduction of azathioprine (6-thioguanine concentrations of approximately 130 pmol/8 $\times$ 10^8) did not have a significant impact on IFX pharmacokinetics compared with patients in cohort A. However, patients in cohort C had a significantly higher rate of low or undetectable IFX levels.[56]

Although less common in clinical practice, withdrawal of anti-TNF agents can also be guided by TDM. It was shown in patients on combination maintenance therapy for IFX and an immunosuppressant that low IFX levels (<2 μg/mL, ELISA) or undetectable concentrations were associated with a lower risk of relapse upon withdrawal of IFX, although the overall risk of relapse remained high.[57,58]

In summary, after 6 to 12 months of combination therapy and adequate anti-TNF concentrations, withdrawal or dose reduction of the immunosuppressive therapy in patients in clinical and endoscopic remission may be considered.

POST–DRUG HOLIDAY

Reinitiation of anti-TNF therapy after a drug holiday can lead to higher rates of anti–drug antibodies, infusion reactions, and delayed hypersensitivity reactions.[59,60] Few studies have explored the role of TDM in this context. In one prospective study of 27 IBD patients, the presence of anti–drug antibodies (ELISA), before reinduction with IFX or ADAL, was not associated with a higher rate of hypersensitivity reactions or of nonresponse (OR 1.5, 95% CI 0.2–11.0, *P*<.7).[61] A retrospective study evaluating clinical outcomes of 128 IBD patients resuming IFX after a median drug holiday of 15 months showed that the presence of anti–drug antibodies (HMSA), after reinitiation (before the second or third infusion), negatively predicted short-term response (HR 0.14, 95% CI 0.026–0.74, *P* = .021), and that trough levels greater than 2 μg/mL were associated with long-term response (HR 2.94, 95% CI 1.18–7.69, *P* = .021).[62] Undetectable antibodies during the induction period were associated with an increased safety of re-initiating therapy (HR 7.7 for infusion reaction with ADAs, 95% CI 1.88–31.3, *P* = .004).[62] Based on this study, TDM during the induction regimen may be considered to identify those patients who can safely restart anti-TNF therapy.

COST-EFFECTIVENESS

The use of TDM has also proven to be a cost-effective strategy in 2 studies. A recent randomized controlled trial out of Denmark of 69 patients with a secondary LOR to IFX showed that treatment based on IFX drug levels and on anti-IFX antibody levels (RIA) incurred lower costs than standard IFX dose intensification (4500 USD vs 10,300 USD, *P*<.001), whereas clinical response in the 2 groups was similar (47% and 53%, respectively, *P* = .78).[63] An American study, using a hypothetical decision analytical model, yielded similar results in terms of efficacy with cost savings.[64] The TAXIT study also assessed cost-effectiveness of TDM in IFX therapy.[52] During the optimization phase, dose deescalation resulted in a 28% decrease in drug cost. In the maintenance phase, TDM was not found to increase drug cost compared with conventional management.[52]

BIOSIMILARS

As patents of existing anti-TNF medications have expired, biosimilars have become widely available in the marketplace. In clinical practice, the arrival of these drugs has been met with some anxiety by both patients and physicians.[65] Available studies suggest pharmacokinetic, immunogenic, and clinical equivalence between biosimilars and the original drugs.[66] However, this evidence comes mostly from patients with rheumatoid arthritis or ankylosing spondylitis, and not specifically IBD patients.[66] A recent study comparing IFX to biosimilar CT-P13 in IBD patients demonstrated cross-reactivity between anti-IFX antibodies and CT-P13 using an ELISA assay ($r \geq 0.98$, 95% CI 0.97–0.99, *P*<.001).[67] Current evidence suggests TDM may be performed for biosimilars in the same way as for original anti-TNF agents, although further studies are needed to validate this practice.[67]

USTEKINUMAB AND VEDOLIZUMAB

Limited data exist to guide the use of TDM with newer biologic therapies. Ustekinumab, an inhibitor of interleukin-12 and interleukin-23, was recently approved for the treatment of CD.[68] The UNITI trials, which demonstrated efficacy of ustekinumab in the induction and maintenance therapy for moderate to severe CD, showed an association between ustekinumab levels (> than 1 μg/mL) measured by a drug-sensitive assay and disease remission during both induction and maintenance therapy.[69] A recent study demonstrated that patients with CD on ustekinumab with trough levels greater than 5 μg/mL (HMSA) were more likely to have a normal CRP compared with those with lower drug levels (63.6% vs 33%, $P = .024$). These investigators also found significant associations between higher ustekinumab levels (>4.5 μg/mL) and endoscopic response (81.3% vs 25%, $P = .008$).[70]

Vedolizumab is a selective adhesion molecule used in the treatment of CD and UC. Data from the GEMINI 2 trial suggest that higher levels of vedolizumab may be associated with higher rates of response and remission in the induction stage and higher rates of remission during maintenance therapy.[71] Although TDM testing is available for both of these biologic medications, data regarding thresholds for adequate drug concentrations are limited.

FUTURE DIRECTIONS

At present, the use of TDM is often limited by local resources, and when available, delays in obtaining results often force clinicians to base their management on other parameters. The upcoming use of point-of-care testing, resulting in immediate availability of drug concentrations, may have an impact on patient care in those with LOR.[72] In fact, the availability of rapid results will help to facilitate studies looking at optimization during induction and maintenance therapy. Further studies need to confirm the upper threshold at which further drug escalation would not be beneficial and what titer of ADAs cannot be overcome with the addition of immunosuppressive therapy or dose optimization. Most importantly, although there is a clear association with drug concentrations and clinical and endoscopic outcomes, there is only limited evidence to demonstrate that proactive adjustments of drug concentrations during induction, maintenance, and LOR to achieve "therapeutic concentrations" improve long-term patient outcomes.

In summary, current evidence supports the use of TDM to guide management after LOR. However, optimal therapeutic targets remain to be established and may vary based on desired clinical outcomes. In addition, the use of TDM in post-induction therapy, dose de-escalation, after a drug holiday and in the withdrawal of immunosuppressive therapy in patients on combination therapy, may be useful. TDM for newer biologics will require further studies to define therapeutic concentrations and to ensure they have the similar pharmacokinetic and pharmacodynamic properties to the anti-TNF medications. Ongoing clinical trials with anti-TNFs and newer biologic medications have already begun to incorporate a TDM component within the trial design to ensure adequate exposure to the drug. With continued study, TDM will become an essential part in personalizing and optimizing the treatment of CD patients on biologic medications.

REFERENCES

1. Colombel JF, Sandborn WJ, Rutgeerts P, et al. Adalimumab for maintenance of clinical response and remission in patients with Crohn's disease: the CHARM trial. Gastroenterology 2007;132(1):52–65.

2. Chaparro MCAD, Panes J, García V, et al. Long-term durability of infliximab treatment in Crohn's disease and efficacy of dose "escalation" in patients losing response. J Clin Gastroenterol 2011;45(2):113–8.
3. Malíčková K, Ďuricová D, Bortlík M, et al. Serum trough infliximab levels: a comparison of three different immunoassays for the monitoring of CT-P13 (infliximab) treatment in patients with inflammatory bowel disease. Biologicals 2016;44(1): 33–6.
4. Baert F, Noman M, Vermeire S, et al. Influence of immunogenicity on the long-term efficacy of infliximab in Crohn's disease. N Engl J Med 2003;348(7):601–8.
5. Kopylov U, Mazor Y, Yavzori M, et al. Clinical utility of antihuman lambda chain-based enzyme-linked immunosorbent assay (ELISA) versus double antigen ELISA for the detection of anti-infliximab antibodies. Inflamm Bowel Dis 2012; 18(9):1628–33.
6. Vaughn BP, Sandborn WJ, Cheifetz AS. Biologic concentration testing in inflammatory bowel disease. Inflamm Bowel Dis 2015;21(6):1435–42.
7. Wang SL, Ohrmund L, Hauenstein S, et al. Development and validation of a homogeneous mobility shift assay for the measurement of infliximab and antibodies-to-infliximab levels in patient serum. J Immunol Methods 2012;382(1–2):177–88.
8. Ordás I, Feagan BG, Sandborn WJ. Therapeutic drug monitoring of tumor necrosis factor antagonists in inflammatory bowel disease. Clin Gastroenterol Hepatol 2012;10(10):1079–87.
9. Blank M, Black S, Chun K, et al. P0942 comparisons of serum infliximab and antibodies-to-infliximab tests used in inflammatory bowel disease clinical trials of remicade. United European Gastroenterol J 2015;2(Suppl 1).
10. Steenholdt C, Ainsworth MA, Tovey M, et al. Comparison of techniques for monitoring infliximab and antibodies against infliximab in Crohn's disease. Ther Drug Monit 2013;35(4):530–8.
11. Hoekman DR, Lowenberg M, Mathôt RA, et al. 536 non-trough IFX concentrations reliably predict trough levels and accelerate dose-adjustment in Crohn's disease. Gastroenterology 2015;148(4):S-107.
12. Stewart MJ, Dubinsky M, Morganstern B, et al. Sa1965 the steady-state pharmacokinetics of adalimumab: do we need to drink from the "trough"? Gastroenterology 2016;150(4):S418–9.
13. Maser EA, Villela R, Silverberg MS, et al. Association of trough serum infliximab to clinical outcome after scheduled maintenance treatment for Crohn's disease. Clin Gastroenterol Hepatol 2006;4(10):1248–54.
14. Bortlik M, Duricova D, Malickova K, et al. Infliximab trough levels may predict sustained response to infliximab in patients with Crohn's disease. J Crohns Colitis 2013;7(9):736–43.
15. Roblin X, Marotte H, Leclerc M, et al. Combination of C-reactive protein, infliximab trough levels, and stable but not transient antibodies to infliximab are associated with loss of response to infliximab in inflammatory bowel disease. J Crohns Colitis 2015;9(7):525–31.
16. Cornillie F, Hanauer SB, Diamond RH, et al. Postinduction serum infliximab trough level and decrease of C-reactive protein level are associated with durable sustained response to infliximab: a retrospective analysis of the ACCENT I trial. Gut 2014;63(11):1721–7.
17. Vande Casteele N, Khanna R, Levesque BG, et al. The relationship between infliximab concentrations, antibodies to infliximab and disease activity in Crohn's disease. Gut 2014;64(10):1539–45.

18. Karmiris K, Paintaud G, Noman M, et al. Influence of trough serum levels and Immunogenicity on long-term outcome of Adalimumab therapy in Crohn's disease. Gastroenterology 2009;137(5):1628–40.
19. Mazor Y, Almog R, Kopylov U, et al. Adalimumab drug and antibody levels as predictors of clinical and laboratory response in patients with Crohn's disease. Aliment Pharmacol Ther 2014;40(6):620–8.
20. Peyrin-Biroulet L, Sandborn W, Sands BE, et al. Selecting therapeutic targets in inflammatory bowel disease [STRIDE]: determining therapeutic goals for treat-to-target. Am J Gastroenterol 2015;110:1324–38.
21. Paul S, Tedesco ED, Marotte H, et al. Therapeutic drug monitoring of infliximab and mucosal healing in inflammatory bowel disease. Inflamm Bowel Dis 2013; 19(12):2568–76.
22. Roblin X, Marotte H, Rinaudo M, et al. Association between pharmacokinetics of adalimumab and mucosal healing in patients with inflammatory bowel diseases. Clin Gastroenterol Hepatol 2014;12(1):80–4.e2.
23. Zittan E, Kabakchiev B, Milgrom R, et al. Higher adalimumab drug levels are associated with mucosal healing in patients with Crohn's disease. J Crohns Colitis 2016;10(5):510–5.
24. Ungar B, Levy I, Yavne Y, et al. Optimizing anti-TNF-α therapy: serum levels of infliximab and adalimumab are associated with mucosal healing in patients with inflammatory bowel diseases. Clin Gastroenterol Hepatol 2016;14(4): 550–7.e2.
25. Colombel JF, Sandborn WJ, Allez M, et al. Association between plasma concentrations of certolizumab pegol and endoscopic outcomes of patients with Crohn's disease. Clin Gastroenterol Hepatol 2014;12(3):423–31.e1.
26. Garcês S, Demengeot J, Benito-Garcia E. The immunogenicity of anti-TNF therapy in immune-mediated inflammatory diseases: a systematic review of the literature with a meta-analysis. Ann Rheum Dis 2012;72(12):1947–55.
27. Baert F, Kondragunta V, Lockton S, et al. Antibodies to adalimumab are associated with future inflammation in Crohn's patients receiving maintenance adalimumab therapy: a post hoc analysis of the Karmiris trial. Gut 2015;65(7):1126–31.
28. Colombel JF, Sandborn WJ, Reinisch W, et al. Infliximab, azathioprine, or combination therapy for Crohn's disease. N Engl J Med 2010;362(15):1383–95.
29. Feagan BG, Mcdonald JW, Panaccione R, et al. Methotrexate in combination with infliximab is no more effective than infliximab alone in patients with Crohn's disease. Gastroenterology 2014;146(3):681–8.e1.
30. Krieckaert CL, Nurmohamed MT, Wolbink GJ. Methotrexate reduces immunogenicity in adalimumab treated rheumatoid arthritis patients in a dose dependent manner. Ann Rheum Dis 2012;71(11):1914–5.
31. Jani M, Barton A, Warren RB, et al. The role of DMARDs in reducing the immunogenicity of TNF inhibitors in chronic inflammatory diseases. Rheumatology 2013; 53(2):213–22.
32. Herfarth HH, Kappelman MD, Long MD, et al. Use of methotrexate in the treatment of inflammatory bowel diseases. Inflamm Bowel Dis 2016;22(1):224–33.
33. Ordás I, Mould DR, Feagan BG, et al. Anti-TNF monoclonal antibodies in inflammatory bowel disease: pharmacokinetics-based dosing paradigms. Clin Pharmacol Ther 2012;91(4):635–46.
34. Yarur AJ, Rubin DT. Therapeutic drug monitoring of anti-tumor necrosis factor agents in patients with inflammatory bowel diseases. Inflamm Bowel Dis 2015; 21(7):1709–18.

35. Ainsworth MA, Bendtzen K, Brynskov J. Tumor necrosis factor-alpha binding capacity and anti-infliximab antibodies measured by fluid-phase radioimmunoassays as predictors of clinical efficacy of infliximab in Crohn's disease. Am J Gastroenterol 2008;103(4):944–8.
36. Ben-Horin S, Chowers Y. Review article: loss of response to anti-TNF treatments in Crohn's disease. Aliment Pharmacol Ther 2011;33(9):987–95.
37. Afif W, Loftus EV, Faubion WA, et al. Clinical utility of measuring Infliximab and human anti-chimeric antibody concentrations in patients with inflammatory bowel disease. Am J Gastroenterol 2010;105(5):1133–9.
38. Yanai H, Lichtenstein L, Assa A, et al. Levels of drug and antidrug antibodies are associated with outcome of interventions after loss of response to Infliximab or Adalimumab. Clin Gastroenterol Hepatol 2015;13(3):522–30.e2.
39. Yarur A, Kanagala V, Stein D, et al. Higher infliximab trough levels are associated with a higher rate of perianal fistula healing in patients with Crohn's disease. Aliment Pharmacol Ther 2017;45(7):933–40.
40. Ungar B, Chowers Y, Yavzori M, et al. The temporal evolution of antidrug antibodies in patients with inflammatory bowel disease treated with infliximab. Gut 2013;63(8):1258–64.
41. Candon S, Mosca A, Ruemmele F, et al. Clinical and biological consequences of immunization to infliximab in pediatric Crohn's disease. Clin Immunol 2006; 118(1):11–9.
42. Nanda KS, Cheifetz AS, Moss AC. Impact of antibodies to infliximab on clinical outcomes and serum infliximab levels in patients with inflammatory bowel disease (IBD): a meta-analysis. Am J Gastroenterol 2012;108(1):40–7.
43. Paul S, Moreau AC, Tedesco ED, et al. Pharmacokinetics of adalimumab in inflammatory bowel diseases. Inflamm Bowel Dis 2014;20(7):1288–95.
44. Ruiz-Argüello BCB, Agua ARD, Torres N, et al. Comparison study of two commercially available methods for the determination of infliximab, adalimumab, etanercept and anti-drug antibody levels. Clin Chem Lab Med 2013;51(12):e287–9.
45. Strik A, Van Den Brink G, Ponsioen C, et al. DOP066. Disappearance of anti-drug antibodies to infliximab and adalimumab after addition of an immunomodulator in patients with inflammatory bowel disease. J Crohns Colitis 2016;10(Suppl 1).
46. Ben–Horin S, Waterman M, Kopylov U, et al. Addition of an immunomodulator to infliximab therapy eliminates antidrug antibodies in serum and restores clinical response of patients with inflammatory bowel disease. Clin Gastroenterol Hepatol 2013;11(4):444–7.
47. Melmed GY, Irving PM, Jones J, et al. Appropriateness of testing for anti–tumor necrosis factor agent and antibody concentrations, and interpretation of results. Clin Gastroenterol Hepatol 2016;14(9):1302–9.
48. Singh N, Rosenthal CJ, Melmed GY, et al. Early infliximab trough levels are associated with persistent remission in pediatric patients with inflammatory bowel disease. Inflamm Bowel Dis 2014;20(10):1708–13.
49. Zittan E, Kelly O, Kabakchiev B, et al. Sa1968 post-induction adalimumab drug levels predict clinical and laboratory remission at week 24 in patients with Crohn's disease. Gastroenterology 2016;150(4):S419.
50. Chaparro M, Guerra I, Iborra M, et al. 538 correlation between adalimumab serum levels and remission after the induction phase in Crohn's disease patients. Gastroenterology 2015;148(4):S-107–8.
51. Vande Casteele N, Gils A, Singh S, et al. Antibody response to Infliximab and its impact on Pharmacokinetics can be transient. Am J Gastroenterol 2013;108(6): 962–71.

52. Vande Casteele N, Ferrante M, Van Assche G, et al. Trough concentrations of Infliximab guide Dosing for patients with inflammatory bowel disease. Gastroenterology 2015;148(7):1320–9.e3.
53. D'Haens G, Vermeire S, Lambrecht G, et al. OP029. Drug-concentration versus symptom-driven dose adaptation of Infliximab in patients with active Crohn's disease: a prospective, randomised, multicentre trial (Tailorix). J Crohns Colitis 2016; 10(Suppl 1).
54. Van Assche G, Magdelaine–Beuzelin C, D'Haens G, et al. Withdrawal of immunosuppression in Crohn's disease treated with scheduled infliximab maintenance: a randomized trial. Gastroenterology 2008;134(7):1861–8.
55. Drobne D, Bossuyt P, Breynaert C, et al. Withdrawal of immunomodulators after co-treatment does not reduce trough level of Infliximab in patients with Crohn's disease. Clin Gastroenterol Hepatol 2015;13(3):514–21.e4.
56. Del Tedesco E, Paul S, Marotte H, et al. OP010. Azathioprine dose reduction in patients with inflammatory bowel disease on combination therapy: a prospective study. J Crohns Colitis 2016;10(Suppl 1).
57. Louis E, Mary JY, Vernier–Massouille G, et al. Maintenance of remission among patients with Crohn's disease on antimetabolite therapy after infliximab therapy is stopped. Gastroenterology 2012;142(1):63–70.e5.
58. Ben-Horin S, Chowers Y, Ungar B, et al. Undetectable anti-TNF drug levels in patients with long-term remission predict successful drug withdrawal. Aliment Pharmacol Ther 2015;42(3):356–64.
59. Hanauer SB, Feagan BG, Lichtenstein GR, et al. Maintenance infliximab for Crohn's disease: the ACCENT I randomised trial. Lancet 2002;359(9317):1541–9.
60. Hanauer SB, Rutgeerts PJ, D'Haens G, et al. Delayed hypersensitivity to infliximab (Remicade) re-infusion after 2-4 year interval without treatment. Gastroenterology 1999;116:A731.
61. Ben-Horin S, Mazor Y, Yanai H, et al. The decline of anti-drug antibody titres after discontinuation of anti-TNFs: implications for predicting re-induction outcome in IBD. Aliment Pharmacol Ther 2012;35(6):714–22.
62. Baert F, Drobne D, Gils A, et al. Early trough levels and antibodies to infliximab predict safety and success of reinitiation of infliximab therapy. Clin Gastroenterol Hepatol 2014;12(9).
63. Steenholdt C, Brynskov J, Thomsen OØ, et al. Individualised therapy is more cost-effective than dose intensification in patients with Crohn's disease who lose response to anti-tNF treatment: a randomised, controlled trial. Gut 2014; 63(6):919–27.
64. Velayos FS, Kahn JG, Sandborn WJ, et al. A test-based strategy is more cost effective than empiric dose escalation for patients with Crohn's disease who lose responsiveness to infliximab. Clin Gastroenterol Hepatol 2013;11(6):654–66.
65. Devlin SM, Bressler B, Bernstein CN, et al. Overview of subsequent entry biologics for the management of inflammatory bowel disease and Canadian Association of Gastroenterology position statement on subsequent entry biologics. Can J Gastroenterol 2013;27(10):567–71.
66. Ben-Horin S, Casteele NV, Schreiber S, et al. Biosimilars in inflammatory bowel disease: facts and fears of extrapolation. Clin Gastroenterol Hepatol 2016; 14(12):1685–96.
67. Ben-Horin S, Yavzori M, Benhar I, et al. Cross-immunogenicity: antibodies to infliximab in Remicade-treated patients with IBD similarly recognise the biosimilar Remsima. Gut 2015;65(7):1132–8.

68. U.S. Food and Drug Administration, Department of Health and Human Services. STELARA (ustekinumab) approval letter. 2016. Available at: http://www.accessdata.fda.gov/drugsatfda_docs/appletter/2016/761044Orig1s000ltr.pdf. Accessed January 22, 2017.
69. Feagan BG, Sandborn WJ, Gaskink C, et al. Ustekinumab as induction and maintenance therapy for Crohn's disease. N Engl J Med 2016;375:1946–60.
70. Battat R, Kopylov U, Bessissow T, et al. Association Among Ustekinumab Trough Concentrations and Clinical, Biomarker, and Endoscopic Outcomes in Patients With Crohn's Disease. Clin Gastroenterol Hepatol 2017. [Epub ahead of print].
71. Sandborn W, Feagan B, Rutgeerts P, et al. Vedolizumab as induction and maintenance therapy for Crohn's disease. N Engl J Med 2013;369(8):711–21.
72. Schuster T, Keller E, Kräuchi S, et al. P242. Performance of the BÜHLMANN Quantum Blue® Infliximab point-of-care assay dedicated for therapeutic drug monitoring of serum infliximab trough levels. J Crohns Colitis 2016;10(Suppl 1).

The Evolution of Treatment Paradigms in Crohn's Disease: Beyond Better Drugs

Reena Khanna, MD[a], Vipul Jairath, MD, PhD[a,b],
Brian G. Feagan, MD[a,b,*]

KEYWORDS

• Crohn's disease • Therapy • Treatment paradigms • Treatment algorithms
• Treat to target

KEY POINTS

- Several new and effective therapies are available for the treatment of Crohn's disease.
- Recent clinical guidelines have advocated for the use of objective markers of inflammation in addition to clinical symptoms to assess response to therapy.
- Early use of effective therapies, prognostication to identify high-risk patients, objective end points, precision medicine, pharmacokinetic/pharmacodynamics factors, and frequent assessment of disease activity are key features of a new treat-to-target algorithm.

INTRODUCTION

Since the pathophysiologic mechanisms responsible for Crohn's disease (CD) have not been fully defined, conventional therapies have been intrinsically based on the use of broad-spectrum immunosuppression. Agents, such as corticosteroids, azathioprine, and methotrexate, suppress the pathologic immune response and control symptoms; but they frequently cause off-target side effects. As our knowledge of immune mechanisms has evolved, drug therapy has moved away from nonspecific immunosuppressives to agents with highly selective activity, such as tumor necrosis factor (TNF) antagonists, vedolizumab, and ustekinumab. Concordant with the availability of these improved therapies, treatment algorithms have also evolved to incorporate a focus on long-term management in distinction to episodic treatment,

Disclosure: See last page of article.

[a] Department of Medicine, University of Western Ontario, 100 Dundas Street, Suite 200, London, Ontario N6A 5B6, Canada; [b] Department of Epidemiology & Biostatistics, University of Western Ontario, 100 Dundas Street, Suite 200, London, Ontario N6A 5B6, Canada
* Corresponding author. Robarts Clinical Trials Inc, 100 Dundas Street, London, Ontario, Canada.
E-mail address: brian.feagan@robartsinc.com

Gastroenterol Clin N Am 46 (2017) 661–677
http://dx.doi.org/10.1016/j.gtc.2017.05.010

increased use of combination therapy, therapeutic drug monitoring, and the earlier introduction of highly effective therapy in patients with a poor prognosis.[1]

To illustrate the potential of an ideal management algorithm that incorporates these principles, consider the results of 2 landmark randomized controlled trial (RCT) algorithms. In the ACCENT I study, which assessed infliximab (IFX) maintenance therapy in patients with an average disease duration of 8 years, a corticosteroid-free remission rate of 29% was observed at week 54.[2] In comparison, the remission rate in the SONIC trial[3] in patients with an average disease duration of 2 years who were assigned combination therapy with IFX and azathioprine (AZA) was 55.6%. Although these studies were performed 8 years apart and were conducted in different patient populations, the magnitude of the observed difference in efficacy supports the use of algorithms that feature early introduction of highly effective therapy. It is notable that SONIC did not exclusively enter high-risk patients, use therapeutic drug monitoring (TDM) to optimize IFX therapy, or use endoscopic healing as a treatment target. These potential strategies to improve management algorithms are discussed later.

HIGHLY EFFECTIVE THERAPIES

The conventional management algorithm for CD is based on step-care, in which treatments are introduced sequentially, starting with the least effective agents and proceeding, based on the symptomatic response to treatment, to more effective drugs (**Fig. 1**). Corticosteroids, which have been the backbone of this approach for more than half a century, are highly effective for controlling symptoms because they down-regulate multiple inflammatory pathways[4,5]; however, this benefit comes at the cost of numerous off-target side effects.[6,7] Furthermore, corticosteroids are ineffective as maintenance therapy. Consequently, the use of corticosteroid-sparing immunosuppressives, such as AZA and methotrexate became established as the next step in the therapeutic pyramid, with AZA being the most widely used agent. However, recent studies have indicated that AZA has little, if any, efficacy as monotherapy.[8,9] Moreover, thiopurine use is associated with an increased risk of lymphoma and nonmelanoma skin cancer.[10] In contrast, TNF antagonists (infliximab, adalimumab, certolizumab) are highly effective for both induction and maintenance of remission in CD[2,11–14] and corticosteroid-sparing and are better tolerated than thiopurines.

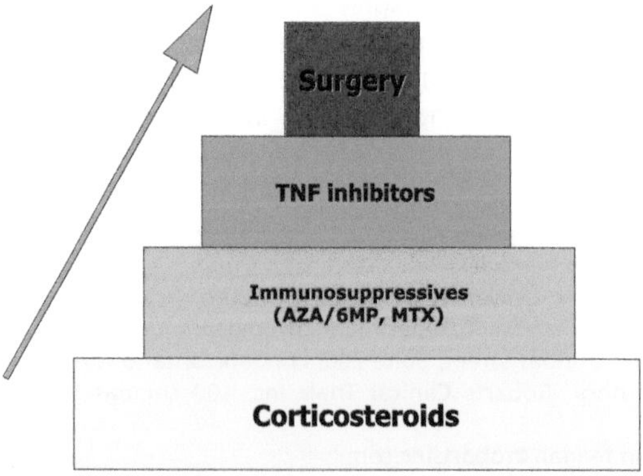

Fig. 1. Conventional therapeutic step-up algorithm. Traditional algorithms have featured the sequential use of therapies based on symptoms, whereby highly effective therapies are reserved for patients who have failed other options. MTX, methotrexate.

Moreover, the SONIC study demonstrated that combined therapy with IFX and AZA is more effective than monotherapy with either agent. These findings have called into question the step-care approach, with several studies demonstrating that the early use of a TNF antagonist in combination with an immunosuppressive is a more effective approach than step-care.[3,15,16] Consequently, many clinicians have abandoned the pyramid algorithm for an approach featuring the early introduction of highly effective therapy in high-risk patients.

Although TNF-antagonist therapy has greatly improved the management of CD, these drugs have some important limitations.[2,14,17,18] Up to one-third of patients do not respond to induction therapy, and an additional 40% lose response over the first year.[19] Treatment with a second TNF antagonist in patients failing these agents has only modest efficacy.[20] In addition, TNF-antagonist therapy is an independent risk factor for serious infection. Thus, a need exists for alternative therapies. A brief description of the recently approved agents follows.

Vedolizumab is a gut-selective therapy that blocks trafficking of a subpopulation of T-lymphocytes to the gut, without affecting their migration to other organs. In the GEMINI 2 study,[21] 368 patients with moderately to severely active CD were randomized to receive 300 mg of intravenous vedolizumab or placebo at weeks 0 and 2. A Crohn's Disease Activity Index (CDAI)–defined[22] response at week 6 was attained in 31.4% and 25.7% of patients in the vedolizumab or placebo groups, respectively (P = .23). In GEMINI 3, remission rates in patients with previous failure to TNF-antagonist therapy were similar between the vedolizumab and placebo groups at week 6; however, significant differences were observed by week 10.[23] In this study, TNF-antagonist naïve patients and those with concomitant use of corticosteroids had higher induction response rates than those with previous failure to TNF-antagonist therapy. In the maintenance phase of GEMINI 2, clinical response was observed at week 52 in 39.0% of patients who received maintenance vedolizumab every 8 weeks (P<.001 for the comparison with placebo), 36.4% who received vedolizumab every 4 weeks (P = .004 for the comparison with placebo), and 21.6% of patients who received placebo. However, it is notable that the patients in this trial had failed conventional therapy, suggesting that this population had refractory disease.[21] In a pooled analysis of 6 studies,[24] vedolizumab demonstrated a favorable safety profile. Although the selectivity of this mechanism minimizes systemic immunosuppression, the efficacy of vedolizumab for the treatment of extraintestinal manifestations and fistulizing CD is a concern.

Given the success of interleukin (IL)-12 and IL-23 inhibition in the treatment of psoriasis,[25] ustekinumab has emerged as a promising new strategy for the treatment of CD. UNITI-1 and -2 were phase 3 RCTs comparing ustekinumab and placebo for induction of remission in patients with moderately to severely active CD.[26] A CDAI-defined clinical response to intravenous induction therapy at week 6 was observed in 34.4%, 33.7%, and 21.5% of patients with prior TNF-antagonist failure who received ustekinumab at a dose of 6 mg/kg, 130 mg, or placebo, respectively (P = .002 and 0.003, respectively). The corresponding values in TNF-antagonist naïve patients were 51.7%, 55.5%, and 28.7% (P<.001). In the IMUNITI maintenance trial,[26] patients with a clinical response to ustekinumab induction treatment were randomized to 90 mg of subcutaneous ustekinumab every 8 weeks, every 12 weeks, or placebo. Clinical remission at week 44 was attained in 53.1%, 48.8%, and 35.9% of patients in these groups, respectively (P = .005 for the comparison of ustekinumab every 12 weeks and P = .040 for the comparison of ustekinumab every 8 weeks, with placebo). Adverse events were similar among the groups. These data led to regulatory approval of ustekinumab for the treatment of CD. Similar to vedolizumab, the role of combination therapy and efficacy in specific patient populations, such as those with fistulizing disease, remains to be determined.

Because of the limitations of the current therapies for CD, development of new drugs is a priority. Additional novel approaches, including IL-23 inhibitors,[27] Sphingosine 1-phosphate receptor modulators,[28] and antisense therapy (SMAD7 inhibitors),[29] are currently under investigation.

In summary, although highly effective new therapies are now available and additional novel agents are in development for the treatment of CD, important questions remain regarding the optimal use of these agents in treatment algorithms. In the immediate future, TNF antagonists are likely to remain the first-line therapy for severe or fistulizing CD.[30] Vedolizumab is a preferred agent for patients with contraindications to systemic immunosuppression or a previous history of malignancy, whereas ustekinumab is a good choice for patients with concomitant psoriasis or TNF-antagonist failure or intolerance. Ultimately, advances in personalized medicine may allow selection of treatment based on laboratory identification of the dominant immune mechanism for individual patients.

Highly Effective Therapies

Early treatment of high-risk patients

Several retrospective analyses have demonstrated a benefit for treatment of CD early in the course of disease.[14,31] In a post hoc analysis of the CHARM study that evaluated adalimumab for the maintenance of remission for moderately to severely active CD, the proportion of patients in remission was inversely proportional to the number of years from diagnosis: 51% of patients who were treated within 2 years of diagnosis, 44% of those treated within 2 to less than 5 years, and 35% of those treated 5 years or more after diagnosis. The corresponding values for patients in the placebo arm were 17%, 11%, and 11%, respectively.[32] Similar results were observed in a post hoc analysis of the PRECiSE 2 trial that evaluated certolizumab for maintenance of remission in patients with moderately to severely active CD. Remission rates were highest in patients with the shortest disease duration (68.4% of patients with a disease duration less than 1 year compared with 44.3% of patients with a disease duration $\geq$5 years).[33] The greater benefit observed in patients with a relatively short disease duration has been attributed to treatment of predominantly inflammatory disease in advance of the development of fibrostenotic or penetrating complications, which are less responsive to medical therapy. This concept is also supported by reviewing results from RCTs performed in different populations. In the ACCENT I study, which assessed IFX monotherapy in patients with an average disease duration of 8 years, a corticosteroid-free remission rate of 29% was observed at week 54.[2] The corresponding remission rate in the SONIC trial[3] in patients with an average disease duration of 2 years who were assigned to receive combination therapy with IFX and AZA was 55.6%. Finally, in the TOP-DOWN[15] study, which compared early combined immunosuppression (ECI) with IFX and AZA with the conventional step-up approach in patients with an average disease duration less than 3 weeks, remission was observed in 60.0% of patients who received combination therapy and 35.9% of patients assigned to conventional care ($P = .0062$) at week 26. Although there are several differences in the design of these trials, a key common feature is initiation of therapy earlier in the course of disease. Earlier initiation of highly effective therapy also limits exposure to corticosteroids, a class of drugs known to increase morbidity and mortality in IBD.[34]

Although highly effective therapy is the goal for all patients, early aggressive therapy is not clinically possible in all patients given safety and cost considerations This situation elevates the importance of identifying high-risk patients.

Risk prognostication

Although a validated prognostic index for CD does not currently exist, several predictive factors have been identified in population-based cohort studies, including perianal disease, fistulas, deep ulceration on endoscopy, previous surgery, corticosteroid use at diagnosis, smoking, diagnosis before 40 years of age, or foregut involvement.[35–41]

In an initial attempt to develop a prediction model for use in individual patients, data from a large referral center cohort[40] identified diagnosis before 40 years of age, perianal lesions, and early requirement for steroids as predictive for severe disease at year 5 of follow-up. However, this St-Antoine's model has been criticized because greater than 85% of the cohort was classified as having severe disease after 5 years,[42] which may be attributed to inclusion of factors such as immunosuppression use in the definition of severe disease. Moreover, this model performed poorly in a second validation cohort.[42]

A second model[42] identified weight loss greater than 5 kg and stricturing disease as predictors of severe disease. However, this model also had relatively poor sensitivity and specificity and led to development of a third risk prediction model derived from a prospective cohort that was largely assembled before the introduction of biologics and followed for up to 10 years.[43] Multiple factors, including age, disease location, disease behavior, and serologic markers, such as anti–*Saccharomyces cerevisiae* antibody (ASCA) seropositivity, were associated with a severe disease course. Nevertheless, the model has not gained clinical acceptance because of poor operating characteristics.

More recently, a tertiary center cohort from Hungary[44] identified the use of AZA within 3 years of diagnosis, disease location, and ASCA seropositivity as predictive factors for advanced disease. The predictive performance has not been defined. In contrast, Siegel and colleagues[45] identified age, sex, diagnosis date, disease location, perianal disease, presence of *NOD2* polymorphism, and multiple serologic markers as predictors of complications (nonperianal intestinal surgery, internal penetrating disease, or bowel stricture) with adequate discrimination (*c*-statistic 0.73).[45]

In the *R*andomized *E*valuation of an *A*lgorithm for *C*rohn's *T*reatment (REACT) study, 2 multivariable models suggested that male sex, lack of previous surgery, low disease activity, remission, and shorter disease duration at baseline were associated with remission at year 2. In contrast, greater disease activity as measured by harvey bradshaw index, perianal or fistulizing disease, corticosteroid therapy, younger age, and treatment in Belgium were associated with an increased risk of major adverse outcomes.[46]

In summary, model development is at an early stage and validated predictive models do not currently exist. As a consequence, predictive models are not widely used in clinical practice. Further research is required to identify groups of patients at high risk of disease complication.

Precision medicine

Given that multiple new drug classes are available, it is conceptually attractive to be able to predict which treatment is most likely to benefit an individual patient. Recent interest has emerged in genetic, epigenetic, metabolomics, and proteomic markers for this purpose.

Etrolizumab (RHuMabβ7, PRO145223, RG-7413; Genentech, San Francisco, USA) is a monoclonal antibody against the β7 subunit of the α4β7 and αEβ7 integrins. This molecule inhibits leukocyte trafficking by preventing the interaction between α4β7 and MAdCAM-1 and also blocks retention of intraepithelial lymphocytes through inhibition of αEβ7–E-cadherin interactions.[47]

In EUCALYPTUS, a phase 2 induction study, 119 patients with moderately to severely active ulcerative colitis were randomized to receive subcutaneous placebo; 100 mg of etrolizumab at weeks 0, 4, and 8 with placebo at week 2; or a 420-mg loading dose at week 0 and 300 mg at weeks 2, 4, and 8.[48] At week 10, clinical remission was observed in 0%, 20.5% (compared with placebo), and 10.3% of patients, respectively ($P = .004$ and $P = .049$ for the comparison with placebo). In a post hoc analysis, patients with higher integrin αE gene expression levels in colonic biopsies were more likely to be in remission compared to patients with low levels of gene expression.[48] This tissue marker is the first that has been identified to predict response to a therapy; however, it requires prospective validation. It is a promising approach to improve the efficacy of drug therapy for individual patients.

Although tissue biomarkers hold potential, additional research is required before use in clinical practice. In future algorithms, assessment of pathologic components of the immune cascade in individual patients will facilitate decisions regarding optimal treatment strategies. In the interim, these decisions are based on disease characteristics and patient profiles.

Treat to Target: What Is the Target?

The traditional treatment target for CD in clinical practice has been control of symptoms. Consistent with this goal, the CDAI, a composite outcome that is dominated by symptom-based items, has been the most commonly used outcome measure in clinical research.[49,50]

Multiple concerns exist regarding the subjective nature of the CDAI and the lack of correlation with objective measures of inflammation, such as endoscopy. High placebo responses in RCTs that exclusively used the CDAI to define adequate disease activity for eligibility have been a significant problem.[2,14,51] In the SONIC trial,[3] 18% of patients who met the CDAI-defined eligibility criterion lacked evidence of objective inflammation (defined either endoscopically or by C-reactive protein [CRP] concentrations). Inclusion of these patients increases the likelihood of a negative trial result. High CDAI scores are also observed with noninflammatory conditions, such as irritable bowel syndrome, bile salt diarrhea, and for patients with strictures.[52] In clinical practice, treatment decisions based on symptoms alone are likely to result in either overtreatment or undertreatment of a substantial proportion of patients.[53]

As a result, both regulatory agencies and clinical guidelines have moved away from exclusive reliance on symptoms for treatment decisions. The recently published Selecting Therapeutic Targets in Inflammatory Bowel Disease (STRIDE) guidelines specifically recommend that "*Resolution of symptoms alone is not a sufficient target. Objective evidence of inflammation of the bowel is necessary when making clinical decisions.*"[54]

Based on these considerations clinical algorithms have shifted toward the combined use of patient-reported outcomes (PROs) and objective measures, such as CRP, endoscopy, magnetic resonance enterography (MRE), and histology to assess response to therapy and to guide next steps.

Patient-reported outcomes

Because a validated PRO for CD does not currently exist,[53] an interim measure has been developed based on the CDAI diary card items.[55] Initially, a 2-item PRO (PRO2), which included stool frequency (SF) and abdominal pain (AP), and a 3-item PRO, which also incorporated general well-being, were developed. However, general well-being was later eliminated as an item because it is not sufficiently specific for CD.[55]

The original version of PRO2 was calculated as the weighted sum of the mean 7-day AP and SF items, with thresholds of an AP score of 1 or less and average daily

SF of 1.5 or less defined for remission in a population with mildly to moderately active CD.[55] However, in patients with more severe disease, an SF threshold of less than 3 has demonstrated greater correlation with CDAI-defined remission.[56]

Several other modifications to the definition of PRO have been proposed, most importantly, removal of the item weights. Current guidance from the Food and Drug Administration advocates use of an unweighted PRO score in conjunction with a measure of endoscopic improvement as coprimary outcomes in CD trials.

There are numerous efforts currently underway to formally develop a validated PRO; however, the process in all cases will take several years to complete. In the interim, AP and SF are recognized as critical components; STRIDE guidelines recommend that *"resolution of abdominal pain and normalisation of bowel habit should be the target"* of treatment of CD.[54]

However, as noted previously, use of objective measures of inflammation, such as biomarkers, endoscopy, MRE, and histopathology, is also considered optimal.

Biomarkers

Erythrocyte sedimentation rate (ESR) and CRP are acute-phase reactants that have been widely used to assess disease activity in CD. Recently, ESR has fallen out of favor because of the lack of standardized measurement techniques and because it is less responsive to change than other inflammatory markers. CRP, an acute-phase reactant produced in the liver in response to IL-6 secretion by activated macrophages and T cells, has generally replaced ESR.[57]

Although measurement of CRP is inexpensive and widely accessible, the lack of sensitivity is a limitation to its use in assessing disease activity. Approximately 15% of patients with endoscopically active CD have normal serum CRP concentrations.[51] The use of this biomarker to determine response to therapy in a diverse outpatient setting would result in undertreatment of a substantial proportion of patients. However, in a patient known to generate a CRP response, this biomarker can be followed to assess treatment efficacy.

In contrast to serum biomarkers, fecal tests theoretically provide direct evaluation of bowel inflammation. Fecal calprotectin (FCP), which is produced by neutrophils, monocytes, and macrophages, is detectable in the stool when these cells transmigrate the intestinal epithelium.[58–63] Calprotectin is resistant to enzymatic degradation and can be measured in the stool for up to 7 days in unprepared samples.

In a meta-analysis of 19 studies that examined 2499 patients,[64] the pooled sensitivity and specificity for FCP to detect endoscopically defined CD were 0.87 (0.82, 0.91) and 0.67 (0.58, 0.75), respectively. The lack of specificity is a problem if the results of the test are to be relied on for treatment intensification.

In summary, although serum and fecal biomarkers are inexpensive and easily accessible, the operating properties may not be sufficiently robust for clinical decision-making. Accordingly, STRIDE recommends, *"Available biomarkers including CRP and fecal calprotectin are not targets. Failure of CRP or fecal calprotectin normalization (below lab-specific cutoff) should prompt further endoscopic evaluation, irrespective of symptoms."*[54] Preliminary results of the CALM study (clinicaltrials.gov: NCT01235689). Show that tight disease control based on biomarker assessments compared with conventional care results in significantly higher rates of endoscopic remission and deep remission.[65]

Endoscopy

Endoscopy is widely recognized as an objective method to assess disease activity in ileocolonic CD. Although routinely used in clinical trials to measure endoscopic CD activity, neither the Crohn's Disease Endoscopic Index of Severity (CDEIS)[66] nor the Simplified Endoscopic Index of Severity (SES-CD)[67] are completely validated indices and, in the authors' opinion, are too cumbersome for use in clinical practice.

Recently, rigorous studies to evaluate the existing endoscopic indices for CD have been undertaken. In an initial study,[68] central reading of both the SES-CD and CDEIS demonstrated high levels of agreement. The most common sources of inter-reader disagreement identified through a consensus process included definitions of stenosis and scoring after balloon dilation, definition of ulcer location when 2 contiguous segments were involved, and differentiation between anal and rectal lesions. Scoring conventions to address these sources of disagreement were then developed.

In a subsequent study, training of nonexpert gastroenterologists on these scoring conventions improved inter-rater reliability as measured by intraclass correlation coefficients for the SES-CD from 0.78 (95% confidence interval [CI] 0.71–0.85) to 0.85 (95% CI 0.79–0.89), a value that is similar to that obtained among expert readers in another study.[69]

Most recently, the responsiveness of the SES-CD and CDEIS to changes in disease activity was assessed in a prospective trial of a treatment of known efficacy in CD.[70] The results indicate that, although both indices are responsive to change, values for both the standardized between group differences and the Guyatt responsiveness statistic were higher for the SES-CD than the CDEIS.

However, concern regarding the complexity of scoring these indices limits their use in clinical practice and clinical trials. This concept was highlighted by Rutgeerts and colleagues[71] in a post hoc analysis of endoscopic videos from the EXTEND[72] study. CDEIS scores were only analyzed from 6 of the 19 participating sites because of improper scoring and calculation of the CDEIS by the remaining 13 sites, suggesting the index is cumbersome and complicated to use. The same study demonstrated that site investigators consistently reported higher scores at all time points (baseline and weeks 12 and 52). The trend for overestimation of lesion severity by site investigators relative to central readers was also observed in the certolizumab MUSIC study, and was more pronounced at enrollment.[73] This discrepancy between site and central readers likely reflects the influence of clinical information available to the site investigator and the knowledge that induction therapy has been received.

Despite these limitations, endoscopic assessment is important for the conduct of CD trials because it reduces placebo rates by excluding patients who lack sufficient disease activity. An endoscopic end point has been mandated by regulatory agencies, and endoscopic improvement is more objective than assessment of pain and diarrhea. However, the ideal time point for assessing endoscopic improvement is unknown. In an endoscopic substudy of the IFX ACCENT I trial, colonoscopy performed at week 10 demonstrated lower rates of mucosal healing than[74] at week 54 (30% and 50%, respectively).[74] Similar results for mucosal healing were observed in the EXTEND adalimumab trial at weeks 12 (27% and 13% for placebo, $P = .06$) and 52 (24% vs 0% for placebo, $P<.001$).[72] Cumulatively, these data suggest endoscopic assessment should take place at a minimum of 12 weeks following initiation of therapy and ideally much later.[75] Accordingly, STRIDE recommends "*absence of ulceration is the target. Endoscopic or cross-sectional imaging assessment should be performed within 6 to 9 months after the start of therapy.*"[54]

In summary, although the use of endoscopy as a treatment target is attractive, conceptually several limitations exist. First, the current endoscopic indices are suboptimal and incompletely validated. Second, the optimal thresholds to define remission or mild, moderate, and severe disease activity are empirically defined and may not be predictive of meaningful clinical outcomes. Third, endoscopy cannot assess isolated small bowel disease. To address the last concern, attention has turned toward cross-sectional imaging. Notwithstanding these considerations, endoscopy is the preferred assessment tool for both clinical trials and clinical practice. The SES-CD is the endoscopic index of choice for RCTs because it is easier to calculate than the CDEIS and may have superior operating properties. In practice, absence of large ulcers is a simple benchmark that clinicians can use.

MRI

In clinical practice, MRE is used in patients with CD to assess active inflammation and for detection of complications, such as strictures, abscess, or fistulas.[76–78] Because failure to intubate the ileum during colonoscopy occurs in up to 25% of patients,[79] MRE can be used to evaluate these patients' bowel wall thickness and intensity of inflammation (through the use of gadolinium contrast). In contrast, endoscopy only assesses the mucosal surface.

Several MRE indices are available to assess disease activity: however, the Magnetic Resonance Index of Activity (MaRIA) and London indices have been most widely used because they were rigorously developed using endoscopy or surgical resection specimens, respectively, as the gold standard for comparison.[80] The components of the MaRIA index include bowel wall thickness, gadolinium enhancement, ulceration, and edema.[80] High correlation between MRE and ($r > 0.80$; $P < .001$) the CDEIS has been demonstrated in 2 studies.[80,81] The components of the London index include wall thickness and mural signal intensity on T2-weighted sequences. The London index has demonstrated a moderate correlation with histopathologic inflammation from intestinal biopsies of the terminal ileum (Kendall tau = 0.40, 95% CI 0.11–0.64, $P = .02$).[82] Both indices have demonstrated adequate reliability and responsiveness following a treatment of known efficacy.[83,84]

The STRIDE guidelines recommend, "*When endoscopy cannot adequately evaluate inflammation, resolution of inflammation as assessed by cross-sectional imaging is a target in CD.*"[54] However, it should be noted the MRE is rater dependent and access in some jurisdictions is limited. In addition, the optimal time to assess improvement is unknown. Furthermore, the resolution of MRE may be inadequate to assess subclinical disease detectable by histology. Finally, neither of the MRE indices has been sufficiently validated to be used as a surrogate outcome in RCTs.

Histopathology

Histopathologic assessment in CD is complicated by the patchy and transmural nature of the disease. In addition, it is difficult to access tissue from certain locations in the gastrointestinal tract and in the case of colitis. Furthermore, none of the currently available histologic indices for CD have been adequately validated.

Consequently, STRIDE opines, "*histologic remission is not a target.*"[54] The development of a validated histopathologic index for use in CD is a research priority.

In summary, multiple options with unique benefits and limitations are available for use as CD treatment targets. PROs are important to evaluate the experience of patients; however, they lack specificity for inflammation. Although attractive from cost and convenience perspectives, the operating properties of serum and stool biomarkers are not sufficiently robust to facilitate critical management decisions. Endoscopy will likely retain a pivotal role in the management and assessment of CD; however, endoscopic indices must evolve and become more user friendly and clinically meaningful. As MRI and histology are validated and the optimal time point for assessment is determined, they may become the metrics of choice. In the interim,

PROs in combination with an objective marker of inflammation should be considered the treatment target of choice.

PHARMACOKINETICS/PHARMACODYNAMICS

The recognition that large variability exists in the clearance of monoclonal antibodies[85–88] has critical implications for optimizing therapeutic algorithms. The pharmacokinetics of TNF antagonists vedolizumab and ustekinumab are variously influenced by development of antidrug antibodies (ADAs), serum albumin concentration, use of concomitant immunosuppressives, body weight, sex, prior biologic therapy, and the degree of systemic inflammation.[89]

TDM, defined as measurement of trough drug and ADA concentrations, enables clinicians to make informed decisions regarding therapy in patients who have lost response to a biologic. Four groups of patients can be identified: those with suboptimal trough drug concentrations without ADAs who may benefit from dose intensification, those with suboptimal trough drug concentrations who are positive for ADAs and who may benefit from a switch to a drug in the same therapeutic class, those with optimal trough drug concentrations and no ADAs who may benefit from a switch to another class of agent; and patients with therapeutic drug concentrations and positive ADAs. It is difficult to make evidence-based recommendations in this last circumstance.

A retrospective analysis from Mayo Clinic[90] identified 2 distinct patient populations: those with subtherapeutic IFX concentrations and those with detectable ADAs. The highest response rates were obtained with dose intensification in the former group (86% compared with 33% who underwent a change in therapy, $P<.02$) and with switching to a second TNF antagonist in the latter group (92% compared with 17% who underwent dose intensification, $P<.004$). This study provided a framework for evidence-based therapeutic decision-making. Subsequently, the cost-effectiveness of TDM-based decision-making for patients with secondary loss of response compared with empirical changes suggested similar rates of remission (66% compared with 63%) for both strategies: however, testing-based therapies were less expensive ($31,266 compared with $37,266).[91] The cost-effectiveness of TDM-based approach was confirmed in an RCT in which 66 patients receiving IFX therapy were randomized to empirical or TDM-based dose intensification. Similar response rates were observed in both groups (53% and 58%, $P = .81$); however, the costs were lower with TDM ($7736 compared with $11,760, $P<.001$).[92]

Data regarding the use of TDM to prospectively guide dosing are quite limited. In the TAXIT study, 270 patients with therapeutic IFX concentrations on long-term maintenance therapy were randomized to dosing changes to sustain drug concentrations between 3 μg/mL and 7 μg/mL or dosing changes based on clinical symptoms.[93] Although no differences were seen with these strategies for 1-year remission rates, lower costs were observed in the TDM group. The lack of difference in remission rates may be attributed to the fact that patients were in remission at baseline.

In summary, TDM has emerged as a potential component of CD treatment algorithms. Point-of-care testing will facilitate the use of this tool in the future. Although clinical experience has endorsed the use of TDM in patients with secondary loss of response to TNF antagonists, the broader use of this modality in treatment algorithms is currently unknown.

CONTROLLED TRIALS OF TREATMENT ALGORITHMS

Over the last 15 years, treatment algorithms for CD have evolved from episodic therapy with a single agent in patients with severe disease to long-term combination therapy initiated earlier in the disease course,[1,94] which has increased the rates of symptomatic remission.[3]

In the TOP-DOWN[15] study, which assessed ECI with IFX and AZA compared with the conventional step-up approach in patients with an average disease duration of less than 3 weeks, remission was observed in 60.0% of patients who received combination therapy and 35.9% of patients assigned to conventional care (P = .0062) at week 26.

Subsequently, REACT,[46] a cluster randomization trial that implemented early combined immunosuppression in real-world practices, was performed. Community practices were randomized to ECI or conventional care, and patients were followed for 2 years. In this study, ECI advocated for routine assessments every 12 weeks, and application of therapeutic changes until clinical remission was attained. Although 12-month site-level remission rates were similar at ECI and conventional care sites (66.0% and 61.9%, adjusted difference 2.5%, 95% CI −5.2% to 10.2%, P = .5169), the 24-month patient-level composite rate of major adverse outcomes defined as occurrence of surgery, hospitalization, or serious disease-related complications was significantly lower at the ECI sites (27.7% vs 35.1%; absolute difference, 7.3%; hazard ratio; 0.73; 95% CI, 0.62–0.86, P = .0003). It is notable that the average disease duration in this trial was 12 years, suggesting that there is a potential for even greater benefit when this algorithm is applied in patients with shorter disease duration.

As a result of this study, interest has emerged in this treat-to-target philosophy to alter the course of disease.[95] Unlike the top-down or bottom-up strategies, this approach individualizes therapy based on response and minimizes steroid exposure by earlier administration of effective therapies (**Fig. 2**).[16]

TOWARDS AN INTEGRATED TREATMENT ALGORITHM FOR CROHN'S DISEASE

Treatment decisions are currently based largely on subjective assessments of disease severity and patient factors. In the future, it is likely that prediction models will identify patients at the greatest risk of developing disease complications. These patients will receive early effective therapies that will be selected using biomarkers. A treat-to-target approach, featuring pharmacokinetic and objective outcomes, will be used to guide therapeutic changes until remission is attained.

Clinical algorithms will continue to evolve in the coming years; in particular, the choice of outcome, timing of end point assessment, and use of information from pharmacokinetic and precision medicine will refine our choice of therapy and our ability to optimize treatments. However, additional information is required regarding therapeutic drug thresholds and methods to predict response in each patient. These areas are active areas of research that will revolutionize the delivery of care in IBD.

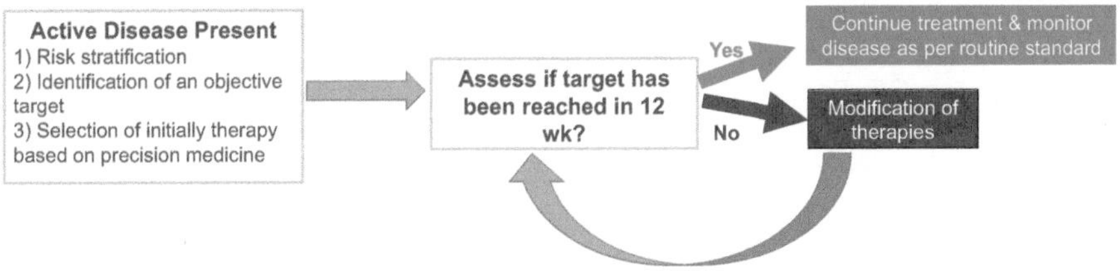
Active Disease Present
1) Risk stratification
2) Identification of an objective target
3) Selection of initially therapy based on precision medicine
Assess if target has been reached in 12 wk?
Yes
No
Continue treatment & monitor disease as per routine standard
Modification of therapies

Fig. 2. Treat-to-target algorithm. A new treat-to-target algorithm of care is based on risk stratification of patients, identification of objective treatment targets, selection of initial therapy based on precision medicine, regular assessment of disease activity, and implementation of therapeutic changes until objective end points are achieved.

DISCLOSURE

Disclosure Statement: R. Khanna has received honoraria from AbbVie, Janssen, Pfizer, Shire, and Takeda Pharma; B.G. Feagan has received grant/research support from Millennium Pharmaceuticals, Merck, Tillotts Pharma AG, Abbott Labs, Novartis Pharmaceuticals, Centocor Inc, Elan/Biogen, UCB Pharma, Bristol-Myers Squibb, Genentech, ActoGeniX, and Wyeth Pharmaceuticals Inc; consulting fees from Millennium Pharmaceuticals, Merck, Centocor Inc, Elan/Biogen, Janssen-Ortho, Teva Pharmaceuticals, Bristol-Myers Squibb, Celgene, UCB Pharma, Abbott Labs, AstraZeneca, Serono, Genentech, Tillotts Pharma AG, Unity Pharmaceuticals, Albireo Pharma, Given Imaging Inc, Salix Pharmaceuticals, Novo Nordisk, GSK, Actogenix, Prometheus Therapeutics and Diagnostics, Athersys, Axcan, Gilead, Pfizer, Shire, Wyeth, Zealand Pharma, Zyngenia, GiCare Pharma Inc, and Sigmoid Pharma; and speaker's fees from UCB, Abbott, and J&J/Janssen; V. Jairath has received scientific advisory board fees from AbbVie and Sandoz and speaker's fees from Takeda and Janssen.

REFERENCES

1. Danese S, Colombel JF, Reinisch W, et al. Review article: infliximab for Crohn's disease treatment–shifting therapeutic strategies after 10 years of clinical experience. Aliment Pharmacol Ther 2011;33:857–69.
2. Hanauer SB, Feagan BG, Lichtenstein GR, et al. Maintenance infliximab for Crohn's disease: the ACCENT I randomised trial. Lancet 2002;359:1541–9.
3. Colombel JF, Sandborn WJ, Reinisch W, et al. Infliximab, azathioprine, or combination therapy for Crohn's disease. N Engl J Med 2010;362:1383–95.
4. Ardite E, Panes J, Miranda M, et al. Effects of steroid treatment on activation of nuclear factor kappaB in patients with inflammatory bowel disease. Br J Pharmacol 1998;124:431–3.
5. Adcock IM. Molecular mechanisms of glucocorticosteroid actions. Pulm Pharmacol Ther 2000;13:115–26.
6. Ford AC, Bernstein CN, Khan KJ, et al. Glucocorticosteroid therapy in inflammatory bowel disease: systematic review and meta-analysis. Am J Gastroenterol 2011;106:590–9 [quiz: 600].
7. Yang YX, Lichtenstein GR. Corticosteroids in Crohn's disease. Am J Gastroenterol 2002;97:803–23.
8. Cosnes J, Bourrier A, Laharie D, et al. Early administration of azathioprine vs conventional management of Crohn's disease: a randomized controlled trial. Gastroenterology 2013;145(4):758–65.e2 [quiz: e14–5].
9. Panés J, López-SanRomán A, Bermejo F, et al. Early azathioprine therapy is no more effective than placebo for newly diagnosed Crohn's disease. Gastroenterology 2013;145(4):766–74.e1.
10. Lichtenstein GR, Feagan BG, Cohen RD, et al. Drug therapies and the risk of malignancy in Crohn's disease: results from the TREAT Registry. Am J Gastroenterol 2014;109(2):212–23.
11. Targan SR, Hanauer SB, van Deventer SJ, et al. A short-term study of chimeric monoclonal antibody cA2 to tumor necrosis factor alpha for Crohn's disease. Crohn's disease cA2 study group. N Engl J Med 1997;337:1029–35.
12. Hanauer SB, Sandborn WJ, Rutgeerts P, et al. Human anti-tumor necrosis factor monoclonal antibody (adalimumab) in Crohn's disease: the CLASSIC-I trial. Gastroenterology 2006;130:323–33 [quiz: 591].

13. Sandborn WJ, Feagan BG, Stoinov S, et al. Certolizumab pegol for the treatment of Crohn's disease. N Engl J Med 2007;357:228–38.
14. Schreiber S, Khaliq-Kareemi M, Lawrance IC, et al. Maintenance therapy with certolizumab pegol for Crohn's disease. N Engl J Med 2007;357:239–50.
15. D'Haens G, Baert F, van Assche G, et al. Early combined immunosuppression or conventional management in patients with newly diagnosed Crohn's disease: an open randomised trial. Lancet 2008;371:660–7.
16. Khanna R, Bressler B, Levesque BG, et al. A cluster randomization trial of early combined immunosuppression for the management of Crohn's disease. Lancet 2015;386:1825–34.
17. Colombel JF, Sandborn WJ, Rutgeerts P, et al. Adalimumab for maintenance of clinical response and remission in patients with Crohn's disease: the CHARM trial. Gastroenterology 2007;132:52–65.
18. Singh JA, Wells GA, Christensen R, et al. Adverse effects of biologics: a network meta-analysis and Cochrane overview. Cochrane Database Syst Rev 2011:CD008794.
19. Danese S, Fiorino G, Reinisch W. Review article: causative factors and clinical management of patients with Crohn's disease who lose response to anti-TNF-alpha therapy. Aliment Pharmacol Ther 2011;34(1):1–10.
20. Sandborn WJ, Rutgeerts P, Enns R, et al. Adalimumab induction therapy for Crohn disease previously treated with infliximab: a randomized trial. Ann Intern Med 2007;146:829–38.
21. Sandborn WJ, Feagan BG, Rutgeerts P, et al. Vedolizumab as induction and maintenance therapy for Crohn's disease. N Engl J Med 2013;369:711–21.
22. Best WR, Becktel JM, Singleton JW. Rederived values of the eight coefficients of the Crohn's Disease Activity Index (CDAI). Gastroenterology 1979;77(4 Pt 2):843–6.
23. Sands BE, Feagan BG, Rutgeerts P, et al. Effects of vedolizumab induction therapy for patients with Crohn's disease in whom tumor necrosis factor antagonist treatment had failed. Gastroenterology 2014;147:618–27.e3.
24. Colombel JF, Sands BE, Rutgeerts P, et al. The safety of vedolizumab for ulcerative colitis and Crohn's disease. Gut 2017;66(5):839–51.
25. Papp KA, Langley RG, Lebwohl M, et al. Efficacy and safety of ustekinumab, a human interleukin-12/23 monoclonal antibody, in patients with psoriasis: 52-week results from a randomised, double-blind, placebo-controlled trial (PHOENIX 2). Lancet 2008;371:1675–84.
26. Feagan BG, Sandborn WJ, Gasink C, et al. Ustekinumab as induction and maintenance therapy for Crohn's disease. N Engl J Med 2016;375:1946–60.
27. Sands BE, Chen JJ, Penney M, et al. Initial evaluation of MEDI2070 (specific anti-IL-23 antibody) in patients with active Crohn's disease who have failed anti-TNF antibody therapy: a randomized, double-blind placebo-controlled phase 2A induction study. Gastroenterology 2015;148:S163–4.
28. Sandborn WJ, Feagan BG. Ozanimod treatment for ulcerative colitis. N Engl J Med 2016;375:e17.
29. Monteleone G, Neurath MF, Ardizzone S, et al. Mongersen, an oral SMAD7 antisense oligonucleotide, and Crohn's disease. N Engl J Med 2015;372:1104–13.
30. Sands BE, Anderson FH, Bernstein CN, et al. Infliximab maintenance therapy for fistulizing Crohn's disease. N Engl J Med 2004;350:876–85.
31. Sandborn WJ, Colombel JF, Rutgeerts P, et al. Adalimumab maintains clinical remission and response in patients with active Crohn's disease: results of the CHARM trial. Am J Gastroenterol 2006;101:S458 [abstract: 1176].

32. Schreiber S, Reinisch W, Colombel JF, et al. Early Crohn's disease shows high levels of remission to therapy with adalimumab: sub-analysis of CHARM. Gastroenterology 2007;132:A147.
33. Schreiber S, Colombel JF, Bloomfield R, et al. Increased response and remission rates in short-duration Crohn's disease with subcutaneous certolizumab pegol: an analysis of PRECiSE 2 randomized maintenance trial data. Am J Gastroenterol 2010;105:1574–82.
34. Lichtenstein GR, Feagan BG, Cohen RD, et al. Serious infection and mortality in patients with Crohn's disease: more than 5 years of follow-up in the TREAT registry. Am J Gastroenterol 2012;107:1409–22.
35. Gower-Rousseau C, Dauchet L, Vernier-Massouille G, et al. The natural history of pediatric ulcerative colitis: a population-based cohort study. Am J Gastroenterol 2009;104:2080–8.
36. Gupta N, Cohen SA, Bostrom AG, et al. Risk factors for initial surgery in pediatric patients with Crohn's disease. Gastroenterology 2006;130:1069–77.
37. Lee JH, Cheon JH, Moon CM, et al. Do patients with ulcerative colitis diagnosed at a young age have more severe disease activity than patients diagnosed when older? Digestion 2010;81:237–43.
38. Van Limbergen J, Russell RK, Drummond HE, et al. Definition of phenotypic characteristics of childhood-onset inflammatory bowel disease. Gastroenterology 2008;135:1114–22.
39. Solberg IC, Vatn MH, Hoie O, et al. Clinical course in Crohn's disease: results of a Norwegian population-based ten-year follow-up study. Clin Gastroenterol Hepatol 2007;5:1430–8.
40. Beaugerie L, Seksik P, Nion-Larmurier I, et al. Predictors of Crohn's disease. Gastroenterology 2006;130:650–6.
41. Pigneur B, Seksik P, Viola S, et al. Natural history of Crohn's disease: comparison between childhood- and adult-onset disease. Inflamm Bowel Dis 2010;16:953–61.
42. Loly C, Belaiche J, Louis E. Predictors of severe Crohn's disease. Scand J Gastroenterol 2008;43:948–54.
43. Solberg IC, Cvancarova M, Vatn MH, et al. Risk matrix for prediction of advanced disease in a population-based study of patients with Crohn's disease (the IBSEN Study). Inflamm Bowel Dis 2014;20:60–8.
44. Lakatos PL, Sipeki N, Kovacs G, et al. Risk matrix for prediction of disease progression in a referral cohort of patients with Crohn's disease. J Crohns Colitis 2015;9:891–8.
45. Siegel CA, Whitman CB, Spiegel BM, et al. Development of an index to define overall disease severity in IBD. Gut 2016. [Epub ahead of print].
46. Khanna R, Bressler B, Levesque BG, et al. Early combined immunosuppression for the management of Crohn's disease (REACT): a cluster randomised controlled trial. Lancet 2015;386:1825–34.
47. Cepek KL, Parker CM, Madara JL, et al. Integrin alpha E beta 7 mediates adhesion of T lymphocytes to epithelial cells. J Immunol 1993;150:3459–70.
48. Vermeire S, O'Byrne S, Keir M, et al. Etrolizumab as induction therapy for ulcerative colitis: a randomised, controlled, phase 2 trial. Lancet 2014;384:309–18.
49. Best WR, Becktel JM, Singleton JW, et al. Development of a Crohn's disease activity index. National cooperative Crohn's disease study. Gastroenterology 1976;70:439–44.

50. Sandborn WJ, Feagan BG, Hanauer SB, et al. A review of activity indices and efficacy endpoints for clinical trials of medical therapy in adults with Crohn's disease. Gastroenterology 2002;122(2):512–30.
51. Sandborn WJ, Gasink C, Gao LL, et al. Ustekinumab induction and maintenance therapy in refractory Crohn's disease. N Engl J Med 2012;367:1519–28.
52. Lahiff C, Safaie P, Awais A, et al. The Crohn's disease activity index (CDAI) is similarly elevated in patients with Crohn's disease and in patients with irritable bowel syndrome. Aliment Pharmacol Ther 2013;37:786–94.
53. Department of Health and Human Services. US Food and Drug Administration (FDA) guidance for industry: patient-reported outcome measures use in medical product development to support labeling claims. Rockville (MD): Department of Health and Human Services (US) FaDA, Center for Drug Evaluation and Research (CDER); 2009. http://www.fda.gov/downloads/Drugs/GuidanceComplianceRegulatoryInformation/Guidances/UCM193282.pdf.
54. Peyrin-Biroulet L, Sandborn W, Sands BE, et al. Selecting therapeutic targets in inflammatory bowel disease (STRIDE): determining therapeutic goals for treat-to-target. Am J Gastroenterol 2015;110:1324–38.
55. Khanna R, Zou G, D'Haens G, et al. A retrospective analysis: the development of patient reported outcome measures for the assessment of Crohn's disease activity. Aliment Pharmacol Ther 2015;41:77–86.
56. Abhyankar B. PRO measures for Crohn's disease: vedolizumab data, 2013. Available at: http://www.great3.org/wp-content/uploads/2015/04/PRO-measures-for-Crohn%E2%80%99s-Disease-Vedolizumab-Data-Dr.-Brihad-Abhyankar-MS-FRCS-MBA-FFPM.pdf. Accessed March 30, 2016.
57. Pepys MB. C-reactive protein: a critical update. J Clin Invest 2003;111:1805–12.
58. Roseth AG, Schmidt PN, Fagerhol MK. Correlation between faecal excretion of indium-111-labelled granulocytes and calprotectin, a granulocyte marker protein, in patients with inflammatory bowel disease. Scand J Gastroenterol 1999;34:50–4.
59. Fagerhol MK, Dale I, Andersson T. A radioimmunoassay for a granulocyte protein as a marker in studies on the turnover of such cells. Bull Eur Physiopathol Respir 1980;16(Suppl):273–82.
60. Poullis A, Foster R, Mendall MA, et al. Emerging role of calprotectin in gastroenterology. J Gastroenterol Hepatol 2003;18:756–62.
61. Poullis AP, Zar S, Sundaram KK, et al. A new, highly sensitive assay for C-reactive protein can aid the differentiation of inflammatory bowel disorders from constipation- and diarrhoea-predominant functional bowel disorders. Eur J Gastroenterol Hepatol 2002;14:409–12.
62. Tibble JA, Bjarnason I. Fecal calprotectin as an index of intestinal inflammation. Drugs Today (Barc) 2001;37:85–96.
63. Tibble J, Teahon K, Thjodleifsson B, et al. A simple method for assessing intestinal inflammation in Crohn's disease. Gut 2000;47:506–13.
64. Mosli MH, Zou G, Garg SK, et al. C-reactive protein, fecal calprotectin, and stool lactoferrin for detection of endoscopic activity in symptomatic inflammatory bowel disease patients: a systematic review and meta-analysis. Am J Gastroenterol 2015;110(6):802–19 [quiz: 820].
65. Colombel JF, Panaccione R, Bossuyt P, et al. Superior endoscopic and deep remission outcomes in adults with moderate to severe Crohn's disease managed with treat to target approach versus clinical symptoms: data from CALM (abstract). Gastroenterology 2017;152:S155.

66. Mary JY, Modigliani R. Development and validation of an endoscopic index of the severity for Crohn's disease: a prospective multicentre study. Groupe d'Etudes Therapeutiques des Affections Inflammatoires du Tube Digestif (GETAID). Gut 1989;30:983–9.
67. Daperno M, D'Haens G, Van Assche G, et al. Development and validation of a new, simplified endoscopic activity score for Crohn's disease: the SES-CD. Gastrointest Endosc 2004;60:505–12.
68. Khanna R, Zou G, D'Haens G, et al. Reliability among central readers in the evaluation of endoscopic findings from patients with Crohn's disease. Gut 2016;65(7): 1119–25.
69. Dubcenco E, Zou G, Stitt L, et al. Effect of standardised scoring conventions on inter-rater reliability in the endoscopic evaluation of Crohn's disease. J Crohns Colitis 2016;10:1006–14.
70. Khanna R, Zou G, Stitt L, et al. Responsiveness of endoscopic indices of disease activity for Crohn's disease. Am J Gastroenterol 2017. [Epub ahead of print].
71. Rutgeerts P, Reinisch W, Colombel JF, et al. Agreement of site and central readings of ileocolonoscopic scores in Crohn's disease: comparison using data from the EXTEND trial. Gastrointest Endosc 2016;83:188–97.e3.
72. Rutgeerts P, Van Assche G, Sandborn WJ, et al. Adalimumab induces and maintains mucosal healing in patients with Crohn's disease: data from the EXTEND trial. Gastroenterology 2012;142:1102–11.e2.
73. Hebuterne X, Lemann M, Bouhnik Y, et al. Endoscopic improvement of mucosal lesions in patients with moderate to severe ileocolonic Crohn's disease following treatment with certolizumab pegol. Gut 2013;62:201–8.
74. Rutgeerts P, Diamond RH, Bala M, et al. Scheduled maintenance treatment with infliximab is superior to episodic treatment for the healing of mucosal ulceration associated with Crohn's disease [see comment]. Gastrointest Endosc 2006;63: 433–42 [quiz: 464].
75. Sands B, Feagan B, Rutgeerts P, et al. Vedolizumab induction therapy for patients with Crohn's disease and prior anti-TNF antagonist failure: a randomized, placebo-controlled, double-blind, multicenter trial. Inflamm Bowel Dis 2012;18: S24–5.
76. Panes J, Bouhnik Y, Reinisch W, et al. Imaging techniques for assessment of inflammatory bowel disease: joint ECCO and ESGAR evidence-based consensus guidelines. J Crohns Colitis 2013;7:556–85.
77. Panes J, Bouzas R, Chaparro M, et al. Systematic review: the use of ultrasonography, computed tomography and magnetic resonance imaging for the diagnosis, assessment of activity and abdominal complications of Crohn's disease. Aliment Pharmacol Ther 2011;34:125–45.
78. Garcia-Bosch O, Ordas I, Aceituno M, et al. Comparison of diagnostic accuracy and impact of magnetic resonance imaging and colonoscopy for the management of Crohn's disease. J Crohns Colitis 2016;10(6):663–9.
79. Jauregui-Amezaga A, Rimola J, Ordas I, et al. Value of endoscopy and MRI for predicting intestinal surgery in patients with Crohn's disease in the era of biologics. Gut 2015;64:1397–402.
80. Rimola J, Rodriguez S, Garcia-Bosch O, et al. Magnetic resonance for assessment of disease activity and severity in ileocolonic Crohn's disease. Gut 2009; 58:1113–20.
81. Rimola J, Ordas I, Rodriguez S, et al. Magnetic resonance imaging for evaluation of Crohn's disease: validation of parameters of severity and quantitative index of activity. Inflamm Bowel Dis 2011;17:1759–68.

82. Steward MJ, Punwani S, Proctor I, et al. Non-perforating small bowel Crohn's disease assessed by MRI enterography: derivation and histopathological validation of an MR-based activity index. Eur J Radiol 2012;81:2080–8.
83. Cohen J. A Coefficient of agreement for nominal scales. Educ Psychol Meas 1960;20:37–46.
84. Ordas I, Rimola J, Rodriguez S, et al. Accuracy of magnetic resonance enterography in assessing response to therapy and mucosal healing in patients with Crohn's disease. Gastroenterology 2014;146:374–82.e1.
85. Fasanmade AA, Adedokun OJ, Blank M, et al. Pharmacokinetic properties of infliximab in children and adults with Crohn's disease: a retrospective analysis of data from 2 phase III clinical trials. Clin Ther 2011;33:946–64.
86. Wade JR, Parker G, Kosutic G, et al. Population pharmacokinetic analysis of certolizumab pegol in patients with Crohn's disease. J Clin Pharmacol 2015;55: 866–74.
87. Rosario M, Wyant T, Milch C, et al. Pharmacokinetic and pharmacodynamic relationship and immunogenicity of vedolizumab in adults with inflammatory bowel disease: additional results from the GEMINI 1 and 2 studies. J Crohns Colitis 2014;8:S42–3.
88. Ternant D, Aubourg A, Magdelaine-Beuzelin C, et al. Infliximab pharmacokinetics in inflammatory bowel disease patients. Ther Drug Monit 2008;30:523–9.
89. Ordas I, Mould DR, Feagan BG, et al. Anti-TNF monoclonal antibodies in inflammatory bowel disease: pharmacokinetics-based dosing paradigms. Clin Pharmacol Ther 2012;91:635–46.
90. Afif W, Loftus EV Jr, Faubion WA, et al. Clinical utility of measuring infliximab and human anti-chimeric antibody concentrations in patients with inflammatory bowel disease. Am J Gastroenterol 2010;105:1133–9.
91. Velayos FS, Kahn JG, Sandborn WJ, et al. A test-based strategy is more cost effective than empiric dose escalation for patients with Crohn's disease who lose responsiveness to infliximab. Clin Gastroenterol Hepatol 2013;11:654–66.
92. Steenholdt C, Brynskov J, Thomsen OØ, et al. Individualised therapy is more cost-effective than dose intensification in patients with Crohn's disease who lose response to anti-TNF treatment: a randomised, controlled trial. Gut 2014; 63(6):919–27.
93. Vande Casteele N, Ferrante M, Van Assche G, et al. Trough concentrations of infliximab guide dosing for patients with inflammatory bowel disease. Gastroenterology 2015;148:1320–9.e3.
94. Panaccione R, Rutgeerts P, Sandborn WJ, et al. Review article: treatment algorithms to maximize remission and minimize corticosteroid dependence in patients with inflammatory bowel disease. Aliment Pharmacol Ther 2008;28:674–88.
95. Bouguen G, Levesque BG, Feagan BG, et al. Treat to target: a proposed new paradigm for the management of Crohn's disease. Clin Gastroenterol Hepatol 2015;13:1042–50.e2.

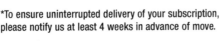

Printed and bound by CPI Group (UK) Ltd, Croydon, CR0 4YY
03/10/2024
01040397-0005